# FORENSIC PATHOLOGY TEXTBOOK



## A Clinical Reference Covering Death Scene Investigation, Wound Interpretation, and Cause-Manner Determination for Candidates

**Ramon C. Henson, MD**

**Trademark Disclaimer**

All brand names, product names, drug names, certification names, and registered trademarks mentioned in this textbook are the property of their respective owners. Their use in this publication does not imply endorsement, affiliation, or sponsorship by the trademark owner, nor does it imply that the trademark owner has reviewed, approved, or is in any way associated with this work. All trademarked names and registered marks appearing in this textbook are used solely for purposes of identification and educational reference, without any intent of trademark infringement.

**Medical Disclaimer**

This textbook is intended solely for educational and informational purposes and is designed to support the continuing professional development of licensed healthcare providers. The clinical content presented herein reflects information believed to be accurate and current at the time of publication; however, medicine evolves rapidly, and readers are advised that new research findings, updated clinical practice guidelines, and revised regulatory approvals may alter or supersede information contained in this work after its publication date.

Nothing in this publication constitutes medical advice, clinical guidance specific to any individual patient, or a substitute for the independent professional judgment of a licensed and qualified healthcare provider. No clinician-patient relationship is established, implied, or intended by the use of this textbook or any portion thereof. All clinical decisions, including but not limited to diagnosis, therapeutic selection, drug dosing, and patient monitoring, must be individualized based on thorough and direct assessment of the patient, the totality of current published evidence, applicable clinical practice guidelines, institutional protocols, and the informed professional judgment of the responsible clinician.

Drug information, dosages, treatment protocols, and therapeutic recommendations presented in this publication are offered for educational reference only and must be independently verified against current prescribing information, pharmacopeial references, and applicable regulatory approvals prior to clinical application. The author and publisher have made every reasonable effort to ensure the accuracy and completeness of the information presented; nevertheless, they expressly disclaim all liability for any adverse outcomes, clinical errors, patient harm, loss, or injury alleged to arise, directly or indirectly, from the use, misuse, or application of any information, recommendation, protocol, or clinical guidance contained in this publication.

## TABLE OF CONTENT

# Contents

# PREFACE

Forensic pathology is a subspecialty organized around a single, exacting question: what happened, and how do we know? Every case that enters the medical examiner's office arrives as a body plus a story, and every case must leave as a certified cause and manner of death that will stand up not only to peer review but to cross-examination in open court. The distance between a decomposed decedent on a bathroom floor and a Cause of Death line on a certificate is not traveled by intuition. It is traveled by disciplined reasoning that begins at the scene, ends at the death certificate, and integrates injury interpretation, autopsy findings, ancillary studies, scene context, and history at every step along the way.

This textbook was written for the physician learning to travel that distance. Its primary reader is the forensic pathology fellow — the anatomic pathologist who has completed residency training, has entered a one-year fellowship, and within twelve months will be expected to sit for the American Board of Pathology's forensic subspecialty examination and to function autonomously in a coroner's or medical examiner's office. The book is also written for the anatomic pathology resident on a forensic rotation who needs a working reference, for the practicing medical examiner who wants a systematic framework to teach to visiting trainees, and for the medicolegal death investigator who benefits from understanding the reasoning the pathologist is doing at the table.

## Why This Book Was Built the Way It Was

Forensic pathology carries a documented problem that the standard reference literature has not solved. Studies of wound interpretation among trained observers consistently show error rates that would be unacceptable in any other diagnostic specialty. In one representative published analysis, correct identification of gunshot wound type was achieved in only about four of every ten cases, and correct interpretation of sharp force wounds in fewer than half. The errors do not cluster among the untrained; they occur among practitioners with formal training who are relying on the traditional macroscopic criteria that the classic textbooks describe. Meanwhile, the National Academies committee reviewing the medicolegal death investigation system has flagged, as recently as 2025, the pressure of undue influence on manner-of-death determinations and the difficulty of protecting cause-and-manner reasoning from bias. And formal, structured preparation for courtroom testimony remains, in most fellowship programs, a mentor-dependent apprenticeship rather than a curriculum.

The fellow inherits all three problems at once. She is expected to interpret wounds under conditions where the published error rate for trained observers is high; to defend a manner determination that may be legally contested; and to testify to that reasoning in a deposition or trial where the language of the courtroom differs from the language of the autopsy suite. What she needs from a textbook is not another encyclopedia of injury photographs. She needs a reasoning scaffold that walks her, case by case, from the death scene to the certified determination — and that names the traps documented in the peer-reviewed literature so she can avoid them before they appear in a deposition.

## The Scene-to-Certification Decision System

The Scene-to-Certification Decision System is the reasoning scaffold this book delivers. It appears twice inside every clinical chapter, and it consolidates at chapter end and again in the back-of-book Master Atlas. Each instance carries the reader through six fields, in a fixed order that mirrors the actual arc of case work: Presenting Death Scenario (the case as it walks in the door — scene, body, circumstances); Autopsy Signature (the defining findings on external, internal, and microscopic examination that anchor this scenario); Cause Determination (the injury or disease that started the lethal chain, with the reasoning that identifies it as such); Manner Determination (natural, accident, suicide, homicide, or undetermined, argued rather than asserted); Trap Logic (the look-alike scenarios and misinterpretation risks documented in the literature); and a Certification Anchor (the one durable rule that locks the determination in a form that survives cross-examination).

The system is not a formula and it is not a checklist. It is a disciplined structure for the kind of reasoning experienced forensic pathologists already do in their heads. Making it explicit lets the fellow see the reasoning, practice it against known scenarios, and carry it into cases where the pattern is new but the discipline transfers. Every scenario in the book — the entrance wound with an unusual soot pattern, the pediatric sudden death with an ambiguous scene, the drug-related death with therapeutic and lethal blood levels superimposed, the death in police custody with restraint marks and cardiovascular disease — is worked through the system in full. The chapter-end Scene-to-Certification Decision Recap ties the chapter's scenarios into a single thematic navigator, and the back-of-book Scene-to-Certification Master Atlas indexes every scenario in the book by death category and cross-references it back to its chapter.

## How the Book Is Organized

Twenty-four chapters cover the working scope of medicolegal death investigation. The book opens with the foundations — the medicolegal system in which the forensic pathologist operates, the death scene, postmortem changes and time-of-death estimation, and the mechanics of the forensic autopsy itself. It then moves through the injury categories that dominate day-to-day casework: blunt force, sharp force, gunshot, asphyxial, and the thermal, electrical, and chemical injuries. A short section on sudden natural death follows, because most cases that enter the medical examiner's office are natural cases even when the scene initially suggests otherwise, and the fellow needs a framework for recognizing them.

The middle of the book turns to the special populations — the pediatric decedent, the abused or neglected child, the elderly with fractures of uncertain origin, the sexual assault decedent, and the death in custody or restraint. These are the cases with the highest legal and emotional stakes, and they are worked through with the same Scene-to-Certification arc as every other scenario, because that discipline is what protects the determination when it is contested. Toxicology and drug-death interpretation, postmortem imaging, human identification, and mass fatality response then round out the technical scope. The final three chapters address death certification itself, autopsy report construction, and courtroom testimony as a distinct clinical skill. The book closes with the Master Atlas.

## What the Book Does Not Contain

There are no practice questions, board-style items, mock examinations, or answer keys anywhere in this book. Not in the chapters, not in the callouts, not in the Master Atlas. The forensic pathologist's daily reality is not multiple choice, and the reasoning discipline the book teaches is degraded by being packaged in that form. When the fellow needs question-format board preparation, that is a separate resource in a separate genre; this book is a clinical reference and it functions as one. Clinical cases in the text are narrative scenarios, walked through in the reasoning sequence the pathologist would follow at the table — never problems posed with five lettered options.

There is also no citation apparatus in the running text. Landmark studies and consensus guidelines are named where they matter — the National Association of Medical Examiners position papers, the National Institute of Standards and Technology work on bloodstain pattern analysis, the American Academy of Pediatrics guidance on sudden unexpected infant death — but they are named in prose, not attached to bracketed reference numbers. The intent is a reference that reads at the speed of clinical work, not a document that reads at the speed of a systematic review.

## A Note on Practice, Scope, and Currency

Drug doses, blood alcohol thresholds, laboratory reference ranges, and specific therapeutic protocols where they appear in this book are given as clinical reasoning anchors rather than as numbers to be applied at the table. Every specific value should be confirmed against current formulary references, current state or jurisdiction statute, and current professional-society guidance before it drives a decision. Medicolegal practice varies substantially by jurisdiction — coroner versus medical examiner systems, statutory reportable death definitions, permissible autopsy scope, and the criminal code that ultimately consumes the pathologist's testimony all differ across state and national lines. The book presents the principles and the reasoning that transfer across jurisdictions; the reader is responsible for the local statutes and institutional protocols that govern her actual practice.

Forensic pathology continues to evolve. Postmortem cross-sectional imaging is displacing selected traditional dissection steps. Molecular autopsy is entering routine sudden-death workup. Novel synthetic opioids and stimulants appear faster than reference laboratories can validate assays for them. The reasoning discipline embedded in the Scene-to-Certification Decision System is meant to outlast the specific findings it currently operates on — to remain workable when the trap logic in a chapter has to be updated with next year's peer-reviewed literature, and to give the reader a stable structure inside which to place whatever comes next.

The intended outcome of a year spent working through this book is a fellow who can approach an unfamiliar case at the autopsy table, execute the arc from scene to certification with discipline, defend the determination in a deposition, and recognize when a case does not fit any established scenario and requires further investigation. That is the standard the fellowship is designed to produce, and it is the standard the book is written to.

# CHAPTER 1: PRINCIPLES OF FORENSIC PATHOLOGY AND THE MEDICOLEGAL DEATH INVESTIGATION SYSTEM

**Learning Objectives**

1. Define forensic pathology and distinguish its scope from anatomic pathology and clinical pathology.
2. Compare the coroner and medical examiner systems in the United States and identify the operational implications of each for the forensic pathologist.
3. Identify the categories of death that are statutorily reportable to the medicolegal system across most jurisdictions and reason about jurisdictional ambiguity.
4. Distinguish cause of death, manner of death, and mechanism of death, and apply the distinction to a death certificate.
5. Recognize sources of undue influence on cause-and-manner determinations and articulate the professional practices that protect the objectivity of the determination.

## Foundations and Scope of Forensic Pathology

Forensic pathology is the medical subspecialty concerned with the investigation of sudden, unexpected, violent, and suspicious deaths. It is a subspecialty of anatomic pathology in the American training system, requiring completion of anatomic pathology residency (or combined anatomic and clinical pathology residency) before entry into a one-year forensic pathology fellowship. The American Board of Pathology certifies forensic pathology as a subspecialty, and certification requires successful completion of the forensic pathology examination administered after fellowship. The workforce this training system produces is small — the number of practicing board-certified forensic pathologists in the United States is estimated at approximately half the number required to serve the country's medicolegal death investigation needs — which places persistent operational pressure on medical examiner and coroner offices and on the fellows who are entering the specialty.

The scope of forensic pathology extends well beyond the autopsy suite. It comprises death scene investigation, external and internal examination of the body, ancillary testing (toxicology, histology, microbiology, molecular studies, and postmortem imaging), integration of scene and medical history with autopsy findings, formulation of cause and manner of death, drafting of the autopsy report, certification of the death, communication with families and law enforcement, and expert testimony in criminal and civil proceedings. The forensic pathologist works at the intersection of medicine and law, and the outputs of the specialty — the autopsy report, the death certificate, and courtroom testimony — have legal consequences for individuals, families, insurance carriers, and the criminal justice system.

### Distinction From Hospital Autopsy and Anatomic Pathology

The forensic autopsy is not merely a hospital autopsy performed on a decedent with a legal question attached. The two differ in authority, purpose, documentation, and scope. A hospital autopsy is performed with family consent, primarily for medical audit and education, and its findings are protected by the physician-patient privilege that extended to the decedent. A forensic autopsy is performed under statutory authority of the medical examiner or coroner, requires no family consent, is documented to a standard that anticipates courtroom challenge, and produces findings that enter the public record via the death certificate and — in many jurisdictions — the autopsy report itself. The forensic pathologist documents injury with a specificity (measurement, orientation, characterization, photographic support) that a hospital pathologist rarely produces, because the eventual audience of the report includes attorneys, investigators, jurors, and appellate judges.

**KEY POINT:** A forensic autopsy is a legal proceeding conducted in a medical setting. Every finding documented is a potential exhibit at trial. Every finding not documented is presumptively absent, whether or not it was actually present at examination.

### Adjacent Specialties and the Team of Medicolegal Investigation

Forensic pathology operates in close working relationship with several adjacent disciplines. Forensic anthropology contributes when the body is skeletonized, incinerated, or fragmented and the pathologist requires expertise in skeletal biology and trauma. Forensic odontology contributes identification through dental comparison and interpretation of bite-mark injury (with the important caveat that bite-mark analysis carries substantial and well-documented interpretive limitations). Forensic toxicology provides the chemical analysis on which drug death and postmortem interpretation depend, and the pathologist must understand the toxicologist's methods and their limitations rather than treating a reported value as a self-explanatory number. Forensic radiology, in the form of postmortem imaging, is entering routine practice, particularly for gunshot wound trajectory work and for pediatric skeletal surveys. Death investigators — medicolegal death investigators certified by the American Board of Medicolegal Death Investigators, or investigators trained under an individual office's protocols — conduct the scene investigation on which the pathologist depends. The pathologist's authority extends to signing the death certificate; her authority does not extend to independently investigating a scene without an investigator, or to interpreting a toxicology chromatogram without a toxicologist, and understanding that division of labor is fundamental to competent practice.

## The Coroner and Medical Examiner Systems in the United States

Medicolegal death investigation in the United States is organized under two structurally distinct systems: the coroner system and the medical examiner system. The distinction matters because it determines who signs the death certificate, what training that person is required to have, and how the forensic pathologist fits into the office. The two systems coexist across states, sometimes within the same state (some jurisdictions operate hybrid systems in which coroners hold statutory authority but employ or contract with forensic pathologists to perform autopsies).

### The Coroner System

The coroner is an elected or appointed public official. In many jurisdictions the coroner is not required to be a physician; the office may be held by a funeral director, a former law enforcement officer, or any citizen meeting statutory eligibility. The coroner holds statutory authority to investigate deaths falling within a defined jurisdictional scope, to determine cause and manner of death, and to sign the death certificate. Where the coroner is not a physician, autopsies are performed by a contracted forensic pathologist whose findings inform — but do not necessarily bind — the coroner's determination. The historical coroner system dates to medieval England and predates the modern medical specialty of pathology. Its persistence in modern American practice reflects the deep entwinement of death investigation with local political authority.

### The Medical Examiner System

The medical examiner is a physician, in almost all jurisdictions specifically a forensic pathologist. The office is appointed rather than elected, typically by a governing body such as a county board or a state health department. The medical examiner holds statutory authority parallel to the coroner's but performs the autopsy and signs the death certificate personally. The medical examiner system emerged in the United States in the twentieth century, first in Massachusetts (1877) and then in New York City (1918), specifically to replace what reformers viewed as an inadequately medicalized coroner system with a system in which death investigation was conducted by professionally qualified physicians.

### SCENE-TO-CERTIFICATION DECISION SYSTEM — Jurisdictional Reporting Arc

**Presenting Death Scenario:** An 82-year-old woman is found deceased in her single-family home by a neighbor who has not seen her for three days. The neighbor calls emergency services. Paramedics pronounce death at the scene. Police secure the residence. There are no signs of forced entry, no signs of a struggle, and no visible trauma to the body. The decedent has a documented history of congestive heart failure and hypertension. She was not enrolled in hospice, and her last physician contact was six weeks earlier for a routine visit.

**Autopsy Signature:** External examination is unremarkable apart from early postmortem changes (mild greenish discoloration of the abdomen, patchy skin slippage). No injury is identified. Internal examination shows severe atherosclerotic coronary artery disease with a 95 percent stenosis of the proximal left anterior descending artery, cardiomegaly at 480 grams, concentric left ventricular hypertrophy, and marked pulmonary edema. Toxicology is negative apart from therapeutic-range levels of the decedent's prescribed antihypertensive medications.

**Cause Determination:** Atherosclerotic and hypertensive cardiovascular disease. The severity of coronary stenosis, the cardiomegaly, the left ventricular hypertrophy, and the pulmonary edema together identify a lethal cardiovascular event of sufficient severity to account for death without requiring an alternative explanation.

**Manner Determination:** Natural. The determination rests on the affirmative finding of natural disease of sufficient severity, integrated with a scene showing no evidence of external injury or third-party involvement, and a body showing no evidence of trauma.

**Trap Logic:** Delayed discovery is not a manner determinant. A body found three days after death, alone, in a locked residence, does not automatically raise suspicion of foul play — nor does it automatically exclude it. The trap is to certify natural manner because the case looks natural rather than because natural disease of sufficient severity has been affirmatively identified. In a moderately decomposed body, obscured skin injury and skeletal fracture must be excluded through full-body radiography and careful external examination under adequate lighting; skin slippage from decomposition can mask patterned injury, and postmortem hypostasis can mimic contusion.

**Certification Anchor:** Natural manner is affirmed by the presence of natural disease of sufficient severity, not by the absence of a suspicious scene. When affirmative natural disease and negative injury findings coexist, natural manner holds. When natural disease is present but injury cannot be adequately excluded (obscured by decomposition, insufficient scene documentation, absent radiographic screening), the determination remains pending until the exclusion is complete.

### Consequences of the Structural Difference

For the forensic pathologist entering practice, the practical consequences of the coroner-versus-medical-examiner distinction are substantial. Under a medical examiner system, the pathologist is both the medical investigator and the certifier of death; her professional judgment binds the death certificate directly. Under a coroner system in which the coroner is a non-physician, the pathologist provides medical findings but the coroner retains certification authority; the pathologist must understand that her autopsy report is an input to the coroner's determination rather than the determination itself, and disagreements between pathologist and coroner over cause or manner are resolved (or unresolved) through the coroner's authority. Neither system is inherently better at protecting the accuracy of death determinations; each has documented failure modes, and each has produced excellent and inadequate practice depending on the individual office. The pathologist's obligation is to understand the system she works within and to structure her documentation and communication to serve professional practice within it.

**CLINICAL PEARL:** In coroner jurisdictions, the pathologist writes the autopsy report as a professional medical opinion. She does not write cause and manner into the death certificate; the coroner does. When the coroner departs from the pathologist's opinion, the autopsy report stands as the medical record of the case regardless of what the certificate ultimately reads.

## Statutory Reportable Deaths and Jurisdictional Framework

Not every death enters the medicolegal system. The great majority of deaths in the United States occur in expected, medically attended circumstances and are certified by an attending physician (a hospital physician, a hospice medical director, a primary care physician). The medicolegal system takes jurisdiction over deaths falling into statutorily defined categories. The categories vary in exact language across states but converge on a common core.

## The Core Categories of Reportable Death

Reportable deaths generally include deaths that are sudden and unexpected in an apparently healthy person; deaths that are violent or traumatic in origin regardless of the interval between injury and death; deaths from suspected or known intoxication or poisoning; deaths in police or correctional custody, or during police contact; deaths of persons whose identity is unknown; deaths occurring under suspicious circumstances or where foul play is suspected; deaths of infants and children where the cause is not immediately evident; deaths of decedents not attended by a physician within a defined period before death; deaths occurring during medical or surgical procedures or from anesthesia; deaths from occupational exposure or workplace injury; deaths that may pose a public health threat (novel infections, environmental exposures); and deaths of decedents whose bodies are to be cremated (many jurisdictions require medicolegal review before cremation to prevent the destruction of evidence).

**Sudden and unexpected death.** Death without warning in an apparently healthy person, or without a diagnosed condition adequate to explain death, enters the medicolegal system for evaluation.

**Violent or traumatic death.** Death from injury — blunt, sharp, gunshot, thermal, chemical, electrical — is reportable regardless of the interval between injury and death and regardless of whether the injury was intentional.

**Suspected intoxication or poisoning.** Death from drug overdose (prescription or illicit), acute or chronic alcohol intoxication, or environmental toxin exposure is reportable.

**Death in custody or during police contact.** Deaths of persons in police custody, in correctional facilities, or occurring during police interaction (including deaths during arrest, restraint, or after use of less-lethal force) are uniformly reportable and require heightened investigative rigor.

**Unattended death.** Death of a person not seen by a physician within a defined period (varying by state, often 20 or 30 days) before death is reportable.

**Suspected infant or child death.** Sudden death in infancy (SUID), unexpected death in childhood, and any child death from suspected abuse or neglect are reportable and generally require full autopsy.

## Jurisdictional Ambiguity and the Duty to Consult

The reporting statutes rarely draw crisp lines. A death from a fall in a nursing home occurring in an 89-year-old with severe osteoporosis and known dementia may or may not be reportable depending on how the fall occurred, whether staff supervision was appropriate, and whether the decedent was under regular medical care. A death from remote gunshot wound in a paraplegic whose immediate cause is urosepsis is reportable as a homicide (assuming the original manner was homicide) regardless of the twelve-year interval. A death from apparent drug overdose in a hospice-enrolled patient with terminal cancer may cross reporting thresholds depending on whether the drug involved was the prescribed hospice medication and whether the dose was consistent with prescribed use. When ambiguity exists, the professional standard is to report; the medicolegal office can decline jurisdiction after review, but a death that should have been reported and was not creates immediate downstream problems for the attending physician who certified it, for the family, and for any subsequent legal proceeding.

**CAUTION:** The decision to report is not the decision to accept jurisdiction. Reporting is a communication that allows the medicolegal office to evaluate; jurisdictional acceptance is the office's determination that the death falls within its statutory authority. The clinician who is uncertain should always report.

## Cause, Manner, and Mechanism of Death

The distinction among cause of death, manner of death, and mechanism of death is the conceptual center of forensic certification. Every trainee learns the three definitions early and every practitioner encounters cases in which the distinction is confused — by the attending physician who certified the death, by law enforcement, by the family, and sometimes by counsel in a deposition. The trainee's task is to hold the distinction with precision, because the death certificate depends on it and because courtroom testimony frequently turns on it.

### Cause of Death

Cause of death is the injury or disease that initiated the sequence of physiological disturbances — the lethal chain — that led to death. The cause of death may be immediate (the event just before death, e.g., ventricular fibrillation), intermediate (an event in the chain, e.g., myocardial infarction), or proximate (the event that started the whole process, e.g., atherosclerotic coronary artery disease). Death certification requires all links in the chain, from immediate through proximate, along with any significant conditions that contributed to death without being part of the direct chain.

The proximate cause is the entry to the chain and often determines manner. A death from urosepsis that traces to chronic urinary catheterization that traces to paraplegia that traces to a remote gunshot wound of the spine has the gunshot wound as its proximate cause, and the manner of death tracks the manner of the original gunshot. This is the "but for" principle: but for the original injury, none of the downstream events would have occurred. The temporal interval between the proximate cause and death, however long, does not sever the chain as long as no efficient intervening event has broken it.

### Mechanism of Death

Mechanism of death is the nonspecific final common pathway by which the cause exerts its lethal effect — the physiological derangement that ends the biological function of the organism. Cardiopulmonary arrest, hypovolemic shock, respiratory failure, septic shock, cardiac arrhythmia, and asphyxia are mechanisms. Every death is preceded by a mechanism, but a mechanism is never a cause. "Cardiopulmonary arrest" as an entry on a death certificate is a certification error, because it names the mechanism (the heart and lungs stopped) rather than the cause (why they stopped). The medicolegal certifier avoids naming mechanisms on the certificate; the mechanism belongs in the discussion of pathophysiology, not on the certification.

**CLINICAL PEARL:** If a proposed cause of death could apply to virtually every fatal case regardless of what actually killed the person, it is a mechanism, not a cause. Cardiopulmonary arrest, cardiac arrest, respiratory arrest, asystole, and multi-organ failure are diagnoses of mode, not of etiology.

### Manner of Death

Manner of death is the classification of how the cause came about. The manner categories used in United States certification are: natural, accident, suicide, homicide, and undetermined. Natural manner is assigned to death caused entirely by disease or by natural degenerative processes. Accident is assigned to death caused by unintended injury or unintended poisoning — the fall from a ladder, the motor vehicle collision without foul play, the accidental drug overdose. Suicide is assigned to death caused by a self-inflicted injury or poisoning with intent to end life. Homicide is assigned to death caused by the volitional act of another person, regardless of intent to kill — the criminal category (murder, manslaughter, negligent homicide) is a legal determination that the manner classification does not attempt to duplicate. Undetermined is assigned when the available information does not support a manner determination to reasonable medical certainty.

### SCENE-TO-CERTIFICATION DECISION SYSTEM — Cause-Versus-Mechanism Distinction Arc

**Presenting Death Scenario:** A 35-year-old man dies in a long-term care facility. He has been paraplegic for twelve years following a gunshot wound to the thoracic spine sustained during a robbery. The original assault was investigated as a homicide, and the assailant was convicted of assault at that time. In the years since the injury, the decedent has had chronic indwelling urinary catheterization, recurrent urinary tract infections, a stage-IV sacral pressure ulcer with underlying osteomyelitis, and progressive functional decline. He dies in the setting of documented pneumonia and clinical sepsis.

**Autopsy Signature:** External examination shows a healed midline surgical scar from the acute injury care, a healed gunshot wound entrance scar on the posterior thorax, and a large sacral decubitus with exposed bone. Internal examination shows bilateral bronchopneumonia with purulent airway exudate, chronic pyelonephritis, and osteomyelitis of the sacrum. Microscopic examination confirms acute-on-chronic infection. Radiographic examination shows the retained bullet fragment adjacent to the T7 vertebral body along the original wound tract.

**Cause Determination:** Remote gunshot wound of the thoracic spine with resultant paraplegia, complicated by chronic urinary catheterization, decubitus ulceration, osteomyelitis, and terminal urosepsis and bronchopneumonia. The cause-of-death chain is documented on the certificate from immediate (bronchopneumonia and urosepsis) through intermediate (paraplegia with chronic infection) to proximate (remote gunshot wound of thoracic spine).

**Manner Determination:** Homicide. The manner tracks the original manner of the proximate cause. The twelve-year interval between injury and death does not sever the causal chain because no efficient intervening event has broken it — every downstream complication is a foreseeable and documented consequence of paraplegia from spinal cord injury.

**Trap Logic:** The trap is certifying urosepsis or bronchopneumonia as the sole cause of death, which certifies the immediate cause without the underlying cause and obscures the homicide origin of the case. A related trap is certifying "cardiopulmonary arrest" or "multi-organ failure" as cause of death — these are mechanisms, not causes, and their appearance on a death certificate is a certification error that will be corrected on review. A third trap is treating the twelve-year interval as evidence that the chain has "run out" and the manner should default to natural; the interval is irrelevant when the chain is unbroken.

**Certification Anchor:** The manner of death tracks the proximate cause. When the proximate cause was a homicide, the manner remains homicide however remote the death, as long as no efficient intervening event has broken the causal chain. Immediate causes and mechanisms do not override proximate cause in manner determination.

## The Forensic Pathologist in the Medicolegal Team

The forensic pathologist is one member of a working investigative team. Understanding the team's structure and the pathologist's role within it protects both the accuracy of the individual case determination and the quality of the pathologist's testimony when the case moves to trial.

### The Death Investigator

The medicolegal death investigator (MDI) conducts the scene investigation on which the pathologist depends. The investigator responds to the scene, photographs the body and its context, interviews witnesses and next of kin, obtains prior medical records, and produces the scene investigation report that the pathologist reads before, during, and after the autopsy. The best pathology practice treats the scene report as an integral part of the case file, not as background. The pathologist who dictates an autopsy report without integrating the scene report is producing a partial document; the pathologist who reads the scene report only after the autopsy is done has missed the opportunity to have scene context inform the internal examination.

### Law Enforcement

Law enforcement officers are frequent contributors to the case file, providing witness statements, evidence collection reports, and case background. The pathologist's professional obligation is to consider law enforcement information as one input among several, not as a directive. Where law enforcement's investigative theory of a case differs from what the autopsy findings support, the pathologist's role is to follow the findings, not to accommodate the theory. This tension — documented as a source of undue influence in the 2025 National Academies review of the medicolegal system — is one of the most challenging elements of forensic practice.

### The Toxicologist

The forensic toxicologist provides the chemical analysis of postmortem specimens and, in many offices, the interpretive framework for reported drug levels. The pathologist must understand the toxicologist's methods sufficiently to know what a reported value means and what it does not mean — a plasma or blood concentration is not a stand-alone determination of cause of death, and postmortem drug redistribution can substantially alter concentrations measured from central versus peripheral blood, a phenomenon addressed in the toxicology chapter.

### The Prosecutor and Defense Counsel

In cases proceeding to criminal trial, the prosecutor and defense counsel become downstream consumers of the pathologist's work. The pathologist is not a member of either legal team; her professional obligation is to the truth of the findings and to the objectivity of the reasoning. She testifies when called by either side. A pathologist who identifies as "the prosecution's expert" or "the defense's expert" has already compromised the professional stance from which competent testimony is delivered.

## Ethics, Objectivity, and Freedom From Undue Influence

The professional obligations of the forensic pathologist are governed by the National Association of Medical Examiners (NAME) position papers and by the ethical standards of the American Academy of Forensic Sciences and the American Society for Clinical Pathology. The core professional obligation is objectivity: the determinations of cause and manner of death are medical opinions reached to reasonable medical certainty based on the available evidence, and they are protected from external pressure to arrive at any particular conclusion.

### Sources of Undue Influence

The 2025 National Academies committee on strengthening the medicolegal death investigation system specifically addressed sources of undue influence on cause-and-manner determinations. Documented sources include: pressure from law enforcement whose investigative theory of a case would be disrupted by a particular determination; pressure from prosecutors preparing for trial; pressure from families whose insurance benefits, litigation posture, or grief response depends on a particular manner classification; pressure from institutional employers whose reputation may be affected (particularly relevant in deaths in custody, deaths in medical settings, and deaths in institutional care); and internal cognitive biases including confirmation bias, availability bias, and anchoring on the initial impression of a case.

**EVIDENCE:** The 2025 National Academies review of the U.S. medicolegal death investigation system identified undue influence on cause-and-manner determinations as a persistent and structurally embedded problem in the American system, particularly in deaths occurring in custody and in institutional settings. Structural protections — independent office authority, protected employment status for medical examiners, transparent case review — are the recommended countermeasures.

### Professional Practices That Protect Objectivity

The pathologist protects objectivity through a small set of durable practices. She documents her reasoning in the autopsy report with sufficient specificity that the determination can be reconstructed and defended without her later verbal explanation. She avoids conclusions that outrun the evidence — the appropriate use of undetermined manner is a professional strength, not a professional weakness. She does not modify determinations in response to pressure that lacks new evidentiary basis; a determination is revised when the evidence changes, not when the audience objects. She discusses difficult cases with colleagues under structures that preserve professional judgment (peer review, morphological consultation, second-opinion consultation from a colleague in another office). And she recognizes the limits of her own expertise — the case that requires forensic anthropology, forensic odontology, or subspecialty pathology consultation is a case where consultation is obtained rather than approximated.

### The Relationship to Law and Legal Standards

The forensic pathologist works in a specialty whose products enter legal proceedings. Cause and manner of death, however, are medical determinations rather than legal determinations, and neither is legally binding on any party. A jury may reach a legal verdict inconsistent with a medical examiner's manner determination; a judge may exclude a pathologist's testimony on a particular point under Daubert or Frye standards; a civil litigation may proceed on a theory of causation that the treating pathologist does not endorse. The pathologist's professional stance is that her determination is a medical opinion given to reasonable medical certainty, offered to inform the legal process, and defensible on cross-examination by the reasoning documented in the autopsy report. She is a witness of professional opinion rather than a witness of fact only, and the objectivity that qualifies her testimony under Daubert or Frye is the practice she has been developing since fellowship.

### Structural Comparison of Coroner and Medical Examiner Systems

The functional differences between the two systems are worth articulating in one place, because the trainee entering fellowship may practice under either or under a hybrid arrangement, and the pathologist's professional posture is calibrated accordingly.

| Attribute | Coroner System | Medical Examiner System |
|---|---|---|
| Selection | Elected or appointed public official | Appointed physician, generally a forensic pathologist |
| Medical training required | Not generally required | Board-certified or board-eligible forensic pathologist |
| Certification authority | Coroner signs the death certificate | Medical examiner signs the death certificate |
| Role of the forensic pathologist | Contracted or employed to perform autopsy; findings inform coroner's determination | Performs autopsy and personally certifies death |

| | | |
|---|---|---|
| Autonomy of pathologist's determination | Pathologist's opinion may be departed from by coroner | Pathologist's opinion IS the determination |
| Historical origin | Medieval English office, imported to colonial America | Twentieth-century American reform (Massachusetts 1877; New York City 1918) |
| Prevalence | Rural counties, smaller jurisdictions in many states | Urban centers, statewide systems in most northeastern and several western states |
| Vulnerability to non-medical influence | Elected office may be subject to political pressure | Appointed office may be subject to institutional pressure |

The lesson embedded in the comparison is that neither system inherently produces better medicolegal death investigation. A well-resourced coroner office with a competent contracted forensic pathologist can produce excellent work, and a poorly resourced medical examiner office with inadequate autopsy volume can produce inadequate work. The pathologist's professional obligation is the same in either setting: perform the medical examination competently, document the findings so they support the determination, and communicate professionally with the certifying authority when that authority is not herself.

## A Working Case in the Foundational Frame

The following narrative case illustrates how the concepts of this chapter operate together in a real determination. It is presented in the sequence a fellow would encounter it — first the call, then the scene, then the autopsy, then the certification.

### The Call and the Scene

A 47-year-old man is brought unresponsive to a police holding cell approximately 25 minutes after being arrested for public intoxication and disorderly conduct in a downtown entertainment district. Officers report that during arrest he was verbally combative and physically resistant. He was placed prone on the ground and handcuffed, then walked to the transport vehicle. In the vehicle he was noted to be quiet; on arrival at the station he was found unresponsive. Cardiopulmonary resuscitation is initiated and he is transported to the emergency department where he is pronounced dead 40 minutes later. The medical examiner's office receives the report from the emergency physician as a death in police custody — unambiguously a reportable death under any statutory framework. The medicolegal death investigator is dispatched to the emergency department and to the arrest scene, and the pathologist is notified as the case will be autopsied on the next scheduled day.

The scene investigator documents the location of arrest, interviews the officers involved (with the pathologist reading these interviews before the autopsy), reviews the body-worn camera footage from the arrest (a critical piece of documentation in modern in-custody death investigation), and identifies any injuries visible on external inspection at the emergency department. The scene report notes that the decedent was on the ground prone for approximately 90 seconds, with an officer's knee on the upper back for a portion of that time; that the decedent verbalized coherently throughout the ground contact; that he was walked to the transport vehicle without apparent distress; and that he was silent in the vehicle for approximately 8 minutes before arrival at the station.

### The Autopsy Findings

External examination shows superficial abrasions to the anterior right shoulder and forehead consistent with prone contact with a paved surface, a small periorbital contusion, and handcuff-associated linear abrasions to both wrists. There is no ligature mark of the neck, no petechial hemorrhage of the conjunctivae or facial skin, and no evidence of significant blunt injury to the neck. Internal examination shows severe cardiomegaly at 520 grams with concentric left ventricular hypertrophy, severe atherosclerotic coronary artery disease with 80 percent stenosis of the proximal left anterior descending artery and 70 percent of the right coronary artery, and moderate hepatic steatosis consistent with chronic alcohol use. There is no cervical soft-tissue hemorrhage. The larynx and hyoid are intact. There are no rib fractures. The lungs show congestion and edema but no aspirated gastric contents. Toxicology reveals a blood ethanol concentration of 0.24 grams per deciliter, a positive urine screen for cocaine, and a confirmatory blood level of cocaine and its metabolite benzoylecgonine consistent with recent use.

### The Reasoning Toward Cause and Manner

The autopsy findings identify severe pre-existing cardiovascular disease of a magnitude that can support sudden death in the setting of physiological stress. Toxicology identifies acute cocaine use and marked ethanol intoxication, both of which contribute cardiovascular stress and both of which are documented triggers of arrhythmic sudden death in the presence of underlying coronary disease. The scene documents physical restraint of relatively short duration without evidence at autopsy of asphyxial mechanism (no petechiae, no ligature, no cervical injury, no fractures). The pathologist's task is to reason from these inputs to a cause and manner determination that is defensible in court — because a death in police custody, in this era, will almost certainly be reviewed by outside experts retained by the family, by civil rights counsel, and potentially by criminal prosecutors.

The cause of death is best formulated as cardiac arrhythmia due to acute cocaine and ethanol intoxication and hypertensive and atherosclerotic cardiovascular disease, with the significant contribution of physical exertion associated with police restraint noted as an additional condition contributing to death. The manner determination is more contested: some experienced pathologists would certify this as an accident (unintended overdose combined with medical disease); others would certify it as undetermined given the contribution of restraint; still others would argue for homicide on the theory that the restraint was a proximate contributor to death. The 2025 National Academies review specifically flagged the manner determination in restraint-associated cardiac arrest as an area where undue influence and inter-office variation are documented. The professional approach is to state the reasoning transparently in the autopsy report, document the manner decision, and be prepared to defend it — including the professional acknowledgement that colleagues in other offices might reason differently on the same facts.

**CLINICAL PEARL:** In a contested death, the strength of the manner determination rests on the transparency of the reasoning, not on the certainty of the conclusion. The pathologist who documents her reasoning — including what she considered and rejected — produces a defensible determination even when others would have decided differently. The pathologist who documents only the conclusion produces a determination that survives only her own testimony and dies with her retirement.

**SCENE-TO-CERTIFICATION DECISION SYSTEM — Foundational Determination Arcs**

---

**Structural Frame of Reference:** The forensic pathologist operates inside a defined statutory system — medical examiner, coroner, or hybrid — that determines who signs the death certificate and how her professional judgment enters the medicolegal record. The first orientation on any case is jurisdictional: does this death fall within the office's authority, and by what mechanism does the professional finding become the certified determination?

**The Reporting Threshold:** Sudden, violent, suspicious, unattended, intoxication-related, custodial, pediatric-unexplained, and identity-unknown deaths are the core reportable categories. Ambiguity resolves toward reporting. The clinician who is uncertain always reports and lets the medicolegal office determine jurisdiction.

**The Cause-Manner-Mechanism Discipline:** Cause is what started the lethal chain (immediate through proximate). Manner is how the cause came about (natural / accident / suicide / homicide / undetermined). Mechanism is the nonspecific final pathway (never a cause on a certificate). Manner tracks the proximate cause; the temporal interval between injury and death is irrelevant unless an efficient intervening event has broken the causal chain.

**The Objectivity Anchor:** The cause-and-manner determination is a medical opinion rendered to reasonable medical certainty and protected from external pressure. Objectivity is preserved through documented reasoning, appropriate use of the undetermined category, refusal to revise determinations in the absence of new evidence, structured peer consultation on difficult cases, and honest recognition of the limits of individual expertise.

## Summary and Key Concepts

Forensic pathology is a subspecialty of anatomic pathology that investigates sudden, unexpected, violent, and suspicious deaths and produces the medical determinations — cause of death, manner of death, autopsy report, and courtroom testimony — that inform the medicolegal system.

The United States medicolegal death investigation infrastructure is organized under coroner and medical examiner systems, which differ in who signs the death certificate and how the pathologist's professional findings enter the record. The pathologist's practice patterns must adapt to the structural system in which she works.

Statutorily reportable deaths converge on a common core across jurisdictions: sudden or unexpected death, violent or traumatic death, suspected intoxication, custodial death, unattended death, pediatric death without evident cause, unidentified decedents, and deaths pending cremation. Ambiguous cases are always reported.

Cause of death is the disease or injury that initiated the lethal chain (immediate through proximate). Manner of death is the classification of how the cause came about (natural / accident / suicide / homicide / undetermined). Mechanism of death is the nonspecific final pathway and is never certified as a cause. Manner tracks the proximate cause across time, provided no efficient intervening event has broken the chain.

The forensic pathologist works within an investigative team and holds professional obligations of objectivity, documented reasoning, and freedom from external pressure. The 2025 National Academies review identified undue influence on cause-and-manner determinations as a persistent problem, and the pathologist protects objectivity through documented reasoning, appropriate use of the undetermined manner, and structured peer consultation on difficult cases.

# CHAPTER 2: THE DEATH SCENE: INVESTIGATION, DOCUMENTATION, AND RECONSTRUCTION

**Learning Objectives**

1. Articulate why scene investigation is a component of the forensic pathologist's reasoning rather than background context.
2. Describe the standard sequence of scene response and the professional roles of the death investigator, law enforcement, evidence technicians, and the pathologist.
3. Apply the principles of scene photography, scene diagramming, and narrative documentation to produce a defensible scene record.
4. Document the body at the scene in a manner that supports subsequent autopsy reasoning — body position, livor and rigor, associated artifacts, and preservation of evidence.
5. Integrate scene findings with autopsy findings to reach a defensible reconstruction and recognize the traps that undermine scene reasoning.

## The Scene as a Component of Case Reasoning

In hospital pathology the specimen enters the laboratory with a clinical history attached, and the pathologist can render an accurate diagnosis on the specimen alone in most cases. In forensic pathology the analogous approach fails. A body arriving at the autopsy suite with no scene context is a body from which certain kinds of injury can be identified but from which many determinations of cause and, especially, of manner, cannot be reliably made. A gunshot wound to the head is a finding on external and internal examination; whether that wound is a suicide or a homicide is answered principally at the scene, by the position of the body, the location and status of the firearm, the presence or absence of a note, the range of fire indicated by soot deposition on skin or clothing, and the trajectory reconstructed from the wound path together with the physical relationship of the body to any surface. The autopsy identifies the wound; the scene answers the question that certifies the case.

This is the reason the forensic pathologist reads the scene report before autopsy, reviews the scene photographs during autopsy dictation, and — in complex cases — responds to the scene personally. The scene is not a separate investigation whose results are handed to her; it is a component of her medical reasoning. When scene documentation is inadequate, the determinations that depend on scene reconstruction cannot be made to reasonable medical certainty, and the manner determination properly moves toward undetermined rather than being extrapolated from findings that cannot support it.

### What the Scene Contributes That the Autopsy Cannot

The scene contributes information the body itself cannot carry. Position of the body relative to a weapon, a ligature, a stairwell, or a body of water indicates the mechanism of terminal event. Environmental temperature, ventilation, and time elapsed since last known contact frame the interpretation of postmortem changes and the estimation of postmortem interval. The presence and character of blood at the scene — pools, drips, spatter, smears, wipe patterns — documents the pattern of bleeding and, sometimes, the sequence of events. Physical evidence at the scene — medications, drug paraphernalia, alcohol, weapons, notes, correspondence, and communication devices — provides context for toxicological findings, for behavioral state, and for intent.

**KEY POINT:** The scene is not context for the autopsy. The scene is part of the case. A forensic pathologist who reads the autopsy findings against the scene report is doing the same integrative work that a clinical pathologist does when she reads a tissue biopsy against the clinical presentation and imaging.

### The Language of Scene Findings

Scene documentation is written for downstream consumers who were not present. The medicolegal death investigator, the police detective, and the pathologist read the scene report; if the case moves to trial, the report may be read years later by attorneys and by a jury. Precise, non-interpretive language is the standard. "Body in supine position on the floor" is documentation. "Victim posed by assailant" is interpretation. The distinction matters because interpretation writes conclusions into the record before the evidence is fully evaluated, and those conclusions become difficult to unwind on cross-examination. Documentation records the observable; interpretation belongs in the reasoning section of the autopsy report, where it is offered as opinion supported by the underlying documentation.

## Scene Response and Team Roles

Scene response is initiated when emergency services or law enforcement identify a death that requires medicolegal jurisdiction. The medicolegal death investigator (MDI) is dispatched. In some jurisdictions, particularly high-density urban systems, MDIs are on call around the clock and respond to every reportable death; in less resourced jurisdictions, the MDI or the pathologist may be reached by telephone and scene investigation is delegated to law enforcement with the pathologist involved by remote consultation. Understanding the local response model is a first task for the entering fellow.

### The Medicolegal Death Investigator

The MDI is the pathologist's principal partner in scene work. In the American Board of Medicolegal Death Investigators (ABMDI) credentialing system, the certified investigator has completed training in death scene investigation, in evidence recognition and handling, in postmortem-change assessment adequate to preserve the pathologist's ability to interpret the body, in family notification, and in written and verbal communication for both medical and legal audiences. The best MDI-pathologist working relationships are characterized by regular case review, shared understanding of what documentation the pathologist requires, and a communication channel that allows the pathologist to request additional documentation, interviews, or scene revisit when the case reasoning requires it.

**Law Enforcement**

Uniformed patrol officers are usually the first professionals on scene. Their responsibilities are to secure the scene, protect the body, identify and manage witnesses, and preserve the physical evidence in place until specialized personnel arrive. When a homicide is suspected or confirmed, homicide detectives assume lead investigative responsibility. Evidence technicians (crime scene analysts) perform detailed photography, evidence collection, and specialized scene work including bloodstain pattern analysis, ballistic reconstruction, and latent print recovery. The pathologist coordinates with the detective and with the evidence technician; the working expectation is that the pathologist informs law enforcement of what she requires to complete the autopsy determination, and that law enforcement informs the pathologist of what they have observed and gathered.

**When the Pathologist Responds Personally**

Personal scene response by the pathologist is standard in some offices and reserved for complex cases in others. It is generally indicated in mass fatality events, in complex homicide scenes where reconstruction depends on physical relationships that photography incompletely captures, in scenes with unusual physical evidence (industrial deaths, deaths in confined space, deaths involving specialized weapons), in high-profile cases where the pathologist will be the eventual witness, and in cases where scene documentation quality is likely to be contested. The pathologist who responds personally documents her own scene observations in her autopsy report and testifies to what she observed directly; the pathologist who does not respond documents that she reasoned from the scene report and the scene photography.

**SCENE-TO-CERTIFICATION DECISION SYSTEM — Scene-Body Discordance Arc**

---

**Presenting Death Scenario:** A 32-year-old woman is found deceased in her second-floor apartment by a family member who had not reached her by phone for two days. The body is supine on the bedroom floor between the bed and the door. There is a small amount of dried blood on the carpet under the head. A prescription bottle of alprazolam is on the nightstand, partially full, with the label intact. The apartment door was locked from the inside with a deadbolt. There are no signs of forced entry. The scene investigator notes that the body position appears "posed" because the arms are extended along the body and the legs are straight.

**Autopsy Signature:** External examination shows a small (1 cm) abraded contusion on the right parietal scalp with underlying subgaleal hemorrhage. There is no depressed fracture, no linear or comminuted skull fracture, and no evidence of ligature or compression injury of the neck. Internal examination shows severe atherosclerotic coronary artery disease that would not be typical for a 32-year-old woman but is documented, cardiomegaly at 380 grams for body habitus, and pulmonary congestion. Livor mortis on posterior body surfaces is fully developed and fixed, consistent with 8 to 12 hours or more since death, but is present on the anterior thorax as well in a pattern indicating the body was moved at least once during the postmortem interval. Toxicology shows an alprazolam level within therapeutic range and a blood ethanol of 0.03 grams per deciliter.

**Cause Determination:** The initial impression suggested a possible fall (subgaleal hemorrhage) with therapeutic-level medication. Detailed review reidentifies the cause as most consistent with cardiac arrhythmia in the setting of underlying cardiovascular disease, with the scalp injury attributed to the fall that occurred as she collapsed. The dual-pattern livor — posterior fixed and anterior partial — documents that she was moved postmortem, from an initial position to the position in which she was found, which is important documentation but does not itself change cause.

**Manner Determination:** Natural. The dual-pattern livor initially raised concern for third-party involvement, but no injuries beyond the scalp abrasion were identified, no ligature or compression, no toxicological explanation for death, and no scene evidence of forced entry or struggle. The family member who discovered the body ultimately acknowledged repositioning the body from a face-down position to supine in an attempt to "make her look peaceful." That single documented repositioning explains the livor pattern.

**Trap Logic:** Scene-body discordance is a signal that something happened between death and discovery, not automatically a signal that the death was homicide. The trap in the opposite direction is to assume that scene-body discordance is always benign and to under-investigate the case. Every discordant finding — livor incompatible with body position, rigor incompatible with body position, injury pattern incompatible with the location of death, blood distribution incompatible with the position of the wound — must be explained before the case is closed. Family repositioning of a decedent is the most common benign explanation and must be actively inquired about, because family members rarely volunteer it out of embarrassment or fear.

**Certification Anchor:** The livor mortis pattern is the timestamp and the position record of the body during the postmortem interval. Livor incompatible with the position of the body at discovery documents intervening movement; identifying who moved the body, when, and why is a scene investigation task that must be completed before certifying manner. Once the movement is explained by non-lethal, non-suspicious circumstance, the cause and manner determinations can proceed on the autopsy findings.

## Scene Documentation: Photography, Diagrams, and Narrative

Scene documentation follows a hierarchy of documentation methods, each with a specific purpose and each with recognized limitations.

### Scene Photography

Photography is the primary documentation method for the scene. Standard practice progresses from overview to mid-range to close-up. Overview photography documents the location and orientation of the scene in the built environment — the address, the exterior of the building, the room in which the body is located, and the relationship of the body to significant features of the room (doorways, windows, furniture, adjacent rooms). Mid-range photography documents the body in its immediate context — the position of the body relative to objects within arm's reach, the pattern of blood or fluid at the scene, the position of any weapon or medication, and the presence and orientation of any other significant physical evidence. Close-up photography documents injuries and evidence at a scale where measurement and identification are possible; close-up shots include a scale ruler and are taken at right angles to the surface being photographed.

The professional standard is to photograph before disturbance and again after each stage of scene processing. Nothing is moved before it is photographed. When the body is turned or the weapon is collected, the moment before and the moment after are documented so that the record shows both the original state and the changed state. Photographs are taken in sequence with metadata (timestamp, camera identification, photographer) recorded, and the sequence is preserved in the case file.

**CAUTION:** Digital scene photographs are subject to the same evidentiary rules as physical evidence. Photographs are authenticated at trial by testimony of who took them, under what circumstances, and whether they fairly and accurately represent the scene at the time. The photographer's contemporaneous notes and the metadata of the image file establish authenticity; edited, cropped, or filter-processed images are contested on cross-examination and may be excluded.

### Scene Diagramming

The scene diagram supplements photography by rendering the spatial relationships in a form that photography cannot fully capture. A room is three-dimensional; a photograph is two-dimensional, and no single photograph shows the full spatial context. The diagram — a hand-drawn or software-generated plan view of the scene — shows the room in outline, the position of the body, the position of relevant objects (weapon, blood pool, furniture, doorways), and measurements from the body to significant features. Diagrams are annotated with the date, time, scene identification, and the identity of the person who prepared them. Modern scene reconstruction in complex cases increasingly uses three-dimensional laser scanning, which produces a spatially precise digital model of the scene that can be interrogated after the physical scene has been released, but the traditional diagram remains the standard documentation form in most cases.

### Narrative Documentation

The narrative scene report is the investigator's written account of what she observed. The narrative captures information that photography and diagramming do not — ambient temperature and lighting, odors present at the scene, the state of the residence (organized, disorganized, evidence of habitation), the account provided by any witnesses or first responders, the identity and location of medication containers and their labels, and the presence or absence of items whose absence is significant (a firearm reported by the family that is not found; an identification document expected in a wallet that is missing). The narrative is the connective tissue that lets a reader who was not on scene understand the scene as it presented to the investigator.

## Documentation of the Body at the Scene

The body itself is documented as an evidence item at the scene, distinct from the eventual autopsy documentation, because the scene provides information about the body that will be lost when the body is moved.

### Body Position and Orientation

The exact position of the body is photographed and diagrammed before any repositioning. Prone versus supine, the position of the head and limbs, and the orientation of the body relative to the room and to any weapon or object are all documented. Small changes in body position have interpretive weight; a hand grasping a firearm, a hand near but not on a firearm, and a hand in a position inconsistent with reaching the firearm at the scene are all different observations that support different reconstructions.

### Postmortem Changes at the Scene

Livor mortis and rigor mortis are documented at the scene because they will progress between scene discovery and autopsy. Livor is described by distribution (which body surfaces), by intensity (developed or minimal), and by fixation (does it blanch on pressure). Rigor is described by extent (present in which muscle groups) and by intensity (partial, complete, breaking). Algor mortis is documented by measurement of ambient temperature and, in cases where postmortem interval matters, by careful measurement of body temperature at a defined anatomical location using a validated method (deep rectal or intrahepatic). These findings, documented at the scene, are the foundation of any subsequent postmortem interval reasoning.

### Preservation of Trace and Fragile Evidence

The hands are protected before transport by paper bags secured at the wrists; plastic bags trap moisture and degrade fingernail and skin evidence and are not used. Loose fibers, hair, or debris on the body are documented in place, then collected before transport when required for the case reasoning. Blood on the body — whether the decedent's own or possibly transferred from another source — is documented photographically and its location described in the narrative before the body is moved. A body that will be moved through a home, down a staircase, and into a transport vehicle will lose evidence in the process; the documentation at the scene is what preserves the record.

**CLINICAL PEARL:** Every action that the death investigator takes at the scene is a choice between documenting the state as found and altering the state to permit the next step. The professional standard is documentation before alteration, every time, without exception. When the body must be moved to reach an underlying surface, the position at rest is photographed first.

## Scene-Body Integration and Reconstruction

Scene documentation and autopsy findings are integrated by the pathologist in the reasoning that supports cause and manner determinations. The integration is where interpretation lives — where the pathologist argues, in the discussion section of the autopsy report, why the findings taken together support the certified cause and manner.

### Reading the Scene Report Before Autopsy

The scene report is read in full before the autopsy begins. The reason is not administrative; it is that the autopsy is a directed examination shaped by the reasoning already underway. A gunshot wound in a decedent found holding a firearm requires different documentation than a gunshot wound in a decedent found with no firearm present. A decomposed body from a locked residence requires attention to organ preservation that a fresh body from a hospital transport does not. A pediatric decedent requires organized documentation of every external surface, of the position and appearance of the diaper if present, and of feeding and sleep environment details that only the scene has captured. The autopsy is guided by scene reasoning; skipping the scene report before autopsy compromises the examination.

### Reading the Scene Photographs During Dictation

The scene photographs are reviewed during autopsy dictation because reconstruction depends on integrating what is found on the body with where and how the body was found. A pattern of livor mortis compatible with the position of discovery is a different finding than a pattern incompatible with that position; the reconstruction of the sequence of events depends on this integration. A pattern of blood on the body that matches the pattern of blood at the scene supports the reconstruction that the decedent bled where she was found; a mismatch between body blood pattern and scene blood pattern documents that death occurred elsewhere and the body was moved.

### The Reconstruction Question

The reconstruction question is the question of what happened, in what order, over what time, at what locations. A well-reconstructed case answers: how did death occur; where did it occur; when did it occur; who or what caused the injuries or exposures that led to death; and what happened between death and discovery. Not every case requires reconstruction — a natural death of an elderly decedent in her own bed does not raise a reconstruction question, and the pathologist's report addresses the case at the level of cause and manner without extensive reconstruction narrative. A homicide, a suspicious death, or a death with scene-body discordance does require reconstruction, and the pathologist's reasoning in the autopsy report addresses each element that the case turns on.

**SCENE-TO-CERTIFICATION DECISION SYSTEM — Resuscitation Artifact Arc**

**Presenting Death Scenario:** A 58-year-old man collapses at home. His wife initiates cardiopulmonary resuscitation and calls emergency services. Paramedics arrive within 8 minutes and continue advanced resuscitation for 25 minutes without return of spontaneous circulation. Death is pronounced at the scene. On external examination in the emergency department — to which the body is transported by paramedics per local protocol — there are multiple contusions across the anterior chest, an intraoral tooth injury, and abrasions on the neck. The paramedics note that the decedent was reportedly "fine" until the moment of collapse. The scene report from the residence documents no signs of struggle, no visible injury on the body before resuscitation began, and no third party present other than the wife.

**Autopsy Signature:** External examination confirms extensive anterior chest contusion in a pattern consistent with the palmar heel of a hand applied at the sternum — the pattern of chest compressions. There is a fractured incisor with underlying oral mucosal abrasion. The neck abrasions are linear and superficial, distributed anteriorly, consistent with tape and adhesive application from an endotracheal tube securing. Internal examination shows severe atherosclerotic coronary artery disease with 90 percent occlusive stenosis of the proximal left anterior descending artery, focal acute myocardial infarction of the anterior wall, and rib fractures at costochondral junctions from resuscitation. There is no cervical soft-tissue hemorrhage, no ligature mark of the neck deep to the tape-related abrasion, and no significant natural or traumatic injury to the neck.

**Cause Determination:** Acute myocardial infarction due to severe atherosclerotic coronary artery disease. The chest contusions, rib fractures, tooth injury, and superficial neck abrasions are all resuscitation-related artifacts, not antemortem injury.

**Manner Determination:** Natural. The autopsy findings identify natural cardiovascular disease of sufficient severity to cause sudden death. The apparent injuries are all attributable to documented resuscitative intervention.

**Trap Logic:** Resuscitation produces predictable patterns of injury that can mimic assault to an examiner unfamiliar with them. Sternal and anterior chest contusion from manual compressions can appear as blunt force chest injury. Bilateral costochondral fractures can appear as forceful chest compression from an assailant. Endotracheal tube adhesive can leave neck abrasions that appear as ligature marks. Intraoral tooth injury from intubation can be misread as blunt oral trauma. The pathologist who does not know these patterns can misinterpret a natural death as a homicide, particularly under time pressure. The countermeasure is knowing what resuscitation looks like on autopsy and confirming that any injury attributed to resuscitation is consistent with the pattern and time course of the resuscitative effort documented in the ambulance and emergency department records.

**Certification Anchor:** Injuries produced by documented resuscitative intervention are attributed to that intervention when their pattern, location, and severity are consistent with the effort described. When a purported resuscitation injury is inconsistent with the documented care — a fingermark contusion at a location not touched during compressions, a laceration in a distribution not caused by intubation — the injury is treated as antemortem until proven otherwise.

## Special Scene Categories

Certain scenes call for specialized approach because the physical environment, the nature of the death, or the population involved introduces documentation demands that go beyond the standard scene protocol.

### Pediatric Scenes

In sudden unexpected infant death (SUID), the scene is a critical element of the determination. Sleep position at discovery, sleep surface, presence of soft bedding or objects, presence of a co-sleeping adult, and ambient temperature are all documented. Doll reenactment — a supervised procedure in which the caregiver demonstrates with an infant doll where the infant was placed to sleep, where the infant was found, and what interventions were attempted — is standard practice in many jurisdictions. Documentation of the feeding history, prior health, and environmental exposures is obtained from the caregiver contemporaneously with the scene work, because delayed accounts drift and because the scene investigation may inform the subsequent determination substantially.

### Scenes With Deceased in Water

Water scenes have specific documentation requirements. The location of the body in the water (surface, submerged, depth), the currents and temperature of the water, the position of the body relative to any structure (dock, boat, riverbank), and the presence of anchoring objects or weighted material on or near the body are documented. Recovery of the body must preserve the pattern of any injuries and the presence of foam cone (a mixture of water, mucus, and pulmonary edema fluid at the mouth and nostrils — a nonspecific finding in drowning but suggestive of vital submersion when present). Water scenes are one context in which forensic response is often delayed and in which postmortem changes complicate interpretation substantially.

### Fire Scenes

Fire scenes require specialized coordination with fire investigators. The position of the body relative to the fire's point of origin, the pattern of thermal injury to the body, and the atmosphere in which the body was found (structural collapse, oxygen depletion, toxic combustion products) all inform the reasoning at autopsy. The distinction between antemortem burn injury and postmortem thermal artifact is a specific interpretive task that depends on scene documentation of fire dynamics as much as on autopsy findings.

### Confined-Space and Occupational Scenes

Deaths in confined spaces (silos, tanks, sewers) and in industrial or occupational contexts (heavy equipment, chemical exposure, agricultural machinery) require scene response by personnel with the safety training and equipment to enter the environment. The pathologist may not be able to respond personally in real time because of confined-space entry requirements; documentation for the pathologist is provided by trained response personnel, and the pathologist supplements it with occupational exposure information from the employer and from state or federal safety agencies as the case proceeds.

### Mass Fatality Scenes

Mass fatality response — a topic developed at length in Chapter 21 — requires activation of an incident command structure that governs the scene through pathologists, investigators, forensic anthropologists, dental identification specialists, DNA analysts, and mortuary personnel. Individual scene documentation is subordinated to the systematic recovery and identification protocol; the standard forensic pathology scene report is replaced by the standardized documentation formats of disaster victim identification.

### Chain of Custody and Handoff to the Autopsy Suite

The transition of the body and physical evidence from the scene to the autopsy suite is governed by chain of custody documentation. Every person who has physical control of the body or of an evidence item between scene and autopsy is documented in a chain of custody record. Breaks in the chain — undocumented handoffs, unlocked storage, unidentified handlers — are among the most common bases on which evidence is challenged at trial. The pathologist inherits the chain of custody at the point the body enters her control at the autopsy suite; she confirms the identity of the decedent by tag or bracelet against the accompanying paperwork, documents the seal status of any evidence transported with the body, and continues the chain with her own documentation as the autopsy proceeds. Photographs of the body as received — including any personal effects, clothing, and adherent debris — constitute the first autopsy documentation step and preserve the integration point between scene and examination.

**EVIDENCE:** Chain of custody challenges at trial are among the most common bases for exclusion or diminished weight of physical evidence, including autopsy specimens and photographs. A chain that documents every transfer, with dated and signed handoffs and secure storage between transfers, is essentially not defeatable on cross-examination. A chain with undocumented gaps is contested and sometimes excluded.

## A Worked Case in Scene-Autopsy Integration

The following case illustrates how scene documentation, autopsy findings, and reconstruction work together in a case that turns on integration.

### Case Presentation

A 28-year-old man is found deceased at approximately 2:00 AM in the driveway of a residence in a suburban neighborhood. Neighbors called emergency services after hearing an argument and, moments later, what one witness described as "shouting and then silence." Police arrive within 6 minutes. The decedent is supine on the concrete driveway with a large pool of blood surrounding the upper torso and head. A folding knife with a 3-inch blade is on the ground approximately 4 feet from the body. The residents of the house are present at the scene. One — a man in his early thirties — has blood on his hands and forearms. He tells officers that he acted in self-defense during an attempted home invasion. The scene is secured, the medicolegal death investigator is dispatched, and the pathologist is notified. She elects to respond personally given the reconstruction implications of the case.

### Scene Documentation

The scene is photographed by an evidence technician in the sequence described above — overview, mid-range, close-up. The body is documented in position. The knife is photographed in place before it is collected. Blood patterns on the driveway are documented; the primary blood pool is at the decedent's upper torso, with radial spatter extending approximately 3 feet on the pavement. A secondary trail of blood extends approximately 12 feet from the primary pool toward the street, decreasing in volume and character consistent with movement of a bleeding source. The scene diagrams document the position of the body, the position of the knife, the extent of the primary blood pool, and the location of the secondary trail. The residence door is documented as unlocked; the exterior of the residence is documented photographically.

The scene narrative documents ambient conditions (approximately 55 degrees Fahrenheit, clear, dry pavement), the account provided by the resident who claims self-defense (which is separated from the scene documentation and preserved as a separate document), the accounts of the neighbors who called emergency services, and the observation that the decedent has no wallet or identification in his pockets. Neighbors identify the decedent by name; family are subsequently notified. The pathologist, on scene, documents her observations of livor mortis (early, developing in dependent surfaces of the body in the position of discovery), rigor mortis (minimal, consistent with 1 to 2 hours since death), and the pattern and orientation of the visible injuries.

### Autopsy Findings

External examination shows two stab wounds to the anterior chest, one in the left mid-clavicular line at the fourth intercostal space and one in the right para-sternal region at the third intercostal space. Both wounds are documented for length, orientation, character of margins, and the pattern of tissue at the wound edges. The left-sided wound is 2.5 cm long, oriented at approximately 10 o'clock to 4 o'clock, with clean margins; internal exploration reveals a wound tract passing posteriorly and slightly downward, terminating in the pericardial sac with an associated 1.5 cm defect in the anterior wall of the right ventricle. The right-sided wound is 2.2 cm long, similarly oriented, with a wound tract passing through the anterior chest wall into the anterior mediastinum without entry into a great vessel or a cardiac chamber. There are three additional wounds to the left forearm consistent with defensive injuries: a stab wound to the volar surface with associated tendon injury, and two incised wounds along the ulnar aspect.

The stabbing pattern — a lethal cardiac wound, a non-lethal chest wound, and defensive wounds to the forearm — documents a struggle rather than a single decisive blow. The trajectories of the cardiac and chest wounds are consistent with an attacker facing the decedent. The defensive wounds to the forearm document that the decedent was conscious and defending during at least some portion of the assault.

### Scene-Autopsy Integration and Reconstruction

The scene documentation and the autopsy findings integrate into a partial reconstruction. The presence of a secondary blood trail extending 12 feet from the primary blood pool documents that the decedent bled while moving, consistent with a period of consciousness after the initial stab wound. The direction of the trail indicates the decedent moved from the residence toward the street; the primary pool at the position of discovery indicates the location where he collapsed. The defensive wounds document a struggle. The pattern is inconsistent with a decedent who intruded on the residence and was immediately incapacitated; it is more consistent with a confrontation of unclear origin followed by an attempt to flee. This reconstruction, alone, does not establish who initiated the encounter, does not identify who was the aggressor, and does not answer the legal question of self-defense. The pathologist's reasoning documents the physical facts — the pattern of injury, the location and direction of blood, the pattern of defensive wounds — and stops at reasonable medical certainty about those facts. The legal determination of self-defense is made by the criminal justice system on the basis of the pathologist's findings, the testimony of the resident, the physical evidence recovered at the scene, and any other available evidence.

**CLINICAL PEARL:** The pathologist reconstructs what the physical evidence supports. She does not reconstruct what she was told at the scene, and she does not incorporate the legal theory of the case into her reasoning. When the physical evidence supports two possible sequences, she documents both and does not choose. The choice between them is made by the fact-finder at trial, not by the medical examiner in the autopsy report.

### Scene Revisit

In cases where scene documentation is inadequate or where new evidence emerges after the scene is released, scene revisit is sometimes necessary. Revisit is a compromised documentation exercise because the scene has changed — blood has been cleaned, the body is gone, objects have been moved, and time has passed. Revisit can nonetheless establish spatial measurements, confirm structural features of the environment, and support the pathologist's testimony by giving her direct familiarity with the location. In cases with the highest reconstruction complexity, three-dimensional laser scanning of the scene at the time of the initial investigation preserves the spatial record in a form that can be revisited without physical return to the location. Where the resources for laser scanning exist, they are increasingly the standard for complex homicide scenes.

## SCENE-TO-CERTIFICATION DECISION SYSTEM — Death Scene Determination Arcs

**The Scene Is Part of the Case:** Scene information is not context for autopsy; it is an integrated element of the case reasoning. The scene report is read before autopsy, the scene photographs are reviewed during dictation, and the reasoning in the autopsy report integrates scene and autopsy findings.

**The Documentation Hierarchy:** Photography documents the visible; diagrams document the spatial; narrative documents everything the visual media miss. The professional standard is documentation before alteration in every case, with photographs authenticated by metadata and contemporaneous notes and with the sequence of the documentation preserved in the case file.

**Body at the Scene:** Body position, livor mortis, rigor mortis, and algor mortis are documented at the scene because they will change between discovery and autopsy. Preservation of trace and fragile evidence — hands bagged in paper, loose materials collected before transport, blood pattern documented before body movement — protects the record that supports the reconstruction.

**Reconstruction Answers the Case Question:** Not every case requires extensive reconstruction. Cases where scene-body discordance exists, where the location of death is contested, where movement of the body during the postmortem interval is documented, or where the manner determination depends on positional reasoning require the pathologist to reconstruct in her autopsy report the sequence of events that the evidence supports.

**Resuscitation and Special-Category Traps:** Resuscitation-related artifacts — sternal contusion, costochondral fractures, endotracheal-tube adhesive marks, intubation tooth injury — are documented patterns that can mimic assault. The pathologist recognizes them as artifacts when the pattern is consistent with documented care and treats them as antemortem when the pattern is not. Pediatric, water, fire, confined-space, and mass-fatality scenes carry documentation requirements beyond the standard protocol; the pathologist knows what each special-category scene requires and confirms it has been obtained before certification.

## Summary and Key Concepts

The scene is an integrated component of forensic pathology reasoning. The autopsy identifies findings; the scene answers questions that the autopsy alone cannot answer, particularly questions of manner determination that depend on position, sequence, and the physical relationship of the body to weapons and objects.

Scene response is a coordinated activity of the medicolegal death investigator, law enforcement, evidence technicians, and the pathologist. Understanding each role, and the local response model that governs which personnel respond to which cases, is a first task for the entering forensic pathology fellow.

Scene documentation follows a hierarchy: photography (from overview to close-up), diagramming (spatial relationships), and narrative (everything the visual media miss). Photographs are authenticated by metadata and contemporaneous notes and preserved unaltered; edited or filtered images are contested at trial.

The body at the scene is documented as an evidence item, including position, orientation, livor mortis, rigor mortis, algor mortis, and the position of the body relative to weapons and objects. Fragile evidence — hands, loose trace materials, blood patterns — is preserved before the body is moved.

Scene-body integration is the pathologist's task. The scene report is read before autopsy, the photographs are reviewed during dictation, and the reasoning in the autopsy report integrates both. Cases requiring reconstruction — scene-body discordance, contested location of death, documented postmortem movement — are addressed with explicit reasoning in the autopsy report.

Special scenes — pediatric, water, fire, confined space, mass fatality — carry documentation requirements beyond the standard protocol. The pathologist confirms that the special-category documentation has been obtained before certifying the death, because in these cases the scene evidence disappears rapidly and is not recoverable after the fact.

# CHAPTER 3: POSTMORTEM CHANGES AND ESTIMATION OF TIME OF DEATH

**Learning Objectives**

1. Explain the physiological and biochemical basis of the postmortem changes seen at the scene and at autopsy.
2. Distinguish livor mortis, rigor mortis, and algor mortis by mechanism, time course, and pattern, and apply each to postmortem interval reasoning.
3. Describe the sequence of decomposition from autolysis through skeletonization and identify the environmental modifiers that accelerate or retard each stage.
4. Estimate a postmortem interval using integrated postmortem-change findings with an appropriate margin of uncertainty, and recognize the limits of interval estimation.
5. Distinguish postmortem artifact from antemortem injury and pathological finding, and articulate the traps that arise when the distinction is missed.

## The Biology of Postmortem Change

Postmortem change is the sequence of physical, chemical, and biological events that transform a body from the state of living tissue to skeletal remains. The sequence is driven by the cessation of oxygenated blood flow at the moment of death and by the loss of the homeostatic and immune mechanisms that ordinarily keep tissue integrity and microbial populations in balance. Understanding the sequence, and understanding the modifiers that accelerate or retard it, is the foundation of any reasoning about time of death and of the recognition of postmortem artifacts that can mimic pathological findings at autopsy.

The biology proceeds in overlapping phases. In the earliest phase, the body cools toward ambient temperature (algor mortis), blood settles in dependent vessels under gravity (livor mortis), and muscle glycogen is depleted with a resulting chemical contracture of muscle fibers (rigor mortis). These early changes are dominated by physical redistribution and by the enzymatic and biochemical shifts within cells that have lost their aerobic substrate. In the intermediate phase, autolysis — the digestion of tissue by its own lysosomal enzymes — and putrefaction — the microbial breakdown of tissue by endogenous flora and by environmental organisms — dismantle the soft tissues. In the late phase, environmental exposure produces the reduction of soft tissue to bone (skeletonization), with or without intermediate states of adipocere formation or mummification depending on conditions.

### The Aerobic-Anaerobic Transition

The biochemical trigger for postmortem change is the loss of oxygenated perfusion. Cells that were metabolizing under aerobic conditions shift immediately to anaerobic metabolism, producing lactic acid and depleting adenosine triphosphate. The intracellular pH falls. Lysosomal membranes destabilize. Cellular potassium leaks into the interstitium. Calcium enters muscle cells uncontrolled from the sarcoplasmic reticulum, initiating the actin-myosin cross-linking that eventually produces rigor. The endothelial integrity of small vessels degrades and blood begins to move by hydrostatic pressure toward dependent tissues rather than by cardiac pumping.

These processes begin within minutes of somatic death, are well established within one to two hours, and progress along time courses that are broadly predictable in a body of standard habitus at temperate environmental conditions. The predictability is degraded, sometimes substantially, by conditions that alter the underlying rate of biochemical or microbial activity — ambient temperature, body habitus, antemortem exertion or febrile illness, wound distribution, and clothing or immersion.

**KEY POINT:** Postmortem interval estimation is not a determination of the time of death. It is a statement of what range of postmortem intervals is consistent with the observed postmortem changes. The range is often wide. Precision is bought by integrating multiple lines of evidence — not by relying on a single finding.

## Early Postmortem Changes: Livor, Rigor, and Algor Mortis

### Livor Mortis

Livor mortis, sometimes termed lividity, is the pooling of blood in dependent vessels under gravity after cardiac arrest ends the maintenance of intravascular pressure. It appears as a purple to violet discoloration of dependent body surfaces. In a supine decedent, livor develops in the posterior surfaces of the neck, trunk, and lower extremities, with contact pallor at points where the body rests against a firm surface and the microvasculature is compressed. Livor is typically first detectable within 30 minutes to 2 hours of death and progressively deepens over the ensuing hours. It reaches maximum intensity by approximately 8 to 12 hours in most cases.

Two properties of livor are exploited in postmortem interval reasoning. The first is blanching. In the early hours, livor blanches when pressure is applied to the discolored skin — the discolored blood is displaced from the compressed capillaries and refills after pressure is released. In the later hours, blanching diminishes and eventually fails, as blood begins to hemolyze and to stain the surrounding tissue rather than remaining intravascular. The transition from blanching to non-blanching livor is termed fixation and typically occurs between 8 and 12 hours after death under temperate conditions, though this window is broad in practice. The second exploited property is repositioning. In the early hours before fixation, moving the body causes the pattern of livor to redistribute; the original pattern fades in the newly non-dependent areas and reappears in the newly dependent areas. After fixation, livor does not fully redistribute; the original pattern persists in part even after repositioning, and a second pattern develops incompletely in the new dependent areas. This is the basis for identifying postmortem movement of the body — the phenomenon illustrated in the previous chapter's Scene-Body Discordance Arc.

The color of livor is diagnostic in specific settings. Bright cherry-red livor suggests carbon monoxide poisoning, in which carboxyhemoglobin substitutes for oxyhemoglobin and produces a color that is retained in the postmortem state. Chocolate-brown livor suggests methemoglobinemia, from either intentional poisoning or from certain drug exposures. Bright pink livor in a body exposed to cold suggests hypothermia (with a similar mechanism of oxygen retention in tissue) or refrigeration; the finding is not specific but is a useful pointer. Bluish livor in dark-skinned decedents may be less prominent than in light-skinned decedents and requires careful examination.

### Rigor Mortis

Rigor mortis is the postmortem stiffening of skeletal muscle produced by the biochemical arrest of the actin-myosin cross-bridging cycle. In life, muscle relaxation depends on adenosine triphosphate, which powers the release of myosin heads from actin filaments. In death, ATP is progressively depleted, calcium enters the sarcoplasm uncontrolled, and the actin-myosin cross-bridges lock in a contracted state. The muscle becomes rigid. This state persists until proteolytic breakdown of the contractile proteins releases the cross-bridges, at which point the muscle relaxes and rigor is said to have passed.

The time course of rigor under temperate conditions follows a general pattern. Rigor is first detectable in the small muscles of the face and jaw, and in the fingers, within 2 to 4 hours after death. It progresses to involve larger muscle groups over the ensuing 6 to 12 hours, reaching full body distribution by approximately 12 hours. It persists at that maximum for approximately 12 to 24 hours, and then begins to pass as decomposition proceeds, resolving progressively over the ensuing 24 to 48 hours. Under temperate conditions, a fully rigid decedent whose rigor has not yet begun to pass is broadly compatible with a postmortem interval between 12 and 36 hours.

Several modifiers alter this course substantially. Rigor develops more rapidly in decedents with high antemortem muscle activity — vigorous physical exertion just before death, seizure activity, or febrile illness — because ATP is depleted at higher baseline rates. In extreme cases, this produces cadaveric spasm, in which rigor is essentially instantaneous and preserves the muscle position at the moment of death. Cadaveric spasm is rare and its recognition has forensic value: an instantaneous rigor gripping a firearm at death, for example, argues against postmortem placement of the firearm in the hand. Rigor develops slowly in cold environments, in decedents with low muscle mass (infants, cachectic elderly decedents), and can be delayed or effectively absent in bodies frozen shortly after death.

**CLINICAL PEARL:** Rigor mortis is broken by physical manipulation — flexing a stiff limb ruptures the acto-myosin cross-links mechanically. A limb whose rigor has been broken does not re-establish rigor. Test rigor by attempting to flex a joint; document the extent and the resistance encountered. Do not test a joint that must remain undisturbed for the reconstruction.

### Algor Mortis

Algor mortis is the cooling of the body toward ambient temperature after death. Living body temperature is maintained by metabolic heat production against passive heat loss to the environment. In death, metabolic heat production ceases and the body loses heat by conduction, convection, and radiation until thermal equilibrium with the environment is reached. In a body of standard habitus at typical indoor ambient temperature (approximately 21 to 22 degrees Celsius), the body cools at approximately 0.8 to 1.0

degrees Celsius per hour during the first several hours after death, then more slowly as the temperature gradient narrows.

The Henssge nomogram is the most widely used method for estimating postmortem interval from body temperature. It integrates measured rectal or intrahepatic temperature, measured ambient temperature, an estimated body weight, and a set of correction factors for clothing and environmental conditions (still air versus moving air; dry versus wet; indoor versus outdoor) to produce an interval estimate with an explicit confidence range. The confidence range is wide — typically plus or minus 2.8 hours for a temperate indoor case at 95 percent confidence — and widens further with departures from the nomogram's baseline assumptions. Application of the Henssge nomogram to a body that has been immersed, buried, or exposed to unusual thermal environments requires additional correction and produces less precise estimates.

The lower limit of usefulness of algor mortis for interval estimation is thermal equilibration with the environment; once the body reaches ambient temperature, further cooling does not occur and algor no longer provides interval information. Under typical indoor conditions, this equilibration is reached at approximately 20 to 24 hours after death and algor is not useful beyond this point. The upper limit of usefulness is the accuracy of the initial measurement; a body temperature measurement made hours after removal from the scene, in a cold storage refrigerator, does not reflect the body's temperature at the scene and cannot be back-calculated to the ambient conditions at the scene.

## SCENE-TO-CERTIFICATION DECISION SYSTEM — Discordant Livor Arc

**Presenting Death Scenario:** A 41-year-old man is found deceased at approximately 4:00 PM in a rural residence by a coworker who came to check on him after he missed a scheduled shift. The body is supine on the kitchen floor. Ambient temperature is 24 degrees Celsius. Livor mortis is visible on both the anterior and the posterior surfaces of the body, with the anterior livor markedly less well developed than the posterior. There is a small amount of blood in the mouth and nostrils. No visible injury is present on external inspection at the scene. Prescription medications, including an opioid analgesic and a benzodiazepine, are present in the residence at various locations.

**Autopsy Signature:** External examination confirms the dual-pattern livor. Rigor mortis is full and beginning to pass in the small muscles of the face and hands, suggesting a postmortem interval in the range of 24 to 36 hours. There are no injuries. Internal examination is unremarkable apart from pulmonary edema and cerebral edema. Toxicology shows a fatal blood concentration of the prescribed opioid together with the benzodiazepine at therapeutic levels.

**Cause Determination:** Combined drug toxicity (opioid and benzodiazepine).

**Manner Determination:** Accident. No evidence of suicidal intent, no note, no communications suggesting self-harm intent. The medications were the decedent's own prescriptions, and the pattern is consistent with unintended overdose of prescribed medication.

**Trap Logic:** The dual-pattern livor documents that the body was in one position for the majority of the postmortem interval and was then moved to a second position that was maintained for less time before discovery. The trap is to assume the movement was suspicious. In this case, the coworker who discovered the body acknowledged, on interview, that he had entered the residence, found the decedent prone on the kitchen floor with the face down in a pool of vomit and airway blood, and turned him over to the supine position before calling emergency services — believing he might still be alive. The dual livor is fully explained by this documented benign movement.

**Certification Anchor:** Any body found with a livor pattern discordant from the position of discovery has been moved during the postmortem interval. The forensic question is who moved the body, when, and why — answered by scene investigation and witness interview. Once the movement is documented and explained by non-lethal, non-suspicious circumstance, the cause and manner determinations can proceed on the autopsy findings without the discordant livor changing the outcome.

## Later Postmortem Changes: Autolysis, Putrefaction, and Decomposition

### Autolysis

Autolysis is the enzymatic self-digestion of tissue by lysosomal enzymes released from the destabilizing cellular architecture. It begins immediately at the cellular level and becomes grossly evident over hours to days. The organs most rapidly affected are those with the highest concentration of lysosomal enzymes — pancreas, adrenal cortex, gastric mucosa — which soften and lose their normal architecture within the first 24 hours. Slower-autolyzing tissues — fibrous tissue, cartilage, arterial media — persist longer. Autolysis is a sterile process that proceeds even in refrigerated storage, although at a substantially slower rate.

### Putrefaction

Putrefaction is the microbial breakdown of tissue by bacterial flora, both endogenous (principally colonic anaerobes) and environmental. Endogenous bacteria escape the bowel wall as the mucosal barrier autolyzes and enter the vascular tree, where they proliferate and produce the visible signs of putrefaction. The classic sequence begins with greenish discoloration of the abdomen (particularly the right lower quadrant, over the cecum) within 24 to 48 hours, followed by marbling of the skin (a superficial pattern of dark discoloration tracking the superficial venous system, produced by hemoglobin degradation and bacterial pigment along vessels), swelling of the face and abdomen from gas production (bloat), and eventual widespread bullae formation and skin slippage.

The time course of putrefaction is highly temperature-dependent. In warm environments (30 degrees Celsius and above), greenish discoloration is often visible within 12 hours, marbling within 24 hours, and generalized bloat within 48 to 72 hours. In cool environments (10 degrees Celsius or below), the same sequence may require weeks. Immersion, burial, and confinement in enclosed spaces further modify the sequence, as discussed below.

### Decomposition and Its Late Endpoints

Progressive putrefaction leads through the stages of active decay and dry decay. Active decay is characterized by liquefaction of soft tissue and by insect activity, which becomes prominent in outdoor bodies within days of death in warm weather. Dry decay follows the loss of most soft tissue mass and is characterized by leathery skin remnants over exposed bone. Skeletonization, the endpoint, is the reduction to bone alone, and depending on environment can require weeks (small body, warm outdoor exposure) to years (large body, cool sealed environment).

Adipocere formation is an alternative late endpoint that develops when bodies are exposed to moist, cool, oxygen-poor environments — immersed in water, buried in wet ground, or confined in humid enclosures. Body fat undergoes hydrolysis and hydrogenation to a firm, waxy substance that preserves body form and can persist for years. Mummification is a second alternative endpoint that develops when bodies are exposed to dry, warm, well-ventilated environments — desert conditions, dry attics. The tissues desiccate rather than putrefying, and the body dries and shrinks with preservation of external form for years to decades. Both adipocere and mummification substantially alter the postmortem interval reasoning because they represent departures from the typical decomposition sequence.

### Forensic Entomology as a Postmortem Interval Tool

Insect colonization of a body follows a predictable succession. Blowflies (Calliphoridae) arrive within hours to days of death and lay eggs primarily at natural orifices and at open wounds. The eggs develop through larval instars, pupate, and produce adult flies over a species- and temperature-dependent timeline that can be back-calculated to give an estimate of the earliest possible colonization time. Later-arriving insect populations — flesh flies, beetles, and eventually skin and hair specialists — provide additional interval markers. Forensic entomological analysis, performed by a specialist, can constrain the postmortem interval in outdoor cases substantially more tightly than any other method and is the standard consultation in cases with unclear time of death and active insect colonization. The pathologist collects representative larvae and pupae at autopsy — both preserved specimens and living specimens for rearing — and provides the entomologist with the ambient temperature history from local weather records for the collection site.

## Modifiers: Environment, Body Habitus, and Antemortem Conditions

### Temperature

Ambient temperature is the dominant modifier of every postmortem process. Elevated ambient temperature accelerates enzymatic autolysis, bacterial putrefaction, and insect development; depressed ambient temperature retards all three. Bodies frozen shortly after death may show minimal postmortem change over months, and postmortem interval estimation in such bodies depends on scene circumstances rather than on body findings. Bodies exposed to fluctuating temperature — warm days, cool nights, or transitions between indoor and outdoor exposure — develop postmortem change at rates that reflect the integrated thermal history rather than either extreme.

### Immersion and Burial

Water immersion slows decomposition compared with terrestrial exposure at equivalent temperature, and cool-water immersion slows it substantially. A body in cool water may show relatively fresh appearance at postmortem intervals that would produce advanced decomposition on land. Bodies recovered from water frequently show adipocere in longer-immersion cases. Burial similarly slows decomposition, with the extent of retardation depending on depth, soil type, and moisture. Shallow burial in warm, moist soil may show near-terrestrial rates; deep burial in cool, dry soil substantially slows the process.

### Body Habitus and Antemortem State

Obese decedents cool more slowly and retain heat that accelerates internal autolysis and putrefaction, producing internal decomposition changes disproportionate to external appearance. Cachectic decedents cool rapidly and may reach ambient temperature within a few hours, limiting the utility of algor mortis. Febrile decedents at death cool more slowly initially because of their elevated starting temperature. Sepsis, particularly with gram-negative organisms already circulating, accelerates putrefaction by seeding the vascular tree with bacteria before death. Trauma with open wounds accelerates local putrefaction at the wound site. Antemortem exercise or seizure accelerates rigor onset.

## Estimation of the Postmortem Interval

### Integrating Multiple Lines of Evidence

Postmortem interval estimation is done by integrating the information available from multiple postmortem-change findings, calibrated by the scene ambient conditions, and expressed as a range with explicit confidence limits. No single finding suffices for a defensible interval estimate. The pathologist reads livor development, livor fixation, rigor extent, rigor onset or passage, body temperature (measured at the scene when possible), and any decomposition stage present. She reads them against ambient temperature at the scene and against the last known contact time and last known evidence of life (a text message sent, a security camera image, a phone call answered). The intersection of the postmortem-change window and the last-known-alive window is the tightest interval estimate the case supports.

| Postmortem Change | Time Course (temperate indoor) | Notes |
|---|---|---|
| Livor first appearance | 30 min to 2 hours | Dependent surfaces, blanches on pressure |
| Livor maximum intensity | 8 to 12 hours | Progressively less blanching |
| Livor fixation | 8 to 12 hours (broad range) | Non-blanching; does not fully redistribute |
| Rigor first detectable | 2 to 4 hours | Face and jaw first, then extremities |
| Rigor full body | 6 to 12 hours | All major muscle groups |
| Rigor persistence | 12 to 24 hours (max) | Fully developed |

| | | |
|---|---|---|
| Rigor passage | 24 to 48 hours | Progressive relaxation as putrefaction proceeds |
| Body temperature equilibration | 20 to 24 hours | In standard habitus at ~21°C ambient |
| Greenish discoloration | 24 to 48 hours | RLQ over cecum; accelerated by warmth |
| Marbling | 48 to 72 hours | Along superficial veins |
| Bloat | 3 to 5 days | Face and abdomen distension |
| Active decay / insect activity | Days to weeks | Highly environment-dependent |
| Skeletonization | Weeks to years | Depends on habitat, insect access, scavenging |

**The Confidence Range and Its Communication**

The postmortem interval estimate is communicated with an explicit confidence range — typically expressed as a window ("the postmortem interval is estimated at 12 to 24 hours") rather than as a single point. The width of the window reflects the honest uncertainty of the estimation. Wider windows are appropriate when environmental modifiers were substantial or unknown, when the postmortem-change evidence is ambiguous, or when the case is at the interface between phases (transitioning from developing rigor to fully developed rigor, or from fresh appearance to early putrefaction). A pathologist who reports "time of death was 4:30 AM on Tuesday" is reporting beyond the evidence unless the case has independent corroboration (an observed collapse, a phone record, a documented last-alive event); the honest medical estimate is almost always a window.

**CAUTION:** Television-style precise time-of-death determination — to the minute or half-hour — is a fictional convention. Real forensic pathology delivers estimates in windows, and the windows are usually hours to days wide. A pathologist who testifies to a narrower window than the evidence supports has overshot her own expertise and will be corrected on cross-examination by any competent opposing expert.

**SCENE-TO-CERTIFICATION DECISION SYSTEM — Long-Interval Postmortem Reasoning Arc**

**Presenting Death Scenario:** A body is discovered in the summer in a wooded area approximately 3 kilometers from the nearest residence. A hiker reports the discovery to law enforcement. The body is skeletonized in part — the head, upper trunk, and upper extremities are largely reduced to bone with attached leathery skin remnants; the lower body and lower extremities retain more soft tissue and show active decay with insect colonization. Clothing is present and largely intact. The decedent's identification cannot be established from documents at the scene.

**Autopsy Signature:** Postmortem examination confirms the differential decomposition — more advanced in the exposed upper body, less advanced in the covered lower body — consistent with either differential insect access, differential scavenger activity, or both. Radiographic examination identifies a healed clavicular fracture and dental restorations that permit odontological identification through dental records comparison. Insect samples are collected from the abdomen and the lower extremities and are submitted to forensic entomology consultation. No injury attributable to a lethal event is identifiable given the soft tissue loss.

**Cause Determination:** Cause of death cannot be determined from the postmortem examination. The soft tissue loss precludes identification of most soft-tissue injury, most soft-tissue disease, and toxicological analysis (although hair may support limited toxicology). Bone is inspected for skeletal trauma, and no fractures beyond the healed clavicular fracture are identified. The case is certified cause undetermined.

**Manner Determination:** Undetermined. Without an identified cause of death and without scene evidence of a specific mechanism, manner cannot be reasoned to reasonable medical certainty. The case remains open pending any additional evidence.

**Trap Logic:** The trap in long-interval cases is to over-reach the postmortem-change evidence — to certify a manner based on the scene location or on circumstantial evidence rather than on findings. A body in the woods without identified injury is not automatically an accident, a suicide, or a homicide. It is a body without an identified mechanism of death, and undetermined is the appropriate manner. A second trap is to overstate the postmortem interval precision — differential decomposition can support a rough interval estimate (weeks to months in this case, refined by entomology) but not a specific date.

**Certification Anchor:** Undetermined is a professional determination, not a professional failure. When cause and manner cannot be reasoned from the available evidence to reasonable medical certainty, the honest determination is undetermined, and the case remains subject to reopening if new evidence emerges. Overreaching to a specific determination compromises the reliability of the entire office.

## Postmortem Change as Evidence

### Distinguishing Artifact From Antemortem Finding

Postmortem changes produce visible findings that can mimic antemortem injury or disease. Skin slippage in early putrefaction produces pale, denuded areas that can resemble abrasion. Marbling produces dark linear patterns that can resemble contusion. Postmortem drying of exposed skin (particularly at the corneas, the tips of the fingers, and any exposed mucosal surface) produces yellow-brown parchment-like areas that can resemble antemortem abrasion. Insect feeding produces punctate skin defects that can resemble puncture injury. Rodent or animal scavenging produces defect patterns that can resemble sharp force injury.

Distinguishing artifact from injury depends on recognizing the characteristic pattern of the artifact and on the absence of vital reaction. Antemortem injury produces vital reaction — hemorrhage into the tissue at the site, inflammatory response if survival was long enough, and demonstration of injury margins consistent with force applied to living tissue. Postmortem artifacts do not produce vital reaction; skin slippage lifts cleanly without underlying hemorrhage, drying artifacts show no dermal or subcutaneous bleeding, and scavenger defects lack the vital tissue response that characterizes injury inflicted on living skin. Histology can support the distinction when it is unclear at gross examination.

### Postmortem Change and Interpretation of Toxicology

Postmortem changes affect the interpretation of toxicological findings substantially. As tissues autolyze and putrefaction proceeds, drugs redistribute from tissue reservoirs into blood. This produces the phenomenon of postmortem redistribution, in which central blood (from the heart) shows drug concentrations substantially higher than the drug's actual concentration at the moment of death, particularly for lipophilic drugs. Peripheral blood (from the femoral vessels) shows less redistribution and is the preferred specimen for interpretation. Advanced decomposition may render toxicological interpretation unreliable altogether, although hair analysis can provide information about drug use across weeks to months prior to death and may support cause reasoning in decomposed cases. These issues are developed in detail in the toxicology chapter.

**CLINICAL PEARL:** Postmortem toxicology from a decomposed body is not a determination of the concentration at death. It is a determination of the concentration in the specimen at the time of analysis. Reasoning from the specimen to the antemortem state requires accounting for redistribution and for decomposition. The peripheral blood specimen, collected before internal examination, is the closest available approximation to the antemortem concentration.

### Vitreous Humor Potassium and Chemical Markers of the Postmortem Interval

Chemical analysis of vitreous humor — the gel-like fluid within the posterior chamber of the eye — provides an additional line of evidence for postmortem interval estimation and remains one of the more useful ancillary techniques in cases where the standard postmortem changes are ambiguous or unavailable. The vitreous is anatomically sequestered, is not subject to putrefactive changes as rapidly as blood, and yields chemistry that can be interpreted with published time-course data. Vitreous potassium concentration rises progressively after death as intracellular potassium leaks across compromised cell membranes and equilibrates with the vitreous compartment. The rise is approximately linear for the first 100 hours postmortem under temperate conditions, and multiple published regression equations (Sturner, Madea, and others) permit an interval estimate from the measured concentration.

The confidence limits on vitreous potassium estimation are wide — typically plus or minus 20 to 40 hours for intervals in the day-to-few-days range — and the method is affected by antemortem hyperkalemia, by hemolysis during specimen collection, and by delayed refrigeration of the specimen. The professional standard is to use vitreous potassium as one of several integrated lines of evidence, not as a stand-alone determinant. Other vitreous analytes — glucose (elevated antemortem in diabetic ketoacidosis, though rapidly falls after death), urea and creatinine (useful in identifying antemortem renal failure), and sodium and chloride (useful in identifying antemortem electrolyte disorder or dehydration) — support cause reasoning independent of postmortem interval questions.

**EVIDENCE:** Vitreous potassium as a postmortem interval marker has been studied since Sturner's work in the 1960s. Modern regression models incorporate ambient temperature and specimen handling variables, but the confidence intervals remain wide compared with the more precise scene-based reasoning available in cases with recent last-known-alive documentation. Vitreous is most useful in cases where scene-based reasoning is unavailable.

### Distinguishing Specific Postmortem Artifacts

Beyond the general principle of vital reaction, several specific postmortem artifact patterns arise in practice with sufficient frequency that they warrant explicit recognition. Postmortem cutaneous lividity in areas of pressure contact can present as pale, contact-pallor patterns that mimic the ligature marks of neck compression or the fingermark contusions of manual assault; the distinguishing feature is the absence of underlying subcutaneous hemorrhage on layered dissection. Postmortem gastric ulceration — a well-recognized artifact in which gastric acid digests the antral mucosa after death — can be misread as an antemortem peptic ulcer with terminal hemorrhage, but the artifact lacks the granulation tissue and vital hemorrhage of a true ulcer. Postmortem intussusception of small bowel segments, particularly in infants, is a benign artifact that must not be misread as a mechanical bowel obstruction contributing to death.

Postmortem changes at the eyes deserve specific attention because ocular findings enter both time-of-death and injury reasoning. Corneal cloudiness begins within 2 to 3 hours after death in an open eye and progresses steadily; a covered eye clouds more slowly. Tache noire — the horizontal dark band across the exposed sclera in an open eye — is a drying artifact rather than a subconjunctival hemorrhage and must not be misread as such. Postmortem tardieu spots — punctate hemorrhages in dependent tissues, particularly the lower extremities — develop from capillary rupture under the pressure of gravity-driven blood pooling and are not equivalent to the antemortem petechiae associated with asphyxial death.

Skin slippage and epidermal loss produce pale, denuded areas that mimic abrasion; the distinguishing features are the clean lifting of the epidermis in sheets rather than the disorganized epidermal loss of true abrasion, and the absence of underlying dermal hemorrhage. Skin slippage in decomposed bodies can produce patterned areas of loss (over pressure points, over sites of clothing contact) that must be interpreted in the context of the position and clothing of the body rather than as evidence of contact injury. Marbling — the dark, branching pattern of superficial vein discoloration in early putrefaction — can be misread as tracking of subcutaneous hemorrhage, but marbling follows the venous anatomy in a pattern that hemorrhage does not, and does not extend into the deeper tissues on layered dissection.

### A Worked Case in Cold-Water Immersion Postmortem Interval

A 55-year-old man is reported missing after failing to return from a solo winter hiking trip. His vehicle is found at a trailhead adjacent to a mountain lake. Search and rescue operations locate his body on the fifth day after his last known contact, submerged approximately 3 meters below the surface of the lake at a location approximately 30 meters offshore. Water temperature at recovery is measured at 4 degrees Celsius; ambient air temperature in the region has ranged between minus 10 and plus 5 degrees Celsius during the interval. The body is recovered, transported to the medical examiner's office, and examined.

External examination shows well-preserved features with no significant decomposition. The skin is pale and cold. There is minimal maceration of the hands and feet, consistent with brief water contact. Livor mortis is faintly visible on the anterior surfaces of the body. There is no facial cyanosis, no foam cone at the mouth, and no significant injury on external inspection. Internal examination shows mild pulmonary edema, congestion of the visceral organs, and no injury to the neck, chest, or abdomen. Toxicology is negative apart from a trace of ethanol at 0.02 grams per deciliter. Vitreous potassium is 12 mEq per liter.

The postmortem interval reasoning must integrate several lines of evidence, none of which alone is precise. The near-absence of decomposition at 5 days after last known contact is fully explained by the near-freezing water temperature, which retards putrefaction dramatically. The absence of rigor is expected — rigor develops slowly in cold environments and passes over the multiple days elapsed. The presence of anterior livor may indicate that the body was face-down for a period after death — consistent with drowning while facing the water surface. The vitreous potassium of 12 mEq per liter is elevated (a value of approximately 12 to 15 corresponds to intervals in the several-day range under temperate conditions) but must be interpreted against the cold-water immersion, which slows the equilibration and may result in an underestimate of interval from potassium alone. The scene reasoning — vehicle at trailhead, last known contact five days prior, no evidence of survival elsewhere — supports an interval estimate consistent with death on or near the last known contact date. Cause is certified as drowning based on the scene, the postmortem findings, and the exclusion of alternative causes; manner is accident. The postmortem interval is stated as consistent with an interval of approximately 4 to 5 days, with the wide confidence range acknowledged in the report.

**CAUTION:** Cold-water immersion preserves bodies to a degree that can mislead an examiner unfamiliar with the phenomenon. A body recovered from cold water with minimal decomposition after weeks of immersion should not be interpreted as recently deceased. The scene ambient conditions, the water temperature history, and the last-known-alive documentation together set the interval; the body findings confirm compatibility rather than establishing the interval independently.

**SCENE-TO-CERTIFICATION DECISION SYSTEM — Postmortem Interval Reasoning Arcs**

**The Biology Behind the Findings:** Postmortem changes are the physical, biochemical, and microbial consequences of loss of oxygenated perfusion at death. Early changes — livor, rigor, algor — dominate the first 24 to 48 hours. Later changes — autolysis, putrefaction, decomposition — dominate thereafter and progress under strong environmental modification.

**The Integrating Discipline:** Postmortem interval estimation integrates multiple lines of evidence — livor development and fixation, rigor extent and passage, body temperature against ambient, decomposition stage, insect activity — with scene ambient conditions and last-known-alive documentation. No single finding suffices for a defensible estimate. The estimate is a range, not a point.

**Environmental Modification:** Temperature is the dominant modifier. Immersion, burial, body habitus, and antemortem state substantially alter the standard time course. A body outside the typical temperate-indoor scenario requires calibration; a body in an unusual environment (frozen, immersed, mummified, adiposed) may not support standard-form interval estimation at all.

**Artifact Discipline:** Postmortem change produces findings that can mimic antemortem injury — skin slippage, marbling, drying artifacts, insect and scavenger defects. Vital reaction (hemorrhage into tissue, inflammatory response, dermal bleeding) distinguishes injury from artifact. Histology supports the distinction when the gross appearance is unclear.

**The Honest Estimate:** The pathologist communicates postmortem interval as a range with explicit confidence limits. Overreaching to a precise time is a testimony failure that competent opposing experts will correct. Undetermined is the appropriate determination when the evidence does not support certification to reasonable medical certainty, and it is a professional strength rather than a professional failing.

## Summary and Key Concepts

Postmortem changes result from the cessation of oxygenated perfusion at death and proceed in overlapping phases: early physical redistribution and biochemical shifts (livor, rigor, algor); intermediate enzymatic autolysis and microbial putrefaction; and late environmental transformations to skeletonization, adipocere, or mummification.

Livor mortis, rigor mortis, and algor mortis each follow characteristic time courses under temperate indoor conditions and are read together for postmortem interval reasoning. Livor blanching and fixation, rigor extent and passage, and body-temperature cooling against ambient temperature are the three principal early findings used.

Later postmortem changes — greenish discoloration, marbling, bloat, active decay, skeletonization — progress under strong environmental modification. Warmth, immersion, burial, body habitus, and antemortem state all alter the time course substantially and require calibration in interval reasoning.

Forensic entomology provides the tightest interval estimation for outdoor cases with active insect colonization. The pathologist collects representative insect specimens at autopsy and provides ambient temperature history to the consulting entomologist.

The postmortem interval is estimated as a range with explicit confidence limits, integrating multiple lines of evidence. Overreaching to a precise time is a testimony failure. The Henssge nomogram and similar temperature-based methods have inherent confidence limits that widen substantially outside standard conditions.

Postmortem changes produce artifacts that can mimic antemortem injury. Vital reaction — tissue hemorrhage, inflammatory response, demonstration of force applied to living tissue — distinguishes true injury from postmortem artifact; histology supports the distinction when gross appearance is unclear.

# CHAPTER 4: THE FORENSIC AUTOPSY: TECHNIQUE, DOCUMENTATION, AND ANCILLARY STUDIES

### Learning Objectives

1. Describe the purpose, statutory authority, and professional scope of the forensic autopsy and distinguish it from the hospital consented autopsy.
2. Perform a systematic external examination, including documentation of identifying features, clothing, injury, and postmortem changes.
3. Describe the standard technique of internal examination, including evisceration approach, organ inspection, and specialized dissections.
4. Select and collect appropriate ancillary specimens for toxicology, histology, microbiology, molecular testing, and specimen retention, driven by the case question.
5. Produce an autopsy report that documents findings and supports the certification of cause and manner of death to a standard that will withstand courtroom challenge.

## Purpose and Authority of the Forensic Autopsy

The forensic autopsy is the systematic examination of a decedent conducted under statutory authority of the medical examiner or coroner to establish the cause of death, the manner of death, the identity of the decedent when unknown, and any medically relevant information required by the investigation. It differs from the hospital consented autopsy in authority (statutory rather than family consent), purpose (medicolegal rather than educational), scope (comprehensive rather than targeted), documentation standard (courtroom-defensible rather than internal record), and audience (attorneys, investigators, courts, and public health rather than the treating team). The forensic autopsy is a legal proceeding conducted in a medical setting.

### Statutory Basis

Statutory authority to conduct the forensic autopsy resides with the medicolegal office holding jurisdiction. In most American jurisdictions the office may proceed with autopsy over family objection when the case falls within the reporting categories, though offices generally accommodate family religious and cultural concerns to the extent compatible with completing the investigation. External religious objections — particularly those associated with Orthodox Judaism, Islam, and certain Christian denominations — are addressed through communication, timely completion of the examination, and, in some cases, use of postmortem imaging to reduce the extent of internal examination. The pathologist should understand the office's policies on family notification, on limited autopsy options, and on the escalation of any family objection to legal counsel or judicial resolution.

### The Scope Decision

Every forensic autopsy is a decision about scope. A full autopsy examines every organ system with dissection and organ-by-organ documentation. A limited autopsy focuses on the systems relevant to the presumed cause. A postmortem imaging examination substitutes cross-sectional imaging for some or all internal dissection. The professional standard in most cases of unclear cause is the full autopsy, because the case question is not always answered by the examination that appears most likely to answer it. In cases with clear cause (an elderly decedent with witnessed cardiac arrest and severe known cardiovascular disease), a limited autopsy may be appropriate; in cases with any complexity, the full autopsy is the default.

**CLINICAL PEARL:** The autopsy that is skipped because "the cause is obvious" is the autopsy in which the obvious cause turns out to be incomplete. The senior forensic pathologist learns to be suspicious of obvious diagnoses at intake, because the full autopsy exists precisely to identify what was not obvious.

## External Examination

External examination is the first phase of the autopsy and, in many cases, the phase that carries the highest interpretive weight. Injuries, evidence of medical care, identifying features, and clothing are all documented before internal examination begins. The professional standard is systematic — the examination proceeds in a defined order from head to feet, from anterior to posterior, and each body region is documented before advancing to the next. This discipline ensures no region is skipped.

### Body Identification and Identifying Features

The body enters the autopsy suite with identification, either presumptive (from scene identification, prior medical records, family) or unknown. The pathologist confirms identification against the accompanying documentation before beginning the examination. In cases where identification is presumptive but not yet forensically confirmed, the pathologist proceeds and identification is confirmed by ancillary methods (dental comparison, fingerprint, DNA, or radiographic comparison) as the case allows. Identifying features are documented systematically — sex, apparent age, race or ethnic appearance, stated versus estimated height and weight, hair color and length, eye color, dentition, and any distinguishing features such as scars, tattoos, congenital anomalies, prior surgical incisions, and prosthetic devices. Photographic documentation of identifying features supports later confirmation and, in unidentified cases, publication of images to solicit identification.

### Clothing

Clothing is documented before removal. Each item is described in position on the body, its condition (intact, torn, soiled, stained, blood-soaked), and any evidence adherent to it (fibers, hair, soil, glass, gunshot residue). Clothing is removed in a controlled sequence, preserving the pattern of any defects (a bullet hole in a shirt, a stab defect in a jacket, tear patterns from a struggle) and photographing the defects both in place and after removal. Clothing items that hold evidentiary value are collected for retention or transfer to law enforcement; the chain of custody continues through the pathologist's documentation.

### External Injury Documentation

External injuries are documented by location, dimension, character, orientation, and photographic support. Location is stated with reference to anatomical landmarks and to standard body coordinates — for example, "on the anterior right chest, 3 cm below the right nipple and 2 cm to the right of the sternal midline." Dimension is measured in centimeters with a ruler in the photographic frame. Character is described in objective language — laceration versus incised wound; abrasion with intact or absent epidermis; contusion with specified color; puncture wound with margin appearance. Orientation is stated when the shape supports directionality — a stab wound is oriented, for example, at "approximately 2 o'clock to 8 o'clock relative to the standard anatomical position." Every injury of forensic interest is photographed in overview (showing location on the body), mid-range (showing pattern and immediate context), and close-up with scale.

**KEY POINT:** External documentation is the primary evidentiary record of injury. Once internal examination begins, external documentation is fixed and not revisitable. A pathologist who advances to internal examination before external documentation is complete has closed the record on the external evidence.

### Evidence of Medical Intervention

Evidence of resuscitation and prior medical care is documented systematically. Endotracheal tubes, intravenous access, chest tubes, orogastric tubes, and defibrillator pads are documented in position before removal. Their presence supports interpretation of injuries produced by the intervention itself (sternal contusion from chest compressions, dental injury from intubation, chest wall injury from chest tube placement) and permits distinction of intervention artifact from antemortem injury. Surgical wounds, prior operative scars, and evidence of chronic vascular access (dialysis fistula, central line ports) inform the medical history reconstruction.

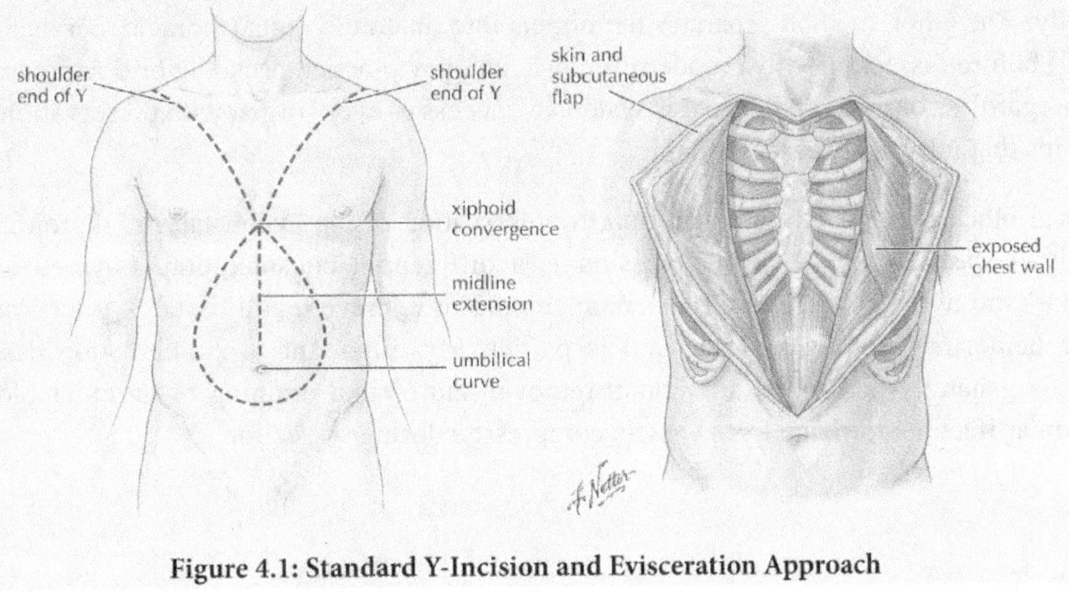


**Figure 4.1: Standard Y-Incision and Evisceration Approach**

## Internal Examination and Evisceration

Internal examination is conducted through a standard Y-incision that permits access to the thoracic, abdominal, and cervical structures. The internal examination proceeds through in-situ inspection, evisceration, dissection of organ blocks, and organ-by-organ examination. The technique described below is the classic Virchow-Rokitansky combined approach with modern modifications and remains the reference method for forensic autopsy in the United States.

### The Y-Incision and Cavity Access

The Y-incision begins at the anterolateral aspect of each shoulder, extends toward the mid-sternum, and converges at the xiphoid before continuing as a midline incision to the pubis, curving around the umbilicus. The skin and subcutaneous tissue are reflected as flaps to expose the anterior chest wall and rib cage. The ribs are transected bilaterally with rib shears or an oscillating saw, and the sternum is removed as a plate with the anterior costal cartilages attached. The pericardial sac is opened first to inspect for hemopericardium; the pleural spaces are opened to inspect for pleural fluid or hemothorax; the peritoneal cavity is inspected for fluid, hemorrhage, or perforation.

### In-Situ Inspection

Before evisceration, in-situ inspection documents the anatomical relationships and identifies findings that may be disturbed by evisceration. Adhesions, position of the heart and great vessels, position of the abdominal organs, presence of hernias, and abnormalities of visceral position are all documented at this stage. Fluid collections are measured by volume where clinically significant. Photographic documentation captures findings in situ before organs are removed.

### Evisceration

Evisceration approaches differ across offices. The classic Rokitansky method removes the organ blocks in situ before separating them into organ groups. The Virchow method removes and examines organs individually. The Ghon method separates the organs into anatomic units (thoracic, cervical, abdominal, urogenital) before dissection. Most modern forensic autopsy practice uses a hybrid approach adapted to the case. Regardless of method, the goal is systematic access to every organ with preservation of anatomic relationships that inform the case reasoning.

The cervical block is removed with attention to preservation of the hyoid, larynx, thyroid, and trachea, particularly in cases where neck compression is a differential consideration. Layered anterior neck dissection — through the strap muscles, sternocleidomastoid, prevertebral tissues — documents cervical soft-tissue hemorrhage or its absence, and is particularly important in strangulation cases. Cervical dissection is generally performed after brain removal and cranial draining of vascular blood to avoid postmortem artifact hemorrhage from vessels compressed during dissection.

## Cranial Examination

The cranial examination begins with reflection of the scalp through a coronal incision from mastoid to mastoid, followed by removal of the calvarium with an oscillating saw. The brain is inspected in situ for gross injury and for dural findings before removal. The brain is removed and inspected externally for subarachnoid hemorrhage, cortical injury, and vascular abnormalities. Standard sectioning demonstrates the ventricular system, the basal ganglia, the deep structures, and the brainstem. Fixation of the brain in formalin for several days before final sectioning is indicated in cases with subtle findings, in pediatric cases, and in cases with suspected diffuse axonal injury; unfixed brain sections have poor structural integrity and can obscure the very findings the examination is intended to document.

## Organ Examination

Each organ is weighed, described externally, sectioned, and inspected. The heart is opened by the inflow-outflow method, following the anatomical direction of blood flow through the chambers, or by short-axis cuts perpendicular to the long axis in cases with suspected coronary or myocardial disease. The coronary arteries are examined for stenosis, thrombus, and dissection; significant lesions are documented by measurement of stenosis percentage and by histologic sampling. The lungs are inspected for consolidation, embolism, and injury; standardized sampling for histology supports later analysis. The liver, kidneys, spleen, adrenals, pancreas, and gastrointestinal tract are all inspected and sectioned. Standardized organ weights are recorded; expected reference ranges vary by body habitus and are documented in autopsy manuals available in every office.

Figure 4.2: Coronary Artery Sectioning at Approximately 3 mm Intervals for Stenosis Assessment

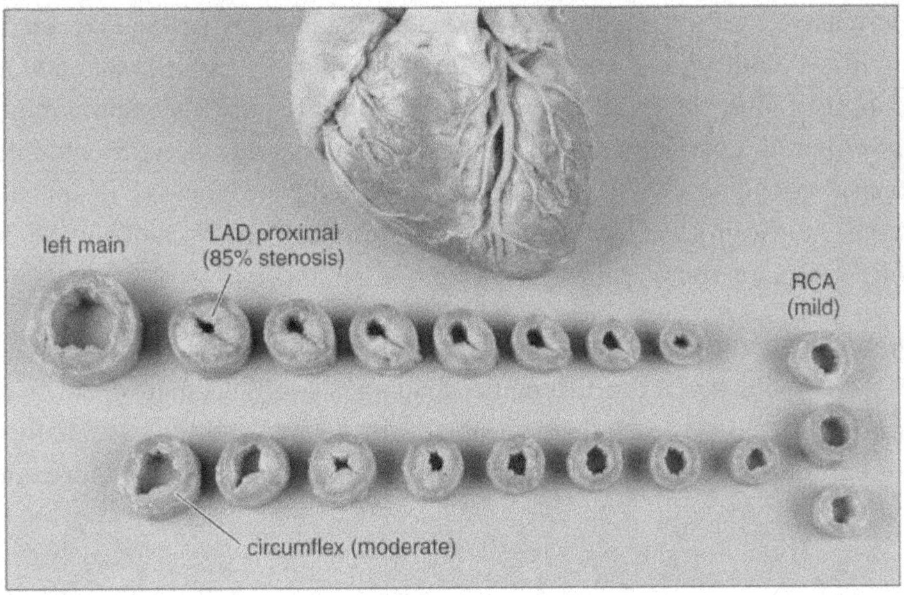

**SCENE-TO-CERTIFICATION DECISION SYSTEM — Autopsy-Directed-by-Scene Arc**

**Presenting Death Scenario:** A 68-year-old woman is found deceased in bed by her adult son. The scene is unremarkable: no signs of struggle, no visible injury, prescription medications on the nightstand consistent with treatment for hypertension and osteoarthritis. The son reports that his mother had been complaining of increasing shortness of breath for approximately 2 weeks and had an appointment with her primary care physician scheduled for the following week. Scene investigator documentation, ambient temperature, and initial external findings suggest a natural death. Prior medical records show hypertension, obesity, and osteoarthritis.

**Autopsy Signature:** External examination is unremarkable apart from mild bilateral lower extremity edema and modest asymmetric calf swelling on the right (right calf 34 cm circumference at 15 cm below the tibial plateau; left calf 31 cm). No injuries. Internal examination is directed by the scene history — in particular the two-week history of progressive shortness of breath and the asymmetric calf swelling — to careful bilateral pulmonary artery inspection and to bilateral deep vein assessment. The right main pulmonary artery contains a large saddle thromboembolus extending into both major branches. The right femoral vein contains organized thrombus consistent with the source. There is no significant coronary disease and no other lethal pathology.

**Cause Determination:** Pulmonary thromboembolism arising from right lower extremity deep vein thrombosis, with contributing conditions of obesity and immobility related to osteoarthritis.

**Manner Determination:** Natural.

**Trap Logic:** The scene appearance of a peaceful death in bed can support an initial impression of arrhythmic or hypertensive cardiovascular death, and a routine autopsy without directed pulmonary artery examination could miss a saddle embolism if the pulmonary arteries are not systematically opened. Small-vessel thromboembolism may be missed entirely without systematic examination. The pattern of asymmetric calf swelling on external examination is the key finding that redirects internal examination toward the pulmonary vasculature. A scene history that includes progressive dyspnea and unilateral leg swelling changes the pretest probability of pulmonary embolism from low (routine autopsy would not systematically look) to high (autopsy is directed to find or exclude it).

**Certification Anchor:** The internal examination is directed by the integration of scene history, external findings, and pretest reasoning about the differential diagnosis. Findings that would be missed on a purely routine examination are identified when the examination is directed by the case history. This is why the scene report is read before autopsy and the external examination is completed before internal examination begins.

## Ancillary Studies and Specimen Retention

Ancillary studies extend the autopsy examination beyond what gross inspection can determine. The selection of ancillary studies is driven by the case question and by the differential diagnosis under consideration at the time of examination. Standard specimen collection at every forensic autopsy includes blood (central and peripheral), vitreous humor, urine when available, gastric contents, and bile; selective collection includes tissue for histology, tissue for toxicology, tissue for microbiology or molecular studies, and specimens for specialized analyses.

### Toxicology Specimens

Toxicology specimens are collected before internal examination whenever practical to avoid contamination and postmortem redistribution artifacts. Peripheral blood — typically from the femoral vein through percutaneous aspiration — is the preferred specimen for interpretation of drug concentrations because it is less affected by postmortem redistribution than central blood. Central blood (from the heart chambers) is collected as an alternative when peripheral collection fails. Vitreous humor is collected from both eyes and is useful for a subset of analytes (ethanol, glucose, electrolytes, urea, potassium) that are less affected by postmortem changes than serum values. Urine when present is collected and is particularly useful for drug screening. Gastric contents document recent oral intake and are examined for undigested tablets or capsules. Bile is a useful matrix for detection of certain drugs excreted through the biliary system. Hair is collected in cases where long-term drug use history is relevant.

### Histology

Standard histologic sampling includes representative sections of the heart (multiple sections showing atrium, ventricle, coronary arteries, and myocardium), lung (multiple lobes), liver, kidneys, spleen, adrenals, pancreas, thyroid, brain (multiple regions), and any organ with gross abnormality. Sections are fixed in 10 percent neutral buffered formalin and are processed to hematoxylin and eosin (H&E) stained slides in the majority of cases; special stains and immunohistochemistry are applied where indicated. Contusion aging, myocardial ischemic injury (which requires characteristic microscopic features and does not become visible on H&E until several hours after the ischemic event), and identification of drowning-related findings (diatoms in tissue sections) are among the specific histological determinations that support the case reasoning.

### Microbiology and Molecular Studies

Microbiologic culture is indicated in cases with suspected infection contributing to death, particularly bacteremia, endocarditis, pneumonia, or meningitis. Postmortem cultures are complicated by rapid endogenous colonization after death; blood cultures from central sites are frequently contaminated and require interpretation against gross findings and histology. Cerebrospinal fluid cultures are more reliable when the meninges are gross-abnormal. Molecular studies are increasingly applied to postmortem tissue: molecular autopsy for suspected inherited arrhythmia syndromes (long QT, catecholaminergic polymorphic ventricular tachycardia), particularly in sudden death of young decedents with negative gross and microscopic examinations; molecular identification of pathogens; and toxicological analysis of tissue specimens when blood is unavailable or inadequate.

### Specimen Retention

Specimen retention policy varies by office. Standard practice retains blood, tissue blocks and slides, and photographs indefinitely; other specimens are retained for defined periods, typically several years, subject to office policy. Retention allows re-examination if new evidence emerges, permits second-opinion analysis by outside experts, and supports legal proceedings that may extend over years. Family requests for return of tissue at case closure are honored where consistent with retention policy and ongoing case needs; family requests for release of tissue for private testing are managed through the office's legal and administrative processes.

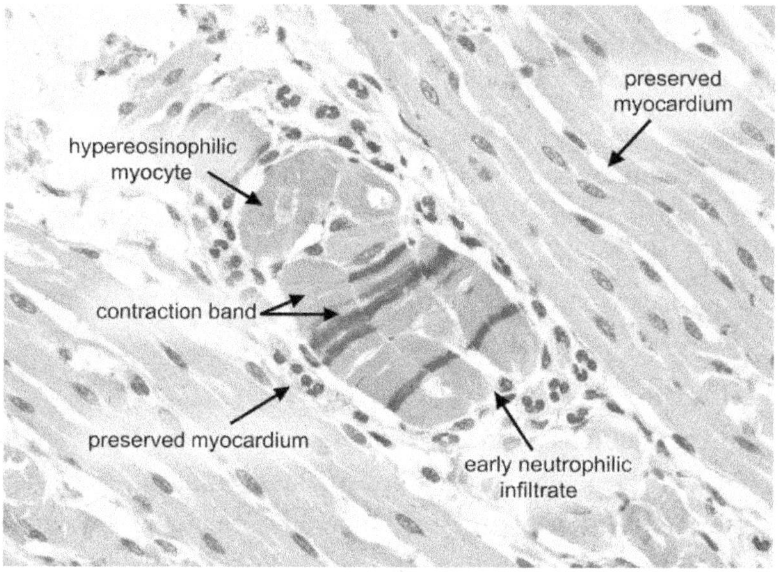


## SCENE-TO-CERTIFICATION DECISION SYSTEM — Ancillary-Study Selection Arc

**Presenting Death Scenario:** A 22-year-old collegiate basketball player collapses during practice, is found in cardiac arrest, and cannot be resuscitated despite immediate bystander CPR and rapid emergency response. He has no known medical history, was cleared for participation on his most recent pre-participation examination, and had no reported prodromal symptoms. Scene documentation is complete; the incident occurred in front of multiple witnesses and video documentation exists. The medical examiner's office accepts jurisdiction on the sudden death of a young adult without known cause.

**Autopsy Signature:** External examination is unremarkable apart from resuscitation-related sternal contusion and rib fractures. Internal examination is directed to comprehensive cardiac evaluation. The heart weighs 380 grams (borderline elevated for body habitus); ventricular walls are of normal thickness; coronary arteries are widely patent without significant atherosclerosis; valves are morphologically normal. Histology of the myocardium shows no fibrosis, no myocyte disarray, no infiltrative disease. The lungs, brain, and other organs are unremarkable. Toxicology is negative. The gross and microscopic examination fails to identify a lethal pathology.

**Cause Determination:** Cause of death is undetermined pending molecular autopsy. Peripheral blood and tissue (myocardium, spleen, liver) have been retained frozen for molecular studies. Postmortem genetic testing for inherited arrhythmia syndromes — long QT syndrome (KCNQ1, KCNH2, SCN5A), catecholaminergic polymorphic ventricular tachycardia (RYR2, CASQ2), Brugada syndrome (SCN5A and associated genes), and hypertrophic cardiomyopathy (MYH7, MYBPC3, and others) — is initiated, and family screening is recommended pending results. Preliminary certification is pending molecular results; if positive, cause will be updated to identified inherited arrhythmia syndrome.

**Manner Determination:** Natural (pending confirmation via molecular studies). The scene, the witness accounts, and the autopsy findings are consistent with sudden natural death; no evidence of trauma, exogenous substance, or third-party involvement supports any other manner.

**Trap Logic:** Sudden death in a young athlete with a structurally normal heart is one of the classic indications for molecular autopsy. Failure to select and retain appropriate specimens at the time of autopsy — frozen tissue for molecular studies, family notification of the possible inherited basis, family screening initiation — misses the opportunity to identify a familial cause with immediate implications for surviving relatives. The trap is to certify the case as "sudden cardiac death, cause undetermined" and close it, when a molecular autopsy is the standard-of-care next step and family screening can prevent additional sudden deaths in surviving siblings and offspring.

**Certification Anchor:** Ancillary studies are selected based on the case question, not the routine panel. In sudden death of a young decedent with a structurally normal heart, molecular autopsy for inherited arrhythmia syndromes is the standard-of-care ancillary study, and appropriate specimens (frozen tissue and blood) must be collected at the primary autopsy. Family notification with recommendation for cardiological evaluation of first-degree relatives is a professional obligation regardless of whether the molecular study result is available.

## The Autopsy Report as Documentation

The autopsy report is the definitive medical record of the case. Its audience includes the certifying pathologist, colleagues who may consult on the case, families, attorneys, investigators, and — in cases proceeding to trial — jurors and appellate courts. Its structure supports the reasoning that leads to certification of cause and manner and preserves the underlying observations in sufficient detail that the reasoning can be reconstructed by a reader who was not present at the examination.

### Report Structure

The standard autopsy report includes identifying information, a case history summary, external examination findings, evidence of medical intervention, internal examination findings organized by anatomical system, results of ancillary studies (toxicology, histology, microbiology, molecular studies as applicable), a discussion of the findings, an opinion section that states the cause and manner of death with supporting reasoning, and the pathologist's signature and credentials. Each section carries specific documentation standards. External and internal findings are stated in objective language; the discussion and opinion sections carry the pathologist's reasoning.

### Objective Description Versus Reasoned Opinion

The report distinguishes between objective description and reasoned opinion. External and internal examination sections describe what was observed — the location, dimension, character of an injury; the weight, appearance, and sections of an organ. These sections are written in objective, non-interpretive language. The discussion and opinion sections carry the interpretation — the integration of findings with case history to reach cause and manner determinations. Blurring the distinction — stating conclusions in the findings sections, or presenting reasoning as fact — undermines the report's defensibility on cross-examination. A finding is what was observed; an opinion is what the observation supports.

**CAUTION:** The autopsy report is the pathologist's testimony in written form. Every sentence is potentially the subject of cross-examination years later. The professional discipline of writing findings as observations and interpretations as opinions is the discipline that produces defensible testimony when the case reaches trial.

### Photographic Documentation Standards

Autopsy photographs are the visual counterpart of the written report and are subject to the same standards of authenticity and defensibility. Every injury of forensic interest is photographed with a scale in frame, at right angles to the plane of the injury, with adequate lighting to demonstrate the pattern. Overview, mid-range, and close-up sequences are standard. Photographs are taken before dissection of a finding, during dissection to document underlying structures, and after dissection to document what was found. Standard practice photographs the body at intake (documenting the state as received), external examination findings in the sequence of examination, in-situ organ relationships, and each organ during examination. Contemporaneous notes on the photograph identifiers link each image to the sequence of the examination and permit reconstruction of the examination flow years later. Digital metadata is preserved unaltered; edited or filter-processed images are not used for documentation purposes because they are contested on cross-examination and may be excluded.

### Autopsy Safety and Infectious Hazards

The forensic autopsy is a hazardous occupational activity and safety practices are non-negotiable. Personal protective equipment for routine autopsy includes gown, waterproof apron, double gloves, sleeve covers, cap, and eye and face protection with splash shield. Standard infectious precautions treat every decedent as potentially bloodborne-pathogen positive; hepatitis B, hepatitis C, and human immunodeficiency virus can persist infectious in postmortem tissue and body fluids. Tuberculosis remains transmissible from postmortem pulmonary tissue and requires respiratory protection (N95 respirator minimum) when tuberculosis is known or suspected. Novel or highly transmissible pathogens — novel influenza, coronaviruses, hemorrhagic fever viruses — require additional respiratory protection and, in some cases, restricted autopsy protocols with reduced dissection and enhanced containment. The pathologist confirms availability and correct fit of all protective equipment before beginning any examination and knows the office's specific protocols for suspected high-consequence pathogens.

Sharps injury is the most common autopsy occupational hazard. Standard practice reduces exposure through the use of controlled dissection techniques, the use of blunt-tip forceps for tissue retraction rather than sharp forceps that hold near the cutting hand, the elimination of hand-passing of sharp instruments (instruments are placed on a designated surface between operators), and the use of protective gloves designed to resist puncture. When sharps injury occurs, the office's exposure protocol is initiated — immediate wound care, source-decedent bloodborne pathogen testing, and provider evaluation for post-exposure prophylaxis as indicated. Documentation of exposure is essential for occupational health follow-up and for any subsequent workers' compensation claim.

**CAUTION:** Sharps injury during autopsy is common enough that every forensic pathology fellow will experience at least one during training. Familiarity with the office's post-exposure protocol before the exposure occurs is essential; a fellow who does not know the protocol will delay initiation of prophylaxis, and the timing of post-exposure prophylaxis to HIV in particular affects its efficacy.

### Documentation of Organ-Specific Findings

Certain organs carry documentation requirements beyond the standard weighing and sectioning. The heart, when a coronary or myocardial process is suspected, is examined by 3 mm serial sections perpendicular to the long axis of the myocardium, with representative sections photographed and sampled for histology from anterior wall, posterior wall, septum, papillary muscles, and each of the four cardiac chambers. Coronary arteries are sectioned at 3 mm intervals and each stenosis is documented for location, percent luminal narrowing, and character (atherosclerotic, thrombotic, dissection). The brain, when a specific pathology is suspected, is fixed for several days before final sectioning and photographed after fixation to document any subtle findings. The neck, when strangulation or compression is under consideration, is dissected in layered fashion — skin and subcutaneous tissue, strap muscles, sternocleidomastoid, prevertebral tissues — with each layer inspected for hemorrhage and photographed as encountered. The larynx, hyoid, and cervical spine are examined separately.

### Organ Weights and Their Interpretation

Standardized organ weights are recorded for every organ during the internal examination. Reference ranges vary by body habitus, age, and sex, and are compiled in autopsy manuals and published reference tables familiar to every practicing forensic pathologist. Adult reference ranges under standard body habitus assumptions include: heart, approximately 250 to 350 grams (men) and 200 to 300 grams (women); each lung, approximately 350 to 500 grams; liver, approximately 1300 to 1800 grams; spleen, approximately 100 to 200 grams; each kidney, approximately 125 to 175 grams; brain, approximately 1300 to 1500 grams. Organ weights outside reference range direct attention to specific pathological processes — an increased heart weight (cardiomegaly) directs attention to hypertension, valvular disease, cardiomyopathy, or infiltrative processes; increased liver weight directs attention to congestion, steatosis, or infiltrative processes; a decreased brain weight in a young decedent suggests remote injury or neurodegenerative process. Organ weights are interpreted in the context of body habitus rather than as isolated absolute values; a heart weight of 400 grams in a decedent weighing 60 kilograms indicates substantial cardiac hypertrophy, whereas the same weight in a decedent weighing 120 kilograms is expected for body size.

Documentation of organ weights carries an evidentiary function beyond the immediate reasoning of the case. A subsequent reviewer — a second-opinion pathologist retained by the family, an opposing expert in litigation, an internal quality review — uses the documented weights to reconstruct the state of the organs at the time of examination. Failure to weigh organs, or failure to document the weights, forecloses this reconstruction and undermines the report on cross-examination. The professional standard is to weigh every organ that is examined and to document every weight.

### Brain Fixation and Delayed Neuropathological Examination

Brain examination in specific cases benefits from formalin fixation before final sectioning. Unfixed brain tissue has poor structural integrity, is difficult to section cleanly, and can obscure findings including diffuse axonal injury, cortical contusion aging, and small vascular malformations. Cases in which brain fixation is standard include pediatric decedents (especially in suspected abusive head trauma, where axonal injury is central to the reasoning), decedents with suspected diffuse axonal injury from mechanical trauma, decedents with suspected cerebrovascular pathology (aneurysm, arteriovenous malformation, spontaneous intracerebral hemorrhage), decedents with subtle findings on initial gross inspection, and any case in which the neuropathological findings will materially affect the certification. The brain is suspended by the basilar artery in a bucket of 10 percent neutral buffered formalin and fixed for a minimum of one week, with two weeks preferred. Final sectioning is then performed and standard sections (multiple coronal cerebral sections, hindbrain and brainstem sections, cerebellar sections) are photographed and sampled for histology. Neuropathology consultation is obtained in cases where subspecialty interpretation is required.

**CLINICAL PEARL:** The brain that requires fixation is the brain that will not be sectioned at the primary autopsy. The professional decision to fix a brain is made during the initial examination, not weeks later when the case has proceeded and re-examination is impossible. When the case history or the initial gross findings suggest that neuropathological detail will matter, fix the brain.

### Body Reconstruction and Family Concerns

The forensic autopsy involves incisions that must be closed for return of the body to the family. Standard reconstruction closes the Y-incision with heavy suture (typically a running lock stitch) that will remain closed under the handling of body preparation for viewing. The cranial incision is closed similarly after replacement of the calvarium. Organs are returned to the body cavity or, per office policy, held for further examination and returned at case closure. When family requests to view the body are anticipated, particular attention to appearance-preserving reconstruction is warranted — minimizing visible incisions on the face and neck, maintaining anatomic contour, and coordinating with the receiving funeral director on the extent of subsequent embalming and cosmetic reconstruction. The pathologist communicates with the family, when appropriate, about what the autopsy involved and about what to expect at viewing; this communication is typically mediated through the death investigator or through office administrative staff, and is calibrated to the case sensitivity.

### Case Conference and Peer Review

Institutional practice in most medical examiner and coroner offices includes some form of regular case conference in which difficult or complex cases are presented to the full staff for peer discussion. The purposes are twofold: to ensure consistency of practice across the office, and to provide the certifying pathologist with the input of colleagues on cases where the reasoning could reasonably support more than one determination. Case conference is not a mechanism for the office to overturn an individual pathologist's judgment; the certifying pathologist retains authority over her cases. It is a mechanism for the professional community of the office to keep its practice calibrated, its reasoning transparent, and its determinations defensible against the eventual scrutiny of external review.

## Special Autopsy Situations

### Decomposed and Skeletonized Remains

Decomposed bodies require adapted approach. Standard organ examination may be limited by autolysis; standardized organ weights become uninterpretable. The examination focuses on injury identification (where soft tissue permits), on skeletal findings (fractures, prior injury), and on any ancillary analyses that decomposition permits (hair for long-term drug analysis; occasionally tissue for molecular studies). Skeletonized remains require consultation with forensic anthropology to interpret skeletal trauma, biological profile (age, sex, ancestry, stature), and identification. Odontological consultation is indicated when dentition is preserved and identification is required.

### Pediatric Autopsy

The pediatric autopsy, particularly in cases of sudden unexpected infant death, requires a specific documentation protocol including full-body radiographic skeletal survey (to identify occult fractures characteristic of abuse), meticulous documentation of external findings, careful cranial and CNS examination, and specific attention to the metabolic autopsy (blood spot for newborn screening metabolic panel, vitreous humor for glucose and electrolytes, tissue for molecular studies where indicated). Standardized pediatric autopsy protocols are developed in Chapter 12.

### Autopsy in the Setting of Postmortem Imaging

Postmortem cross-sectional imaging — CT and, less frequently, MRI — is entering routine forensic practice at offices with the resources to support it. Imaging supplements autopsy in gunshot wound trajectory reconstruction, in identification of skeletal injury, and in cases where family religious objection restricts full internal examination. Imaging does not replace autopsy in the majority of cases because injury and disease that require direct inspection (contusion aging, small vessel disease, subtle organ pathology) are not reliably identifiable on imaging. The integration of postmortem imaging with autopsy is developed further in Chapter 19.

### The Autopsy in Contested Cases

Cases that are likely to be contested at trial — homicides, deaths in custody, cases with civil litigation potential, high-profile cases — warrant particular documentation rigor. Photographic documentation is more extensive; specimen retention is more conservative; second-review by a colleague at the time of autopsy is often obtained; and the report is written with the anticipation that opposing experts will scrutinize every finding and every reasoning step. This is not different in kind from routine autopsy, but it is different in degree — the discipline of thorough documentation in every case is what permits confident practice when the case turns out to be contested.

## SCENE-TO-CERTIFICATION DECISION SYSTEM — Forensic Autopsy Reasoning Arcs

**The Autopsy Is a Directed Examination:** The forensic autopsy is directed by the scene history, the external findings, and the differential diagnosis under consideration. Systematic completeness is preserved, but the depth of examination in each system is calibrated to what the case question requires.

**External Before Internal:** External examination carries interpretive weight that cannot be recovered once internal examination begins. Identification, clothing, injuries, evidence of medical care, and postmortem changes are all documented systematically before the Y-incision. The discipline of full external documentation is what preserves the injury record.

**Ancillary Studies Match the Question:** Toxicology, histology, microbiology, and molecular studies are selected based on the case question, not applied as a fixed panel. Peripheral blood for toxicology, representative histologic sections, cultures when infection is suspected, and molecular studies in sudden death of the young are the standard selections. Specimen retention protects the case for later re-examination and second opinion.

**The Report Documents Reasoning:** The autopsy report separates objective findings from reasoned opinion. Findings sections describe what was observed; discussion and opinion sections carry the interpretation. The distinction is what supports the report on cross-examination and preserves professional credibility across years.

**Special Situations Require Adapted Approach:** Decomposed and skeletonized remains, pediatric cases, cases proceeding with postmortem imaging, and contested cases each require documentation adaptations. The core discipline — systematic examination, careful documentation, and reasoned integration — transfers across situations even when the specific techniques vary.

## Summary and Key Concepts

The forensic autopsy is the systematic examination of a decedent conducted under statutory authority to establish cause of death, manner of death, and any related information required by the investigation. It differs from the hospital autopsy in authority, purpose, scope, documentation standard, and audience.

The examination proceeds through external examination (identification, clothing, injury, medical intervention), internal examination through the Y-incision (in-situ inspection, evisceration, organ-by-organ examination, cranial examination), and ancillary studies (toxicology, histology, microbiology, molecular studies). Each phase carries specific documentation standards.

Toxicology specimens are collected before internal examination when practical; peripheral blood is preferred over central blood because of postmortem redistribution. Standard histologic sampling includes representative sections of every organ system; special stains and immunohistochemistry are applied where indicated by the case question.

The autopsy report distinguishes objective description from reasoned opinion. Findings sections state observations; discussion and opinion sections carry the interpretation that supports cause and manner determinations. The distinction preserves the report's defensibility on cross-examination.

Special situations — decomposed remains, skeletonized remains, pediatric autopsy, cases with postmortem imaging, and contested cases — require documentation adaptations but preserve the core discipline of systematic examination and reasoned integration.

# CHAPTER 5: BLUNT FORCE INJURY AND TRANSPORTATION FATALITIES

**Learning Objectives**

1. Describe the biomechanical mechanisms by which blunt force produces the four principal wound categories (abrasion, contusion, laceration, fracture) and reason from wound morphology back to the mechanism of injury.
2. Distinguish antemortem abrasions from postmortem drying artifact and postmortem pressure marks, and apply the distinction to case reasoning.
3. Interpret contusion patterns for weapon identification, age estimation, and distinction from postmortem artifact, and articulate the documented limits of contusion aging.
4. Interpret blunt force head injury — scalp laceration, skull fracture, subdural hemorrhage, epidural hemorrhage, contusion, and diffuse axonal injury — in the context of impact biomechanics and injury sequence.
5. Reconstruct transportation fatalities (pedestrian struck by vehicle, motor vehicle occupant, motorcycle rider) from injury pattern, and use the reconstruction to inform manner determination.

## Mechanisms and Categories of Blunt Force Injury

Blunt force injury is the category of injury produced by impact of a firm object against the body without penetration of the skin surface by the object itself. It is the most common category of traumatic death encountered by the practicing forensic pathologist, and it dominates the caseload of every medical examiner and coroner office. Blunt force is the mechanism of the fall, the motor vehicle collision, the pedestrian struck by a car, the blow from a fist or a bat, the crush injury, and the impact from a fall from height. The unifying biomechanical principle is the application of force distributed across a contact area sufficient to produce tissue disruption without discrete penetration.

The wound categories produced by blunt force are traditionally classified as abrasion, contusion, laceration, and fracture. These categories reflect the tissue that fails first under the applied force. Skin fails superficially to produce an abrasion when force is applied in a tangential or scraping direction. Vascular tissue fails to produce a contusion when force is applied over a wider area with sufficient magnitude to disrupt small vessels. Full-thickness skin and subcutaneous tissue fail to produce a laceration when force overcomes the tensile strength of dermis and connective tissue. Bone fails to produce a fracture when force exceeds the mechanical strength of the skeletal element. In practice, most significant blunt injuries produce combinations of these categories, and the pattern of combination is often more informative than any single wound taken in isolation.

### Biomechanical Principles

The tissue effect of blunt impact depends on four principal variables. Force is the product of mass and acceleration; a small mass at high velocity may deliver as much force as a large mass at low velocity, and the injury pattern reflects the total impulse rather than either factor alone. Contact area determines the pressure at the site of impact; a given force distributed over a small area (a hammer strike) produces a different injury than the same force distributed over a large area (a fall against a broad flat surface). Direction of force relative to the tissue determines whether the injury is compressive, shearing, or tangential. Duration of contact influences the energy transfer to underlying structures; a brief impact deposits energy at the surface, whereas a sustained compression transmits energy deep to underlying organs.

The biomechanics also depend on the properties of the tissue itself. Elastic tissue (skin, superficial vessels) recovers partially after impact; rigid tissue (bone) fails abruptly when its yield point is exceeded. Tissue supported by bone (scalp over the skull) is more resistant to laceration than tissue over soft tissue (skin over the abdomen). Age changes tissue properties substantially: an infant's skull is thin and elastic and fractures with less force than an adult skull, but the underlying brain has substantial water content and can withstand deformation that would produce cortical injury in an adult. An elderly decedent has fragile skin, atrophic subcutaneous tissue, and osteopenic bone; even modest force produces skin tears, deep contusion, and fracture at levels that would be unremarkable in a younger decedent.

**KEY POINT:** The severity of blunt force injury depends on the biomechanics of the impact and on the tissue properties of the decedent. The same force applied to a 25-year-old and to an 85-year-old produces different injuries because the tissue is different. This is not evidence that the force was different; it is evidence that tissue vulnerability varies across the population.

## Abrasions

An abrasion is a superficial injury produced by tangential force that removes or displaces the epidermis without penetrating the dermis. Abrasions are the most superficial category of blunt force injury and are frequently underappreciated because they do not extend deep to underlying structures. Their forensic value lies in their capacity to preserve the pattern of the contacting surface, in their utility for reconstruction of the direction of force, and in the antemortem-versus-postmortem distinction that they support.

### Morphology and Classification

Abrasions are classified by mechanism. A scrape abrasion is produced by tangential motion of a firm surface across the skin, with the epidermis dislodged in the direction of motion; the leading edge of the scrape is usually smoother and the trailing edge shows heaped-up epidermis. This asymmetry documents the direction of force. A pattern abrasion (also termed an imprint abrasion) preserves the pattern of the contacting surface — the tread pattern of a tire, the weave of a fabric, the meshwork of a screen, the surface texture of a paved road. Pattern abrasions have the highest forensic value because they support identification of the object that produced them. A pressure abrasion is produced by compression of the skin against a firm underlying surface (a ligature abrasion of the neck, an abrasion at the site of contact between a body and the pavement in a supine decedent left on the ground). Pressure abrasions do not require tangential motion and often lack the directional asymmetry of scrape abrasions.

### Antemortem Versus Postmortem Abrasion

The distinction between antemortem and postmortem abrasion is one of the classic problems of forensic examination. Antemortem abrasions occur in living tissue with intact circulation; they produce a vital reaction of erythema and mild inflammation, and on histologic examination they show hemorrhage into the dermis and, if survival is prolonged, an inflammatory infiltrate. Postmortem abrasions, produced by dragging or handling of the body after death, occur in tissue without circulation; they produce no vital reaction, no dermal hemorrhage, and no inflammatory response. On gross examination, antemortem abrasions have a moist, reddish appearance in the early hours and a yellow-brown to reddish-brown appearance in the days that follow (scab formation). Postmortem abrasions have a pale, parchment-like appearance from the drying of the exposed dermis. Postmortem drying artifact — the desiccation of any exposed skin surface, particularly at the lips, penis, and any point where the epidermis has been displaced — can mimic antemortem abrasion, but it lacks any vital reaction and is characteristically located at sites of postmortem exposure rather than distributed in patterns consistent with antemortem trauma.

**CLINICAL PEARL:** The parchment-like brown-yellow appearance of a postmortem abrasion is characteristic and often distinguishable from antemortem abrasion at gross examination. When distinction is unclear, histologic examination for vital reaction — dermal hemorrhage and inflammatory infiltrate — supports the determination.

Figure 5.1: Blunt Force Wound Categories: Comparative Wound-Pattern Morphology

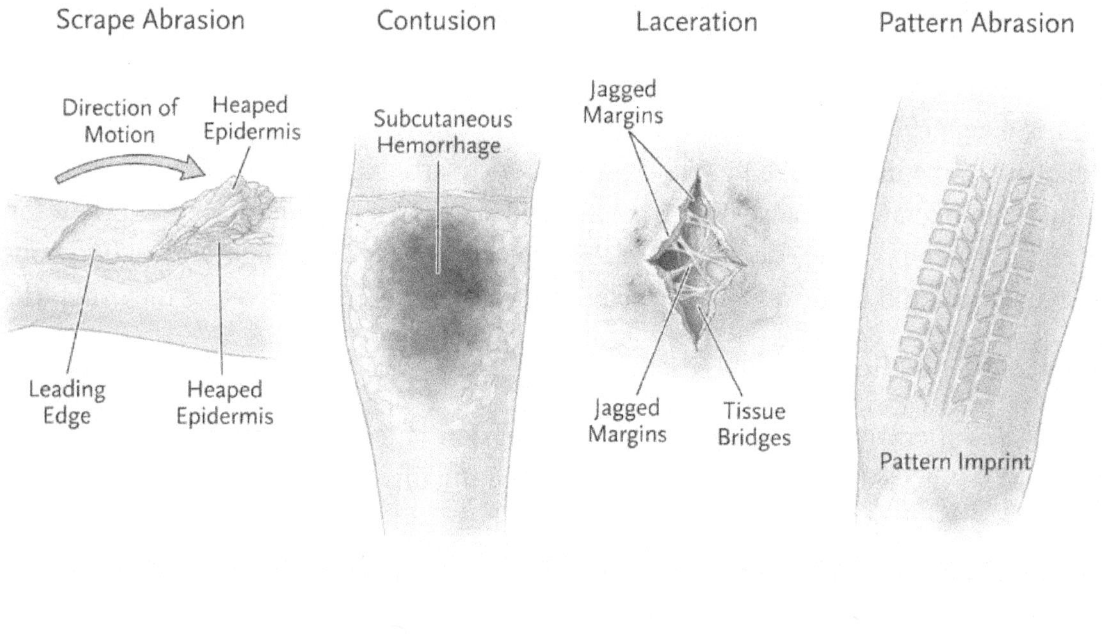

## Contusions

A contusion is a subcutaneous or deep-tissue collection of extravasated blood produced by rupture of small vessels under blunt impact, without breach of the overlying skin. Contusions are commonly termed bruises in lay language, and the terminology has entered clinical usage; the forensic report typically retains the more precise term "contusion" for professional clarity. Contusions carry substantial forensic weight because they preserve the pattern of some impacting objects, they permit rough estimation of the timing of injury within recognized limits, and they document force applied to the body at a level insufficient to lacerate but sufficient to disrupt vasculature.

### Morphology and Pattern Recognition

Contusion morphology varies with the magnitude and character of the applied force. Most contusions are relatively diffuse with central intensity and fading margins, corresponding to blunt impact from a broad object such as a fist or a fall. Some contusions preserve the pattern of the impacting object with sufficient fidelity to permit identification. Linear contusions with tramline (double-line) morphology are classic for a cylindrical impacting object such as a rod, bat, or belt; the tramlines reflect the biomechanics of the impact, in which the outer margins of the contact area are compressed and rupture vessels while the central compression area is less injured. Circular or oval contusions with a central pale area suggest an object with a curved contact surface. Patterned contusions preserving the imprint of a specific object — a shoe sole, a belt buckle, a ring pattern from a knuckle — have very high forensic value when they can be documented and preserved photographically.

### Contusion Aging

The color of a contusion changes with time as extravasated blood is enzymatically degraded. The classic sequence proceeds through red to blue-violet in the first day, blue-green to green over days two to five, yellow-brown through the second week, and fading to normal skin color over subsequent weeks. This color-based aging is a familiar clinical framework and is described in medical training. It is, however, only crudely accurate and is documented in peer-reviewed studies to be substantially unreliable for the purposes of establishing a specific time of injury. Individual variation in metabolism, contusion depth, body region, and skin pigmentation all affect the color evolution. Contusions of similar age in the same decedent may show different colors depending on the depth and location. Multiple studies have demonstrated that even experienced examiners cannot reliably distinguish contusions differing in age by hours from contusions differing in age by days on visual inspection alone.

The professional standard is to document contusion color without overinterpreting the age. A contusion may be described as "recent" (still red or blue-violet), "intermediate" (blue-green to yellow-green), or "resolving" (yellow-brown fading to normal). More precise age assignment is not defensible on cross-examination. Histologic examination provides more objective age markers than gross color — the sequence from acute hemorrhage through hemosiderin deposition to fibroblastic organization occurs over predictable time courses — and is used when age determination materially affects the case.

**CAUTION:** Testimony that a contusion was "approximately X hours old" based on visual color alone is not defensible to reasonable medical certainty. The published literature documents wide variation and inter-observer disagreement. Testimony should be limited to broad age ranges, and when precise timing is critical, histologic examination should be pursued.

### Postmortem Contusion Artifact

Contusions produced after death are limited in extent because they require intravascular blood pressure to force vessel rupture and tissue infiltration. Compression of a dependent surface after death may produce a small amount of pooled blood in tissue that mimics contusion at gross examination — the finding termed livor mortis with tardieu spots. These postmortem findings lack the substantial dermal hemorrhage of true antemortem contusion and do not extend into the deeper subcutaneous tissue. Histologic examination distinguishes true contusion (with infiltration of blood between tissue planes and vital reaction) from postmortem pooling (with blood limited to superficial vessels and no vital reaction).

### SCENE-TO-CERTIFICATION DECISION SYSTEM — Patterned Contusion Arc

**Presenting Death Scenario:** A 3-year-old child is brought to the emergency department by her mother in cardiac arrest. Resuscitation is unsuccessful. The mother reports that the child fell down a flight of stairs while playing unattended. The child is transferred to the medical examiner's office. On external examination, multiple bruises are present on the trunk, back, and extremities, in various apparent stages of resolution, and a pattern of linear paired contusions is noted along the posterior left flank, with tramline morphology and orientation suggesting impact from a cylindrical object approximately 2 cm in diameter.

**Autopsy Signature:** External examination confirms the tramline contusions on the flank, additional patterned contusions on the right thigh and left buttock with a curved margin suggesting a shoe or blunt curved object, and multiple abrasions to the extremities and back. Full-body radiographic skeletal survey identifies three healing rib fractures in different stages of callus formation, a metaphyseal corner fracture of the distal tibia (classic for infant abuse), and a healing distal ulnar fracture. Internal examination shows blunt abdominal trauma with hepatic laceration and hemoperitoneum, subdural hemorrhage of variable ages, and retinal hemorrhages bilaterally on postmortem ophthalmologic examination. Histology of representative contusions demonstrates hemorrhage in various stages of organization, consistent with injuries of multiple different ages.

**Cause Determination:** Blunt force injury of the trunk with hepatic laceration and hemoperitoneum. Contributing conditions include acute and chronic subdural hemorrhage and multiple healing fractures of various ages consistent with prior blunt force injury.

**Manner Determination:** Homicide. The pattern of injuries — patterned contusions consistent with linear objects and curved surfaces, injuries in multiple different stages of healing, classic radiographic findings of infant physical abuse (metaphyseal corner fracture, rib fractures at different stages, retinal hemorrhages), and internal injuries of a severity inconsistent with the reported mechanism of a fall down stairs — all support the manner determination of homicide.

**Trap Logic:** The reported history of a fall must be evaluated against the injury pattern. Falls down stairs typically produce injuries concentrated on prominent points of impact (elbows, knees, head) with distributions consistent with a tumbling body; they do not typically produce patterned linear contusions with tramline morphology, and they do not produce injuries of multiple ages consistent with repeated events. The trap is to accept the caregiver history as the mechanism when the injury pattern is inconsistent with that history. The countermeasure is systematic documentation of the pattern of contusions (with photography, measurements, and preservation of adjacent skin for histology), documentation of the skeletal survey findings (with radiographic images preserved), and integration of all findings with the reported history — identifying inconsistency rather than accepting the history uncritically.

**Certification Anchor:** Patterned contusions carry high forensic value because they document the shape of the impacting object. In pediatric death investigation, patterned contusions inconsistent with the reported mechanism, particularly when combined with skeletal survey findings characteristic of abuse (metaphyseal corner fracture, rib fractures at multiple ages, healing fractures without documented prior care), support the manner determination of homicide. The full pediatric protocol — skeletal survey, retinal examination, histology of contusions, brain fixation — is essential for the case reasoning.

## Lacerations

A laceration is a full-thickness disruption of the skin produced by blunt force that exceeds the tensile strength of dermis. The morphological distinction between laceration (a blunt injury) and incised wound (a sharp injury) is one of the classic distinctions of forensic pathology and is central to reasoning about mechanism. The distinction is developed here in the context of blunt force; sharp force injury is developed in Chapter 6.

### Morphological Features of Laceration

Lacerations differ from incised wounds in several morphologically important ways. Laceration margins are irregular and jagged rather than clean and linear. Laceration walls show bridging fibrous tissue strands — tissue bridges — in which small filaments of connective tissue span the wound cavity because the underlying tissue has not been cut but has failed heterogeneously under the applied force. Laceration margins are typically abraded, reflecting the tangential component of the impacting object as it delivered the force. Underlying deep tissue is contused rather than cleanly cut, and the wound often communicates with underlying subcutaneous hemorrhage. The classic incised wound, by contrast, has clean linear margins, no tissue bridges, no marginal abrasion, and cleanly divided underlying tissues.

### Location and Reconstruction

Lacerations occur preferentially at sites where skin is tightly stretched over underlying bone or where the underlying tissue provides no cushioning. The scalp lacerates readily because it is tightly opposed to the calvarium; the forehead, the occipital region, and the parietal region are common sites. The eyebrow region, the chin, and the malar prominences are similar sites of preferential laceration. Extremity lacerations over the shin or the extensor surface of the forearm reflect the same principle. The presence of a scalp laceration in a decedent with head trauma always warrants layered dissection to identify underlying skull fracture and intracranial injury, because the force that lacerated the scalp is usually sufficient to produce underlying injury even when the intracranial injury is not immediately apparent on gross inspection.

## Blunt Force Head Injury

Blunt force head injury is the most consequential category of blunt force trauma in most caseloads. It causes the majority of deaths in falls, in transportation fatalities, and in blunt assaults, and it accounts for a substantial fraction of all forensic autopsies. The injuries produced by blunt head impact form a characteristic constellation that reflects the biomechanics of the impact and the anatomy of the skull and brain.

### Scalp and Skull Injury

The scalp, as noted above, lacerates readily under blunt impact; scalp lacerations are frequently the visible surface finding that documents head impact. Layered scalp dissection is performed in every autopsy where head impact is suspected. The scalp is reflected to expose the underlying skull, and the pattern of underlying subgaleal hemorrhage documents the location and extent of impact even when the surface scalp injury is limited. Skull fractures follow characteristic patterns determined by the location and character of the impact. Linear fractures radiate from the point of impact along the least resistant direction of the skull. Depressed fractures, in which a segment of bone is driven inward relative to the surrounding calvarium, are produced by impact with a small contact area and higher pressure. Basilar skull fractures involving the base of the skull follow characteristic patterns — the hinge fracture across the middle cranial fossa; the ring fracture around the foramen magnum from severe axial loading. Comminuted fractures involving multiple fragments indicate high-energy impact and are common in transportation fatalities and in falls from height.

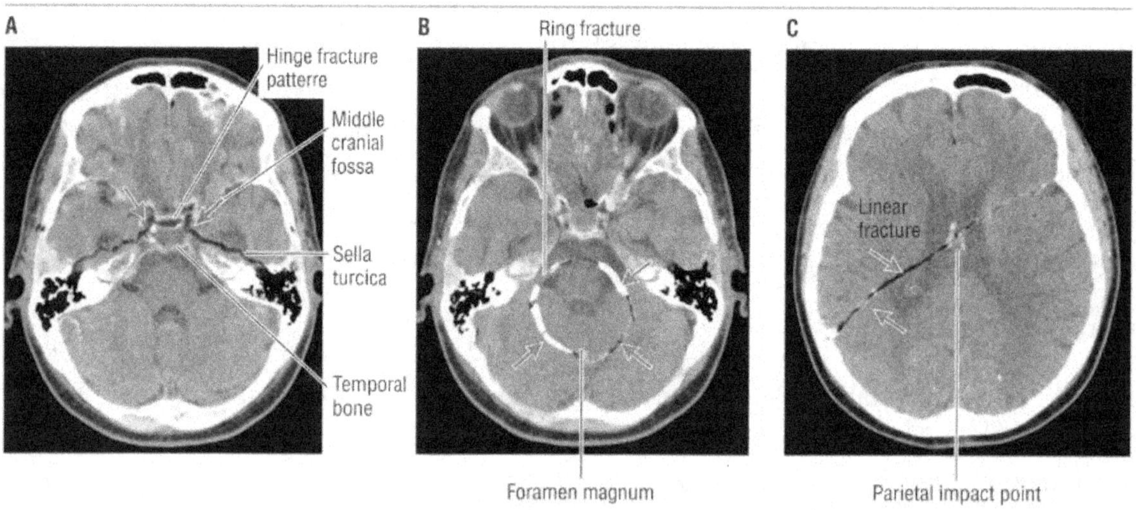


Figure 5.2: Basilar Skull Fracture Patterns on Postmortem CT

## Intracranial Hemorrhage

Blunt head impact produces intracranial hemorrhage in patterns that reflect the underlying anatomy. Epidural hematoma — blood between the dura and the calvarium — typically arises from disruption of the middle meningeal artery and is associated with an overlying fracture of the temporal bone. The classic clinical picture of an epidural hematoma includes a lucid interval between initial loss of consciousness and secondary decompensation as the hematoma expands. Subdural hematoma — blood between the dura and the arachnoid — arises from disruption of bridging veins as the brain moves relative to the dural attachments. Acute subdural hematomas are dense and dark; chronic subdural hematomas over weeks develop a membrane and become progressively encapsulated. Subarachnoid hemorrhage may be traumatic (from cortical vessel disruption) or spontaneous (from a ruptured berry aneurysm); the distinction depends on the pattern and on the presence or absence of underlying disease. Intracerebral hemorrhage from blunt trauma is usually associated with cortical contusion at the site of impact or contrecoup opposite the site of impact.

## Cortical Contusion and Diffuse Axonal Injury

Cortical contusions from blunt impact follow characteristic distributions. Coup contusions occur at the site of impact and reflect direct compression of cortex against the calvarium at the point of contact. Contrecoup contusions occur diametrically opposite the site of impact and reflect the rebound of the brain against the calvarium on the opposite side. The classic pattern in falls, in which the occipital region strikes a surface, is a small occipital coup contusion together with a larger frontal or bilateral frontal contrecoup contusion; the contrecoup contusion often dominates the clinical picture. Diffuse axonal injury is a distinct pattern produced by shear forces during angular acceleration of the head, most commonly in high-energy transportation fatalities.

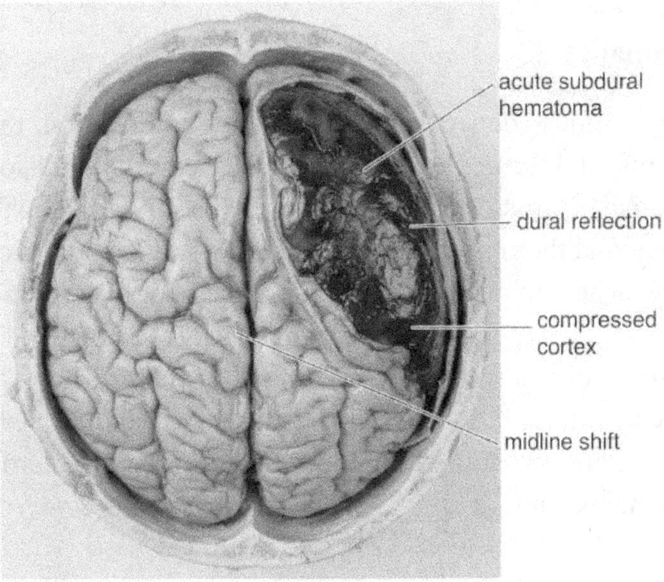


**Figure 5.3: Acute Subdural Hematoma at Autopsy.** Superior view showing a large, dark red-brown subdural hematoma over the right cerebral convexity, causing significant compression of the underlying cortex and midline shift.

It appears grossly as scattered petechial hemorrhage in the corpus callosum, deep white matter, and rostral brainstem; on microscopy, it shows disruption and swelling of axons that can be highlighted on beta-amyloid precursor protein (beta-APP) immunohistochemistry when survival was at least several hours. Diffuse axonal injury is a devastating injury that can produce persistent vegetative state or death without any single dramatic gross finding.

## Transportation Fatalities

Transportation fatalities account for a large fraction of the blunt force caseload in most jurisdictions. The reconstruction of transportation fatalities — pedestrian struck by vehicle, motor vehicle occupant, motorcycle rider — depends on integration of injury pattern with scene information from law enforcement traffic investigators. The pathologist's task is to describe the injury pattern in a way that supports the reconstruction; the reconstruction itself typically involves collaborative work with traffic investigators and, in complex cases, with accident reconstruction engineers.

### Pedestrian Struck by Vehicle

The pedestrian struck by a vehicle presents a characteristic injury pattern that reflects the biomechanics of the impact. Primary impact injuries at the level of the vehicle bumper produce lower extremity injuries — tibia-fibula fractures, femur fractures, ligamentous knee injury — that document the height of the impacting surface and can be measured against the vehicle for reconstruction. Secondary impact injuries occur as the pedestrian is thrown onto the vehicle hood or windshield; these injuries characteristically involve the trunk, upper extremities, and head. Tertiary impact injuries occur as the pedestrian falls to the ground after the vehicle passes; these injuries frequently involve the contralateral side of the body from the initial vehicle contact and produce characteristic road-surface abrasions and injuries to the extremities and head. The pattern of primary, secondary, and tertiary injuries permits reconstruction of the direction of vehicle travel relative to the pedestrian and, in many cases, the vehicle speed at impact.

### Motor Vehicle Occupant

Motor vehicle occupant injury depends on the direction of collision, the position within the vehicle, the use of restraint systems, and the deployment of airbags. Frontal collision produces characteristic injuries including seatbelt bruising across the sternum and abdomen (a diagonal linear contusion), airbag-related facial injury (chemical and thermal irritation from airbag deployment, along with impact injury from the airbag itself), steering wheel impact injuries in unrestrained drivers, and severe head and cervical injury when restraint is inadequate. Lateral collision produces injuries on the side of impact including chest wall injury, pelvic fracture, and head injury with impact on the door or window frame. Rear-end collision produces cervical hyperextension injury (whiplash pattern) and, in severe cases, brainstem injury from severe cervical hyperextension. Rollover produces varied injury patterns including partial ejection injury when the restraint is inadequate.

## Motorcycle and Bicycle Fatalities

Motorcycle riders and bicycle riders sustain characteristic injury patterns that reflect the absence of the protective shell of a car. Head injury dominates the picture in unhelmeted riders; helmet use substantially reduces but does not eliminate head injury risk. Direct impact injuries to the pelvis, extremities, and trunk occur as the rider strikes the road surface or impacted vehicles. Roadway abrasion, often severe, is characteristic; distinguishing roadway abrasion from other tangential injury requires attention to the pattern (widespread, following body contact surfaces) and to the associated foreign material (asphalt particles, road debris). The helmet, when worn, is examined for damage that documents impact points.

## Falls From Height

Fatal falls from height produce injury patterns that reflect the direction of impact, the height of fall, the character of the impacted surface, and the position of the body at impact. The classification of falls into feet-first, head-first, buttocks-first, and lateral impacts is a useful framework for reasoning about the injury pattern. A feet-first fall of substantial height produces characteristic injuries starting at the point of ground contact and transmitting force upward through the axial skeleton — comminuted calcaneal fractures, tibial plateau fractures, femoral neck fractures, vertebral compression fractures, and in the most severe cases atlanto-occipital dissociation or basilar skull ring fracture as force is transmitted through the spine into the skull. A head-first fall produces catastrophic head injury with skull fracture, extensive intracranial hemorrhage, and cervical spine injury. A buttocks-first or seated fall produces pelvic fracture, lumbar spine fracture, and, when the fall is from sufficient height, transmitted injury to the trunk. A lateral fall produces a pattern of chest and pelvis injury on the side of impact with head impact often but not invariably present.

The height of the fall determines the severity of injury within broad limits. Falls from ground level to standing (as in a syncopal collapse) typically produce limited injury — forehead or occipital scalp laceration, occasional skull fracture in elderly decedents, subdural hematoma in decedents with cerebral atrophy allowing bridging vein stretch. Falls from height between one story and two stories produce moderate injuries with a strong dependence on landing position. Falls from three stories or higher produce severe multi-system injury including transection of the aorta at the ligamentum arteriosum from deceleration, hepatic laceration from the impact of the diaphragm on the liver, splenic laceration, pulmonary contusion, and severe pelvic and lower extremity injury in feet-first landings. Falls onto soft surfaces (grass, snow, water) modify the injury pattern by extending the deceleration time; falls onto hard surfaces (concrete, packed earth, roof tile) produce more severe injury at the same height.

The reconstruction of a fall depends on the scene documentation — the height, the character of the landing surface, and the position of the body relative to the point below the fall origin. Suicide falls from height typically show a body position consistent with a self-initiated jump (feet-first or head-first, distributed away from the building base) and a scene that documents a decision point at the fall origin (an open window, an accessible roof edge, personal effects at the top). Accidental falls typically show body position consistent with loss of balance (uncontrolled lateral or backward) with a scene consistent with the reported mechanism (a stairwell, an unprotected work surface, an intoxicated decedent at a fall origin). Homicidal falls — rare but documented — may show inconsistency between body position and stated mechanism, evidence of prior altercation, or injuries inconsistent with the fall itself. The reconstruction integrates the fall physics, the injury pattern, and the scene evidence to support the manner determination.

**CLINICAL PEARL:** The height of the primary impact point on the body against the fall height and landing surface constrains the physics of the fall. A pattern of injuries inconsistent with the reported fall mechanism — for example, a head impact injury without any lower extremity or trunk injury in a reported jump — argues against the reported mechanism and warrants investigation of alternative mechanisms including physical assault before the fall.

### Craniocervical Junction and Cervical Spine Injury

The craniocervical junction — the transition from skull to cervical spine at the atlanto-occipital and atlantoaxial joints — is uniquely vulnerable in blunt trauma and warrants specific examination in transportation fatalities, in falls, and in cases with severe head impact. Atlanto-occipital dissociation is a catastrophic injury produced by severe distraction, hyperflexion, or hyperextension of the neck. The ligamentous attachments between the occipital condyles and the atlas are disrupted, and the skull is effectively separated from the cervical spine at the level of the joint. The injury is typically immediately fatal because it disrupts the brainstem-spinal cord junction, and it is diagnosed at autopsy by dissection of the ligamentous complex or by postmortem CT documentation of the disrupted joint. The injury is more common in pediatric decedents than adults because the ligamentous complex is relatively weaker in the developing spine.

Cervical spine injury below the craniocervical junction includes vertebral fracture, ligamentous injury, and cord injury. Hangman fractures — bilateral pedicle fractures of the axis — are classically associated with judicial hanging but also occur in motor vehicle collisions when the head is thrown forward against the windshield or dashboard with the neck extended. Odontoid (dens) fractures are common in falls in elderly decedents. Cervical spine injuries lower in the axis produce cord injury patterns that correspond to the level of injury — high cervical cord injury (C1-C4) produces immediate respiratory arrest and death; lower cervical cord injury produces quadriplegia with variable survival depending on respiratory function. The examination of the cervical spine in blunt trauma cases requires layered dissection and, in cases with high suspicion for craniocervical injury, careful preservation of the joint capsule for direct inspection before disruption by dissection.

### Blunt Chest and Abdominal Injury

Blunt chest injury produces characteristic patterns depending on the mechanism. Rib fractures follow the pattern of applied force; anterior-posterior compression (as in chest compression during CPR, or in motor vehicle collision with steering wheel impact) produces fractures at the costochondral junctions and along the mid-axillary line as the ribs bend outward. Lateral compression produces fractures at the anterior and posterior points of maximum curvature. Multiple rib fractures at the same site on adjacent ribs produce flail chest, in which the chest wall segment moves paradoxically with respiration. Cardiac injury from blunt force ranges from myocardial contusion (with characteristic patchy hemorrhage in the myocardium and, in severe cases, myocardial rupture with hemopericardium) to commotio cordis (arrhythmic death from precordial impact during a vulnerable phase of the cardiac cycle, most classically documented in young athletes struck in the chest by a projectile such as a baseball). Aortic injury — partial or complete transection at the ligamentum arteriosum from severe deceleration — is the classic aortic injury of high-speed motor vehicle collision and of fall from height.

Blunt abdominal injury produces a similar spectrum. The liver is the most commonly injured abdominal organ from blunt force, particularly in falls from height where the diaphragm is driven downward against the liver at impact. Hepatic laceration produces hemoperitoneum and, if extensive, exsanguination. Splenic injury is common in blunt trauma to the left upper quadrant. Pancreatic injury is uncommon but characteristic when it occurs — usually from a focal impact against the vertebral column at the level of the pancreas, as from a handlebar or steering wheel injury. Renal injury from blunt trauma follows a similar pattern. Bowel injury from blunt trauma is relatively uncommon but may include mesenteric tears with peritoneal hemorrhage, seat-belt-associated small bowel injury, and traumatic diaphragmatic rupture.

**SCENE-TO-CERTIFICATION DECISION SYSTEM — Pedestrian Impact Reconstruction Arc**

**Presenting Death Scenario:** A 42-year-old woman is struck by a vehicle while crossing a street at approximately 6:30 PM. Multiple witnesses report seeing a vehicle traveling at high speed strike the pedestrian and continue without stopping. Emergency response is immediate; the pedestrian is transported to a trauma center where she is pronounced dead approximately 45 minutes after the impact. The medical examiner's office accepts jurisdiction. Traffic investigators identify a vehicle recovered several miles away with front-end damage and human tissue in the grille.

**Autopsy Signature:** External examination documents primary impact injuries at the level of the right lateral lower extremity: a linear pattern abrasion across the right lateral thigh at approximately 55 cm above heel; underlying comminuted fracture of the right femur; and displaced fractures of the right tibia and fibula. Secondary impact injuries are documented on the trunk and head: extensive contusion of the right chest wall with underlying rib fractures; a large scalp laceration over the right parietal region with underlying comminuted parietal skull fracture; acute subdural hematoma over the right cerebral hemisphere. Tertiary impact injuries include extensive left-sided abrasions and contusions with embedded road debris, consistent with contact with pavement after the vehicle impact.

**Cause Determination:** Blunt force injuries of head, chest, and lower extremity due to pedestrian-motor vehicle collision. The dominant lethal injury is the acute subdural hematoma with associated cerebral injury.

**Manner Determination:** Homicide. The manner is homicide because the vehicle operator did not stop at the scene (leaving the scene of a fatal collision may itself be a criminal act) and because the criminal investigation may support charges beyond the manner classification. The manner classification is medical; the specific charges are legal. Alternatively, if the criminal investigation had determined the collision was purely accidental with no criminal component, the manner would be accident. The medical examiner's manner determination reflects the circumstances known at the time of certification and can be amended as the investigation develops.

**Trap Logic:** The reconstruction of pedestrian impact depends on measurement of primary impact injury height against the vehicle. The height of the primary impact abrasion (55 cm above heel in this case) can be measured against the vehicle bumper height to confirm consistency of the vehicle with the collision. When measurement is not documented, this reconstruction is not possible. The pathologist must measure and document the height of primary impact injuries in every pedestrian fatality. A related trap is the failure to distinguish primary, secondary, and tertiary impact injuries in the report; without this distinction the reconstruction cannot be reproduced from the record.

**Certification Anchor:** Pedestrian struck by vehicle produces a characteristic pattern of primary (bumper level), secondary (hood or windshield level), and tertiary (roadway impact) injuries. Systematic documentation of each level, with measurements referenced to standard anatomical landmarks, supports reconstruction of vehicle speed and direction and permits matching of the pedestrian injury pattern to a suspect vehicle.

## SCENE-TO-CERTIFICATION DECISION SYSTEM — Blunt Force Determination Arcs

**The Wound Categories and Their Mechanism:** Blunt force produces four principal wound categories reflecting which tissue fails first: abrasion (superficial epidermis), contusion (subcutaneous vessels), laceration (full-thickness skin), and fracture (bone). Most significant blunt injuries produce combinations that document the mechanism more reliably than any single wound taken in isolation.

**The Antemortem-Postmortem Discipline:** Antemortem injuries produce vital reaction (dermal hemorrhage, inflammatory response, tissue infiltration); postmortem changes and artifacts do not. Histologic examination distinguishes ambiguous gross findings. The distinction is fundamental to reasoning about mechanism and manner.

**The Aging Limits:** Contusion aging by gross color is unreliable beyond broad ranges (recent, intermediate, resolving). Precise time-of-injury estimation from visual inspection is not defensible on cross-examination; histologic examination is required when specific timing is critical. This is a documented limit of the specialty.

**Head Injury Integration:** Blunt head injury produces a characteristic constellation — scalp laceration, skull fracture, epidural or subdural hematoma, cortical contusion (coup and contrecoup), and diffuse axonal injury — that reflects the biomechanics of impact. Layered scalp dissection, brain fixation for detailed examination, and integration with the scene reconstruction are the standard techniques.

**Transportation Fatality Reconstruction:** Transportation fatalities are reconstructed from the pattern of primary, secondary, and tertiary impact injuries integrated with scene information from traffic investigators. Systematic documentation of injury height at primary impact, of the pattern of secondary trunk and head injury, and of tertiary roadway contact permits matching of the injury pattern to the vehicle and to the mechanism of the collision.

## Summary and Key Concepts

Blunt force injury is the most common category of traumatic death encountered in forensic pathology practice. It is characterized by four principal wound categories — abrasion, contusion, laceration, and fracture — each reflecting the tissue that fails first under the applied force.

Abrasions preserve the pattern of the impacting surface in pattern abrasions and support reconstruction of the direction of force in scrape abrasions. The distinction between antemortem abrasion (with vital reaction) and postmortem drying artifact is fundamental and often requires histologic examination when unclear at gross inspection.

Contusions preserve the pattern of some impacting objects, permit crude age estimation within acknowledged limits, and document force applied at levels insufficient to lacerate but sufficient to disrupt small vessels. Contusion aging by gross color alone is unreliable for precise time estimation and testimony must reflect this limit.

Lacerations are morphologically distinguished from incised wounds by irregular margins, tissue bridges, marginal abrasion, and contusion of underlying tissue. The distinction is central to reasoning about mechanism of injury.

Blunt force head injury produces a characteristic constellation of scalp laceration, skull fracture, epidural or subdural hematoma, cortical contusion (coup and contrecoup), and diffuse axonal injury. Systematic examination with layered scalp dissection, brain fixation, and integration with scene reconstruction supports the case reasoning.

Transportation fatalities are reconstructed from the pattern of primary, secondary, and tertiary impact injuries. Systematic documentation of injury height at primary impact, of the pattern of secondary trunk and head injury, and of tertiary roadway contact permits matching of the injury pattern to the vehicle and mechanism of the collision.

# CHAPTER 6: SHARP FORCE INJURY

**Learning Objectives**

1. Distinguish stab wounds, incised wounds, and chop wounds by mechanism, morphology, and forensic significance.
2. Document a sharp force injury with the specific measurements and observations required for wound reconstruction and weapon characterization.
3. Reconstruct a sharp force event from the pattern of wounds, integrating defensive injury, wound tract, and scene evidence.
4. Distinguish sharp force homicide, suicide, and accident from the pattern of wounds and their distribution, and articulate the traps that undermine this distinction.
5. Recognize the documented limits of blade identification from wound characteristics and apply the appropriate degree of certainty in reporting and testimony.

## Categories and Mechanisms of Sharp Force Injury

Sharp force injury is the category of injury produced by an object with a cutting edge, a pointed tip, or both. The wound categories are stab wound (produced by a pointed object with force delivered along its long axis, penetrating the body to a depth greater than the wound length on the skin surface), incised wound (produced by a cutting edge drawn tangentially across the skin, with wound length greater than depth), and chop wound (a hybrid produced by a heavy object with a cutting edge delivered with substantial force, combining features of blunt force and sharp force). The distinction among these categories, and the distinction between sharp force wounds and blunt force lacerations, is one of the central diagnostic skills of forensic pathology and one on which the published literature documents substantial rates of misinterpretation.

The forensic importance of sharp force injury reflects both its frequency (sharp force is second only to firearm injury as a cause of homicidal death in most American jurisdictions and is the most common non-firearm mechanism of homicide) and its potential for reconstruction. A stab wound preserves information about the weapon that produced it — the width of the blade, the length of the blade (partially, and with important limits), the character of the cutting edge (single-edge or double-edge), and the direction of the strike. Systematic documentation and analysis of these features supports courtroom testimony about the character of the weapon and the mechanism of the event.

### The Sharp Force / Blunt Force Distinction

The distinction between sharp force injury and blunt force laceration is the foundational skill, because the two categories look superficially similar at gross examination and the misinterpretation of one for the other is one of the classic errors of the specialty. Incised wounds and lacerations both present as full-thickness disruptions of skin with underlying tissue defect. The distinguishing features favor sharp force injury when wound margins are clean and linear, when there are no tissue bridges in the wound cavity, when there is no marginal abrasion from tangential impact, and when the underlying tissue is cleanly divided. The distinguishing features favor blunt force laceration when wound margins are irregular and jagged, when tissue bridges span the wound cavity, when the margins show tangential abrasion, and when underlying tissue is contused rather than cleanly cut. Peer-reviewed studies of examiner performance in distinguishing these categories have documented substantial error rates — in one representative published analysis, correct identification of wound type was achieved in fewer than half of stab wound cases at the level of the individual examiner. The trainee must be aware of this documented interpretive uncertainty and cultivate the discipline of systematic examination that reduces it.

**EVIDENCE:** Published studies of examiner interpretation of skin wounds document error rates for gunshot wound type identification averaging approximately 4 out of 10 correct assessments, and error rates for stab wound interpretation with fewer than half correct across observer panels. The literature identifies systematic examination against defined criteria — not intuitive pattern recognition — as the countermeasure. The trainee cultivates the systematic discipline and does not overestimate the reliability of visual gestalt.

## Stab Wounds

A stab wound is produced by the introduction of a pointed weapon into the body along the long axis of the weapon, with the depth of penetration greater than the length of the surface wound. Stab wounds are the classic sharp force injury of the assault case and the classic self-inflicted injury of suicide by stab. Their forensic value derives from the information they preserve about the weapon and about the direction of the strike.

### Morphology of the Skin Wound

The skin wound produced by a stab reflects the cross-sectional shape of the weapon at the depth of the wound edge. A knife blade with a single cutting edge (the standard kitchen knife or utility knife) produces a wound with one sharp angle (the edge of the blade) and one blunted or square-cut angle (the back of the blade). This asymmetry documents which side of the blade was oriented in which direction relative to the body. A double-edged blade (a dagger, some hunting knives) produces a wound with two sharp angles. A serrated blade may produce visible serration marks on the skin margins if the wound was inflicted with tangential motion, though the serrations of most kitchen serrated knives are too fine to imprint reliably on skin. A round-cross-section penetrating object (an awl, a screwdriver) produces a wound with round or slit-like morphology depending on the depth.

The length of the skin wound is not the same as the width of the blade. When a knife is withdrawn along the axis of the strike without tangential motion, the wound length approximates the blade width at the depth of penetration. When the knife is withdrawn with tangential motion (a slicing withdrawal), the wound is extended and its length exceeds the blade width. When the skin is under tension at the time of the stab (the abdomen of a standing individual, for example), skin retraction after wound production shortens the apparent wound length. When the skin is redundant, the wound may show as a gape wider than the blade width. These modifications must be considered in reasoning from wound length to blade width; skin wound length is a rough approximation of blade width, not a precise measurement.

## The Wound Tract

The wound tract — the path of the weapon through the tissue — is documented by dissection of the wound in layered fashion, following the tract from skin through subcutaneous tissue, through any bone or cartilage encountered, and into the deep tissue and organs. Documentation of the wound tract includes the depth of penetration measured from skin surface to deepest point of injury, the direction of the tract described in three dimensions (superior-inferior, anterior-posterior, medial-lateral), and the structures traversed with any injury to each. Depth of penetration constrains the blade length, with important qualifications: the blade may not have been introduced to its full length (the penetration may be less than blade length); the blade may have penetrated with compression of soft tissue, allowing penetration deeper than blade length; and the geometry of the tract may not correspond precisely to the blade length if the weapon was moved during the strike.

**Figure 6.1:** Stab Wound Morphology and Blade Characteristics

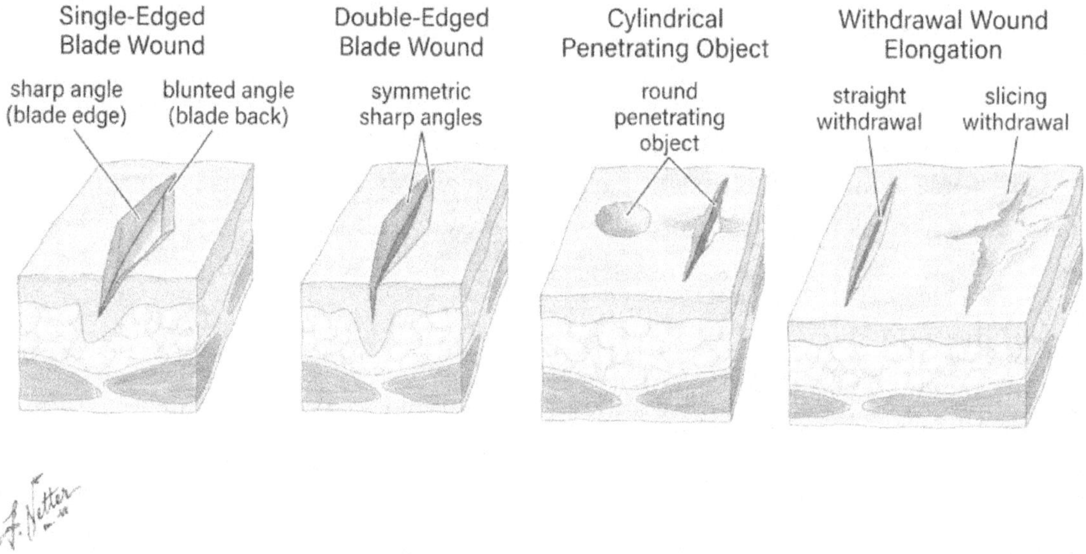


## Documentation Requirements

Every stab wound is documented for location (with reference to anatomical landmarks and body coordinates), length on the skin surface, orientation (using clock-face reference — for example, "oriented from 2 o'clock to 8 o'clock" — or in terms of the anatomical axis), margin characteristics (sharp or blunted at each angle), and any associated marginal abrasion. Photographic documentation includes overview showing the location of the wound on the body, mid-range showing the wound and adjacent anatomy, and close-up with a scale for measurement. Wound tract dissection is photographed in layered fashion showing the path of the wound at each successive tissue layer. Depth of penetration is measured with a probe passed along the natural line of the wound tract without forcing the tissue, and the depth is documented with the probe in place.

**CLINICAL PEARL:** The skin wound tells the pathologist about the blade cross-section; the wound tract tells the pathologist about the blade length and the direction of the strike. Both must be documented for reconstruction; documentation of only the skin wound is not sufficient for testimony about the weapon.

### Multiple Stab Wounds and Reconstruction

Cases with multiple stab wounds require documentation of every wound with the same precision as a single wound. The pattern of wounds — their distribution, the direction of each, and any temporal sequence that can be inferred — supports reconstruction of the event. A cluster of parallel wounds in a single anatomic region suggests a rapid series of strikes without repositioning; a distribution of wounds across multiple regions suggests a struggle with the victim in motion; wounds inflicted through clothing show a pattern of skin and clothing defects that must be integrated. Defensive wounds — wounds on the palms, ulnar aspects of the forearms, and dorsa of the hands — document conscious defense against the strikes and support the reconstruction that the victim was aware during at least part of the assault.

### SCENE-TO-CERTIFICATION DECISION SYSTEM — Stab Wound Reconstruction Arc

**Presenting Death Scenario:** A 34-year-old man is found deceased in his home by a coworker who came to check on him after he did not appear for work. The body is in the living room, prone on the carpet, in a large pool of blood. There is no forced entry to the residence. A folding knife with a 4-inch single-edged blade is on the floor approximately 6 feet from the body, with blood on the blade. Multiple stab wounds are visible on the anterior chest, back, and forearms. The scene investigator documents the body position, the pool of blood, and the position of the knife; the body is transported to the medical examiner's office.

**Autopsy Signature:** External examination documents 14 stab wounds. Seven are on the anterior chest, distributed from the sternal region to the lateral chest wall bilaterally, with the deepest wound on the left mid-clavicular line at the fifth intercostal space (2.5 cm long, oriented from 1 to 7 o'clock, with sharp lower angle and blunted upper angle indicating single-edged blade oriented with cutting edge downward at the strike). Four are on the back, distributed across the left thoracic region. Three are on the left forearm and both hands, with morphology characteristic of defensive wounds. Layered dissection of the anterior chest wound at the fifth intercostal space demonstrates a wound tract passing posteriorly and medially through the fourth intercostal space, penetrating the pericardium, and terminating in the left ventricular anterior wall with an associated 1.5 cm defect. Depth of penetration approximately 8 cm. Wound tract dissection of remaining wounds documents penetration of variable depth into subcutaneous tissue, chest wall musculature, and, in two anterior wounds, the pleural space with associated hemothorax.

**Cause Determination:** Multiple stab wounds of the chest, back, and upper extremities, with lethal cardiac wound. The dominant lethal injury is the stab wound of the left ventricle with hemopericardium and cardiac tamponade.

**Manner Determination:** Homicide. The pattern of 14 wounds distributed across the anterior and posterior body, the presence of defensive wounds on the hands and forearms, and the absence of any pattern consistent with self-infliction (no hesitation wounds, no clustering in accessible sites, wounds inflicted on the back which are not self-accessible) all support homicide. The scene evidence — no forced entry — is consistent with either an attack by a known assailant or with the decedent admitting the assailant, and does not itself change the manner determination.

**Trap Logic:** The number of wounds is not by itself a determinant of manner; occasional cases of suicide involve multiple wounds. The trap is to reason from wound count alone. The countermeasure is systematic reasoning from wound distribution, defensive injury, hesitation wound presence or absence, and accessibility of the wounded sites. Wounds on the back and defensive wounds on the hands are strongly against self-infliction. A related trap is failure to document each wound with sufficient precision to reconstruct the direction of the strike; a report that describes "multiple stab wounds" without individual documentation cannot support courtroom testimony about the mechanism of any specific wound.

**Certification Anchor:** Sharp force injury manner determination rests on the integration of wound distribution, defensive injury, hesitation wound presence, accessibility of wounded sites, and scene evidence. Wounds on the back, defensive wounds on the hands, and absence of hesitation wounds are strong evidence against self-infliction. The pattern is documented systematically in the autopsy report so the reasoning can be reconstructed by a reader who was not present at examination.

## Incised Wounds

An incised wound is produced by a cutting edge drawn tangentially across the skin, with wound length greater than depth. The classic incised wound is the razor cut, the scalpel wound, and the wound produced by a knife drawn across the skin rather than driven into it. Incised wounds carry distinct forensic significance from stab wounds because their pattern reflects a different mechanism and their distribution supports different reconstructions.

### Morphology and Location

The incised wound has clean linear margins without tissue bridges or marginal abrasion. Its depth is greatest at the beginning of the cut (where the blade enters the skin at an angle) and typically shallowest at the end (where the blade tapers off the skin surface); this asymmetry supports reconstruction of the direction of the cut. The classic location of incised wounds in self-inflicted injury is the flexor surfaces of the wrists (where the vessels of the wrist are readily accessible), the anterior neck (where the carotid and jugular vessels can be reached), and the antecubital fossae. The classic location of incised wounds in defensive injury is the ulnar aspect of the forearms (as the victim raises the arms to shield the head and face) and the palms of the hands (as the victim grasps at the blade).

### Hesitation Wounds

Hesitation wounds are shallow, non-lethal incised wounds distributed near the deeper wound in self-inflicted injury. They reflect the decedent's incomplete initial attempts to inflict the fatal wound and are characteristic of suicide by incision at the wrist or the neck. Hesitation wounds are typically superficial, parallel to the fatal wound, and clustered at the site of the fatal wound. Their presence is strong evidence of self-infliction; their absence does not exclude self-infliction (some suicide decedents produce a single decisive wound without hesitation), but their absence in an incised wound death warrants specific consideration of homicide as the alternative. The forensic pathologist documents hesitation wounds as they are found and integrates their pattern with other reconstruction evidence.

### Defensive Wounds

Defensive wounds are wounds sustained during conscious defense against an assault. The morphology of defensive wounds reflects the position of the defender — the arms raised to shield the head and face, the hands raised to grasp at a weapon. Incised defensive wounds cluster on the ulnar aspect of the forearms and on the palms; stab defensive wounds occur in similar locations with the added feature of penetrating wounds through the hands as the victim grabbed the blade. The presence of defensive wounds documents that the victim was conscious during at least part of the assault and supports homicide as the manner determination in cases where self-infliction might otherwise be considered.

Figure 6.2: Defensive Wounds of the Hands and Forearms

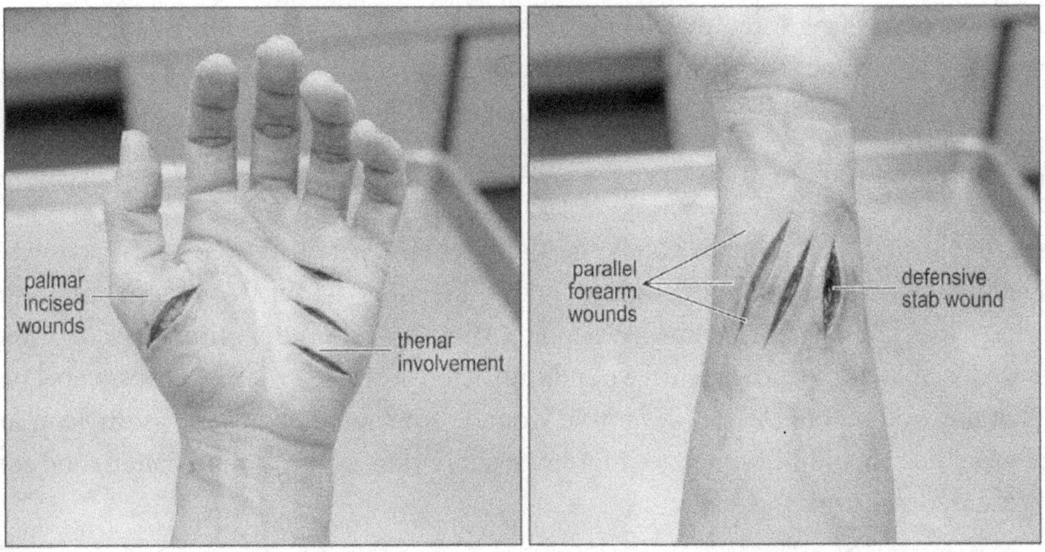


## Chop Wounds

A chop wound is produced by a heavy object with a cutting edge delivered with substantial force — an axe, a hatchet, a machete, a meat cleaver, a large kitchen knife wielded with significant momentum. Chop wounds combine features of sharp force and blunt force: the cutting edge produces a linear wound with relatively clean margins, but the substantial force delivered by the heavy weight produces underlying fracture, deep tissue disruption, and marginal contusion that resemble blunt force injury. Chop wounds are relatively uncommon in most American forensic caseloads compared with stab and incised wounds but are highly characteristic when they occur.

### Morphology and Reconstruction

Chop wounds typically show a linear wound with sharp margins at the cutting edge, underlying bone fracture with a linear fracture line matching the wound orientation, and adjacent contusion from the mass of the impacting weapon. The depth of the wound reflects both the sharpness of the cutting edge and the force of the strike. Cases involving multiple chop wounds distributed across the head, neck, or trunk are often characterized by high blood loss, severe underlying skeletal injury, and a pattern consistent with a specific weapon type when the wound characteristics are integrated with scene evidence.

### Distinction From Stab and Incised Wounds

Chop wounds are distinguished from stab wounds by their length-to-depth ratio (chop wounds have wound length approximating or exceeding depth, whereas stab wounds have depth exceeding length) and by the associated bone fracture (chop wounds characteristically involve underlying bone injury; stab wounds may involve bone but do so with penetrating rather than fracturing pattern). Chop wounds are distinguished from incised wounds by the substantial underlying tissue disruption and by the associated bone injury (incised wounds typically involve only superficial tissue).

## Reconstruction of Sharp Force Events

The reconstruction of a sharp force event integrates the wound pattern, the wound characteristics, the scene evidence, and any witness accounts. The pathologist's contribution is the systematic documentation of the wounds and the reasoning about mechanism that the wound pattern supports.

### The Sequence of Wounds

In some cases, the sequence of wounds can be partially reconstructed. Wounds inflicted while the victim was still bleeding to a large volume produce heavy bleeding at the wound; wounds inflicted after substantial blood loss show less bleeding. Wounds inflicted while the victim was conscious and active produce blood distributed by movement; wounds inflicted after the victim was incapacitated produce blood pooled at the wound. In practice, definitive wound sequencing at autopsy is difficult and testimony about wound sequence should be limited to inferences supported by the wound pattern and scene evidence rather than presented as certain.

### The Direction of Strike

The direction of the strike is reconstructed from the wound tract. The three-dimensional path of the wound documents the direction from which the weapon was applied. In a decedent standing at the time of the wound, a strike from directly in front produces a horizontal wound tract; a strike from above (from a taller assailant or from an assailant standing while the victim is seated or on the ground) produces a downward tract; a strike from below produces an upward tract. Integration of the wound tract direction with the position of the body at the time of the strike (reconstructed from other evidence) supports reasoning about the relative positions of the assailant and victim.

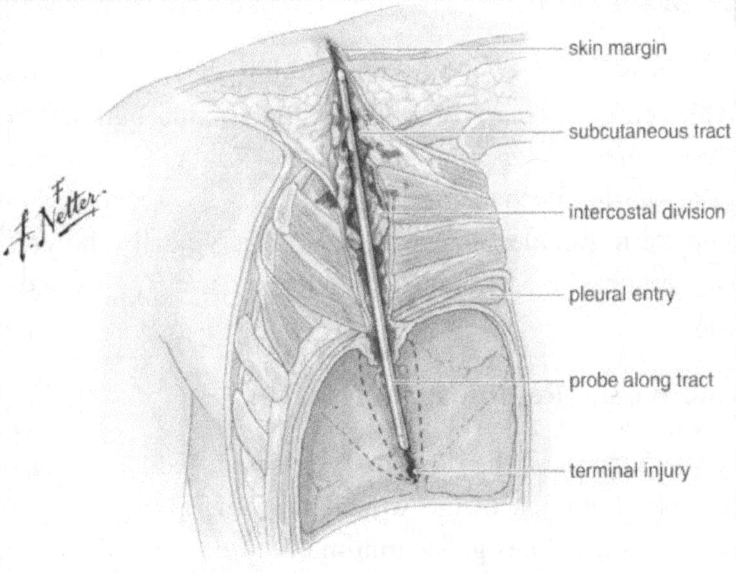

Figure 6.3: Layered Wound Tract Dissection Technique

## Suicide, Homicide, and Accident in Sharp Force Deaths

The manner determination in sharp force death is one of the highest-stakes decisions in the specialty because the misclassification of a homicide as a suicide or the reverse has immediate legal consequences. The determination rests on integration of the wound pattern with the scene evidence and the reasoning about self-infliction versus assault.

### Sharp Force Suicide

Suicide by sharp force typically shows a characteristic pattern. Wounds are located at accessible sites for the dominant hand of the decedent — the wrist, the neck (especially the anterior neck), the antecubital fossa. Hesitation wounds are frequently present clustered near the fatal wound. Wounds are inflicted through skin without clothing intervening (clothing is typically removed or drawn back at the wound site). Weapons are found at the scene near the decedent or, in some cases, remain in the wound. Notes may be present. Wounds inflicted at multiple non-accessible sites, wounds on the back, defensive wounds, and wounds inflicted through clothing are all inconsistent with suicide and shift reasoning toward homicide.

### Sharp Force Homicide

Homicide by sharp force typically involves multiple wounds, wounds distributed across the body including sites not accessible for self-infliction, defensive wounds, wounds inflicted through clothing, and often signs of struggle at the scene. The pattern of homicide varies widely with the mechanism of the assault (single-blade attack, multiple-strike attack, controlled versus frenzied), and the reconstruction must accommodate the variability. The essential discipline is systematic documentation of every wound with sufficient precision that the reasoning about the mechanism can be reconstructed from the report.

### Accidental Sharp Force Death

Accidental sharp force death is uncommon but occurs. Industrial injuries involving cutting equipment, transportation injuries with vehicular sharp force (through glass, through metal), and household accidents with kitchen or garden equipment all account for a small number of forensic caseloads annually. The manner determination rests on the mechanism documented at the scene and on integration of the scene evidence with the wound pattern. Accidental sharp force death typically shows a single wound or a limited pattern consistent with the reported mechanism, without the defensive wounds or multi-site distribution characteristic of homicide.

### Skin Fold Alignment and Wound Reconstruction Nuance

The apparent length of a stab wound on the skin surface is modified by the tension state of the skin at the time of the strike and by the alignment of the wound with the Langer lines of skin tension. A wound inflicted parallel to the local Langer lines gapes minimally after the blade is withdrawn and appears as a slit approximating the blade width. A wound inflicted perpendicular to the Langer lines gapes substantially as the skin retracts along the tension axis and appears wider than the blade width. In cases where blade width is being reconstructed from wound length, the pathologist repositions the skin margins toward their natural alignment before final measurement and documents the wound length as "length when margins are approximated" rather than as the gape width. Failure to appreciate this modifier is a documented source of overestimation of blade width in the literature.

The direction of the strike is further constrained by the shape of the wound tract in three dimensions. A straight tract with uniform width along its length is consistent with a single straight strike without repositioning of the weapon. A curved or angulated tract is consistent with repositioning of the blade during the strike, either by movement of the assailant, movement of the victim, or both. A tract with variable width along its length may indicate multiple strikes through the same skin defect or use of a blade with variable width along its long axis. Documentation of the tract in three dimensions — typically through layered dissection with photography at each layer — permits later reconstruction of these features by an outside expert reviewing the case.

### Postmortem Sharp Force Injury and Its Recognition

Sharp force injuries inflicted after death occur in several contexts and must be distinguished from antemortem injury in the reasoning. Autopsy incisions themselves are sharp force injuries and are documented as such in the autopsy report, distinguished from antemortem injuries by their standard position (Y-incision, cranial incision, evisceration-related incisions) and by the absence of vital reaction. Sharp force applied by the responder or the assailant after death — in dismemberment cases, in attempts to conceal the body, in staged suicide scenes — shows the same absence of vital reaction as any postmortem injury: no bleeding at the wound margins beyond the small amount of pooled blood displaced by the cut, no infiltration of blood into the surrounding tissue, and no inflammatory response. Histologic examination distinguishes antemortem sharp force injury (with dermal hemorrhage and vital reaction) from postmortem sharp force injury (with clean margins and no vital reaction).

Dismemberment cases represent a particular reasoning challenge. The cutting surfaces used in dismemberment produce characteristic wounds — typically at joint spaces (with disarticulation rather than through-bone cutting) or at long bones (with saw marks or hatchet-like cutting patterns). Postmortem dismemberment shows no vital reaction and typically minimal bleeding because the vasculature is empty; antemortem dismemberment, which is rare but does occur in some criminal cases, would show substantial bleeding and vital reaction. The reconstruction of a dismembered case requires integration of the wound pattern, the surface used for cutting, and any tool marks preserved on the bone. Consultation with a forensic anthropologist is standard in dismemberment cases with skeletal cut marks.

**CAUTION:** Sharp force injuries with no vital reaction are postmortem. Sharp force injuries with vital reaction are antemortem. Sharp force injuries at the boundary — with minimal but present vital reaction — are perimortem, inflicted at or immediately after death when tissue reaction is still developing. The distinction has substantial reconstruction implications and must be made on the basis of both gross and histologic findings, not on gross appearance alone.

### Broken Blades, Retained Fragments, and Weapon Recovery

In a small but non-trivial subset of sharp force cases, the blade breaks during the strike and a fragment remains in the wound tract. The retained fragment is a piece of physical evidence with direct forensic value — it can be matched to the parent weapon if the weapon is recovered, and it constrains the identification of the class of weapon used. Retained blade fragments are identified by careful layered dissection with attention to any foreign material along the wound tract, and by radiographic examination of the affected body region either before or during autopsy. Postmortem CT can identify metallic fragments with high sensitivity and is increasingly used as a screening tool in sharp force cases at offices with the resources. Recovered fragments are photographed in place, then removed and preserved with intact chain of custody for transfer to law enforcement.

The weapon itself, when recovered at the scene, is examined for consistency with the wound pattern. Blade width and blade cross-section are compared against the wound length and skin wound morphology. Blood on the blade is examined for consistency with the decedent (typically through DNA comparison performed by the crime laboratory rather than the pathologist directly). Weapon recovery is coordinated with law enforcement chain of custody; the pathologist does not typically retain the weapon itself but does document her examination of it in the autopsy record.

### Documentation Standards Specific to Sharp Force Cases

Sharp force cases have documentation standards specific to the category. Every wound is numbered systematically (typically in a defined sequence such as anterior to posterior, or by body region) with the numbering preserved in the autopsy report and in the photographic record. Each wound is described by number with its location, length, orientation, margin characteristics, and tract characteristics if dissected. Photographic documentation includes overview of each body region showing all wounds in that region, mid-range showing individual wounds with adjacent anatomy, and close-up of each wound with a scale. Layered dissection photography shows the tract of each significant wound. In cases with many wounds, a body diagram with the numbered locations of each wound is a standard supplement to the narrative description — the diagram permits the reader of the report to visualize the distribution at a glance without reconstructing it from the descriptions.

### Wounds Through Clothing

Sharp force wounds inflicted through clothing produce defects in both the clothing and the underlying skin, and the integrated documentation of both is essential. The clothing defect approximates the blade width at the outer surface of the garment and may show additional features characteristic of the strike — for example, thread displacement direction can suggest the direction of blade motion, and superimposed defects in multiple layers of clothing document that the strike was inflicted through the layered garment rather than through a naked chest with the clothing subsequently arranged. The skin defect beneath a clothing defect may differ slightly in orientation, in length, and in the sharpness of the margins because the clothing modifies the blade's contact with skin. Photography documents each clothing item in place, then removed, with the skin defects photographed both through the intact clothing (where possible) and after clothing removal. Any correspondence between clothing defect and skin defect is documented for later reconstruction, and clothing is preserved as evidence with intact chain of custody.

The distinction between wounds through clothing (in an assault case) and wounds through skin with clothing removed (in a suicide) is one line of reasoning that supports the manner determination. A suicide by neck incision typically shows the wound inflicted through skin — the decedent removed or drew back the clothing at the wound site — while a homicidal neck wound may be inflicted through a shirt or collar, producing an integrated defect through fabric and skin. The pattern is not diagnostic in itself but contributes to the reasoning.

### Sharp Force Injury to Bone and Skeletal Cut Marks

Sharp force injury that involves bone — through direct contact with a blade during a strike, through deep penetration to underlying skeletal elements, or in dismemberment — preserves tool marks on the bone that can support weapon identification. Cut marks on bone show characteristic features related to the class of tool used: a knife blade produces a V-shaped or shallow cut with a smooth interior surface; a saw produces parallel striations along the cut with a rectangular cross-section; a hatchet or axe produces a deeper cut with characteristic bevel patterns; a serrated blade may produce visible serration marks along the cut. The forensic anthropologist is the specialist in bone cut mark analysis, and consultation is standard in cases where the cut mark pattern is a central element of the case reasoning. Preservation of the affected bone — in fixed or fresh state per anthropology protocol — permits detailed analysis that a routine autopsy examination would not accomplish.

### Sharp Force Injury in Pediatric Decedents

Sharp force injury in pediatric decedents follows the same principles as in adults but with important modifications reflecting pediatric anatomy and the case context. The infant or young child has a smaller body with less redundant skin, so the same blade tends to produce relatively larger wounds proportional to body size. The infant chest and abdomen offer less bone protection to underlying organs than the adult, so wounds of relatively shallow depth may nonetheless produce lethal internal injury. Sharp force injury in a young child is almost always homicidal (accidental sharp force death in a young child is uncommon), and the case is worked with pediatric protocols including full skeletal survey, integration with any medical history, careful documentation of every wound, and attention to any co-existing evidence of chronic abuse or neglect. The pediatric protocol overlaps substantially with the general child abuse investigation developed in Chapter 13.

**SCENE-TO-CERTIFICATION DECISION SYSTEM — Homicide-Versus-Suicide Sharp Force Arc**

---

**Presenting Death Scenario:** A 46-year-old man is found deceased in the bathtub of his residence by his wife when she returned home from work. There is substantial blood in the bathtub water. A single deep incised wound is present on the left anterior neck. A straight razor is on the tile floor beside the tub. The wife reports that the decedent had been depressed since a recent job loss and had made suicidal statements in the preceding weeks. She reports no prior suicide attempts. The scene shows no signs of forced entry, no signs of struggle, and no defensive wounds visible on external inspection at the scene. The medical examiner's office accepts jurisdiction.

**Autopsy Signature:** External examination documents a deep incised wound of the left anterior neck extending from the left mastoid region across the anterior neck to the right mid-clavicular region, approximately 15 cm long, with wound depth reaching the vertebral column and dividing the left carotid artery, the left internal jugular vein, and the trachea. Three parallel superficial hesitation wounds are present immediately superior to the fatal wound, each 3 to 5 cm long, involving only the skin and superficial subcutaneous tissue. No defensive wounds are present on the hands or forearms. No injury elsewhere on the body. Toxicology shows blood ethanol 0.15 grams per deciliter and no other substances.

**Cause Determination:** Exsanguination due to incised wound of the anterior neck with transection of the left carotid artery and internal jugular vein.

**Manner Determination:** Suicide. The pattern of the wound is consistent with self-infliction: single deep wound at an accessible site, hesitation wounds clustered near the fatal wound, no defensive injury, no signs of struggle at the scene, alcohol-facilitated (a common finding in impulsive suicide), and documented antecedent history of depression and suicidal ideation. The weapon is present at the scene consistent with self-infliction.

**Trap Logic:** The absence of a suicide note does not exclude suicide; most suicide decedents do not leave notes. The presence of a spouse who reports the decedent's history does not itself compromise the determination, though the report must be evaluated independently of the reporter and integrated with the physical findings. The trap in the opposite direction is to certify suicide based on the report of history and the general appearance of the scene without careful documentation of the physical findings that support (or contradict) the determination — the hesitation wounds, the absence of defensive injury, and the accessibility of the wound site. Every determination of suicide by sharp force must document the specific physical findings that support the determination, so the reasoning is defensible when challenged.

**Certification Anchor:** Sharp force suicide is supported by wound accessibility, hesitation wound presence, absence of defensive injury, absence of scene struggle evidence, and integration with antecedent history. The reasoning is documented in the autopsy report with reference to each supporting finding, so a reader who reviews the case later can reconstruct the determination from the record. The absence of any single element does not automatically shift the determination, but a case with multiple elements against suicide (multiple wounds, defensive injury, non-accessible sites, wounds through clothing) requires reasoning through the alternative manner.

## SCENE-TO-CERTIFICATION DECISION SYSTEM — Sharp Force Determination Arcs

**The Sharp Force Wound Categories:** Stab wounds (depth greater than length, produced by penetrating blade along its long axis), incised wounds (length greater than depth, produced by cutting edge drawn tangentially), and chop wounds (heavy cutting instruments producing hybrid sharp-blunt injury with underlying fracture) form the sharp force spectrum. Each category has distinct morphological features that document mechanism and constrain weapon identification.

**The Skin-Tract-Weapon Discipline:** The skin wound documents the cross-section of the blade at the depth of the wound edge (single-edge, double-edge, cylindrical). The wound tract documents the depth and direction of the strike. Neither the skin wound length precisely equals blade width nor does tract depth precisely equal blade length; both are rough approximations subject to specific modifiers. Systematic layered dissection with probe placement documents the tract for reconstruction.

**Defensive and Hesitation Injury:** Defensive wounds on the palms and ulnar forearms document conscious defense during assault and shift the reasoning toward homicide. Hesitation wounds clustered near a fatal wound document incomplete initial self-infliction and shift the reasoning toward suicide. Both are actively looked for and documented in every sharp force case.

**The Documented Interpretive Limits:** Peer-reviewed literature documents wound-interpretation error rates for trained observers at levels that require systematic examination against defined criteria rather than intuitive pattern recognition. Testimony must reflect the actual reliability of the reasoning; overconfidence about blade identification, wound sequencing, and time-of-injury estimation is not defensible on cross-examination.

**Manner Determination Integration:** Sharp force manner determination integrates wound pattern, wound characteristics, defensive and hesitation injury, scene evidence, and antecedent history. Suicide is supported by accessibility, hesitation wounds, absence of defensive injury, and absence of struggle. Homicide is supported by multiple wounds, non-accessible sites, defensive injury, and wounds through clothing. Accidental sharp force death is documented by mechanism consistent with reported cause.

## Summary and Key Concepts

Sharp force injury comprises stab wounds (depth greater than length), incised wounds (length greater than depth), and chop wounds (hybrid sharp-blunt injury with underlying fracture from heavy cutting instruments). The distinction among these categories, and the distinction between sharp force and blunt force laceration, is fundamental and is documented to have substantial published error rates without systematic examination discipline.

Stab wound morphology reflects the cross-section of the blade at the wound edge — asymmetric wound margins for single-edged blades, symmetric for double-edged, and round for cylindrical penetrating objects. The wound tract documents the depth and direction of the strike. Wound length is a rough approximation of blade width; wound depth is a rough approximation of blade length; both are subject to modifiers.

Incised wounds carry the classic locations of self-infliction (wrist flexor surfaces, anterior neck) and the classic locations of defense (ulnar forearms, palms). Hesitation wounds cluster near a fatal self-inflicted wound; defensive wounds document conscious defense during assault. Both are actively looked for and documented.

Chop wounds combine sharp force and blunt force features with associated underlying fracture. They are less common than stab and incised wounds in most caseloads but characteristic when present.

Reconstruction of sharp force events integrates wound pattern, wound tract, defensive and hesitation injury, scene evidence, and antecedent history. The manner determination — suicide, homicide, or accident — rests on the integration and is documented in the autopsy report with reference to the specific findings that support the determination.

The documented limits of blade identification, wound aging, and wound sequencing require testimony calibrated to the actual reliability of the reasoning. Systematic examination and honest expression of uncertainty preserve the credibility of the specialty in the courtroom.

# CHAPTER 7: GUNSHOT WOUNDS AND FIREARM INJURY

**Learning Objectives**

1. Describe firearm fundamentals — handgun versus long gun, cartridge components, and the physics of wound ballistics — as the foundation for wound interpretation.
2. Recognize the morphological features of gunshot entrance wounds by range of fire (contact, near-contact, intermediate, distant) and interpret soot, powder, and searing patterns.
3. Reconstruct a gunshot wound tract, identify entrance and exit wounds, and articulate the reasoning that supports the direction of fire.
4. Distinguish handgun, rifle, and shotgun wound patterns and reason from the wound pattern to the class of firearm involved.
5. Reason systematically toward manner determination in firearm death and recognize the traps documented in the published literature.

## Firearm Fundamentals and Wound Ballistics

Firearm injury is the most consequential category of traumatic death in the American forensic caseload, responsible for the majority of homicides and a substantial fraction of suicides in most jurisdictions. Every forensic pathologist must possess working knowledge of firearm mechanics, ammunition, and wound ballistics because the interpretation of gunshot wounds depends on integrating the wound morphology with the physics of the projectile that produced it. This does not require the pathologist to become a ballistics expert; it does require sufficient understanding to select the correct interpretive framework for a given case and to recognize when a case requires input from a firearms specialist.

The essential distinction among firearm classes is handgun (short barrel, one-handed operation, moderate muzzle velocity), long gun / rifle (long barrel, shoulder-fired, high muzzle velocity), and shotgun (long barrel, shoulder-fired, discharging multiple projectiles or a single slug). Each class produces characteristic wound patterns reflecting the physics of the projectile and the mechanism of discharge. Handgun cartridges are typically pistol calibers such as .22, .38, 9 mm, .40, and .45; typical muzzle velocities range from approximately 250 to 400 meters per second. Rifle cartridges are typically higher-velocity calibers such as .223, .30-06, or .308; typical muzzle velocities range from approximately 700 to 1000 meters per second. Shotguns discharge shells containing either multiple pellets (shot) or a single large projectile (slug); shot loads produce distinctive wound patterns that spread over distance.

### Wound Ballistics

The tissue effect of a projectile is determined by the projectile mass, velocity, shape, and behavior upon tissue entry. Kinetic energy — the classic physics description — is proportional to mass and to the square of velocity, so high-velocity projectiles carry disproportionately greater energy than low-velocity projectiles of the same mass. Handgun projectiles at typical muzzle velocity deposit their energy relatively locally along the wound tract; rifle projectiles at high velocity deposit energy over a wider region because their higher velocity produces a temporary cavity in the surrounding tissue that is substantially larger than the projectile itself. This temporary cavity, which forms and collapses within milliseconds, produces tissue disruption at some distance from the projectile path in high-velocity injury; it explains why rifle wounds cause more extensive internal injury than handgun wounds through comparable body regions.

Projectile behavior after tissue entry depends on projectile design. Full metal jacket projectiles retain their shape through tissue and typically pass through the body with less energy deposition than hollow-point or expanding projectiles. Hollow-point projectiles expand on tissue entry, presenting a larger cross-sectional area and depositing greater energy over a shorter tract; they are frequently retained in the body rather than exiting. Fragmenting projectiles (used in some hunting and military applications) break apart on entry and produce multiple secondary projectiles within the body. The pathologist documents the character of any retained projectile as it is encountered and preserves it for ballistics comparison.

**KEY POINT:** The morphology of a gunshot wound reflects the physics of the projectile that produced it. Handgun and rifle wounds through the same body region produce fundamentally different injury because the projectiles behave differently in tissue. The pathologist reads the wound in the context of the class of firearm involved, when the class can be identified.

## Entrance Wounds and Range-of-Fire Determination

The entrance wound is the point at which the projectile enters the body. Its morphology preserves information about the range of fire and about the position of the muzzle at the moment of discharge. Range of fire is one of the most important interpretations the pathologist makes in a firearm case, because it constrains the reconstruction of the event. Contact, near-contact, intermediate, and distant ranges each produce characteristic entrance wound morphology, and the systematic examination distinguishes them.

### The Abrasion Rim

Every gunshot entrance wound is characterized by an abrasion rim — a marginal band of denuded skin around the wound where the projectile scraped or contused the epidermis as it entered. The abrasion rim is present in virtually every entrance wound and its absence in a suspected entrance wound should prompt reconsideration of which wound is entrance and which is exit. The abrasion rim is typically concentric and symmetrical when the projectile enters perpendicular to the skin surface. When the projectile enters at an oblique angle, the abrasion rim is asymmetric and wider on the side away from the entry angle — a feature that documents the angle of entry.

### Contact Wounds

A contact wound is produced when the muzzle of the firearm is pressed against the skin surface at the moment of discharge. The propellant gases enter the wound tract along with the projectile and produce characteristic findings. Loose contact wounds show a circular entrance defect with a surrounding zone of soot deposition on the skin. Tight contact wounds — where the muzzle is firmly pressed against skin —

produce all propellant gases into the wound tract with less external soot, but the gases expand within the wound cavity and can produce a stellate (star-shaped) tear of the skin as the trapped gases blow the tissue outward. Contact wounds over bone (the temple, the roof of the mouth) may show a characteristic muzzle imprint — a bruised or abraded pattern on the skin reproducing the shape of the firearm muzzle. Contact wounds are strongly associated with self-inflicted injury but do occur in homicide.

### Near-Contact and Intermediate Range

Near-contact wounds are produced when the muzzle is close to but not touching the skin — typically within a few centimeters. Soot is deposited on the skin around the wound in a characteristic pattern, and the pattern of soot deposition can support estimation of the distance. Intermediate-range wounds occur at distances typically between a few centimeters and approximately 60 to 90 centimeters (depending on the firearm and load). At this range, unburned or partially burned powder grains from the propellant strike the skin and become embedded in the epidermis or superficial dermis — a pattern termed powder tattooing or stippling. Powder tattooing is a highly specific finding for a gunshot wound in the intermediate range and is not reproducible after death by any known artifact. Its presence documents that the muzzle was within intermediate range at the moment of discharge and that the skin was living at the moment of entry.

The pattern of soot and powder tattooing constrains the distance more precisely than most other observations available to the pathologist. Test firing of a candidate firearm with the same type of ammunition at known distances against target material produces a comparison series that can be matched to the wound pattern by a firearms examiner. This test firing analysis — typically performed by the crime laboratory rather than by the pathologist — produces range estimates with useful precision for reconstruction. The pathologist documents the soot and powder pattern on the skin so that the firearms examiner can perform the comparison.

### Distant Range

Distant-range wounds are produced when the muzzle is beyond the range at which soot and powder can reach the skin — typically beyond approximately 60 to 90 centimeters for handguns, and further for rifles. At distant range, only the projectile itself strikes the skin, and the entrance wound shows the projectile defect with abrasion rim but no soot deposition or powder tattooing. Distant range does not preclude a specific distance estimate, but the estimate is much less precise than at closer ranges because only the trajectory of the projectile can be reconstructed.

**CLINICAL PEARL:** Powder tattooing on skin is not reproducible artifactually and is not present when the muzzle is far from the skin. Its presence documents intermediate range and living tissue at the moment of the strike. Its absence in an entrance wound documents either distant range or, in some cases, contact range where the propellant enters the wound cavity rather than depositing on the skin surface.

Figure 7.1: Gunshot Entrance Wound Morphology by Range of Fire

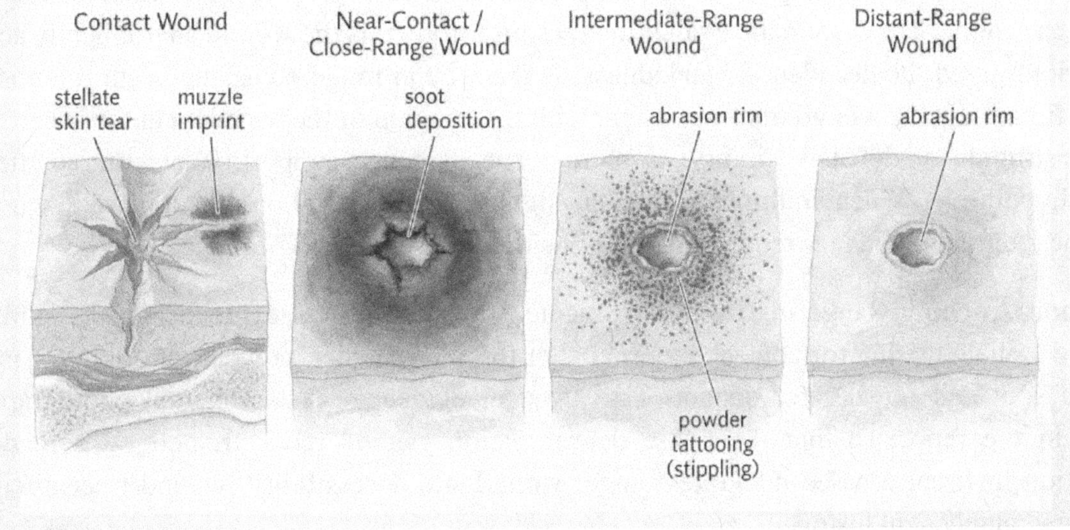


## SCENE-TO-CERTIFICATION DECISION SYSTEM — Range-of-Fire Determination Arc

**Presenting Death Scenario:** A 29-year-old man is found deceased in an apartment stairwell with a single gunshot wound to the right temple. A .38 caliber revolver is on the floor beside his right hand. The scene investigator notes the position of the body against the stairwell wall, the location of the firearm, and blood spatter on the wall consistent with the position. The decedent has a documented history of major depressive disorder and had been discharged from an inpatient psychiatric admission three days prior to death. The decedent was right-handed.

**Autopsy Signature:** External examination documents a single gunshot entrance wound at the right temple, 3 cm anterior to the right external auditory meatus. The entrance wound is a stellate defect with a circular central component and radiating tears in the skin extending outward from the central defect. A well-defined muzzle imprint pattern (a hexagonal outline) is present on the skin surrounding the wound, reproducing the shape of the firearm muzzle. There is no external soot deposition on skin adjacent to the wound (consistent with tight contact where propellant enters the wound cavity). Internal examination shows a wound tract passing from the right temporal region horizontally and slightly posteriorly through the right temporal lobe, the midbrain, and terminating in the left temporal region with a corresponding exit wound. A retained portion of the projectile is recovered from the left temporal soft tissue. Cause of death is gunshot wound of the head with brainstem injury.

**Cause Determination:** Gunshot wound of the head.

**Manner Determination:** Suicide. The determination integrates: contact-range entrance wound (documented by stellate skin tearing and muzzle imprint pattern), accessibility of the wound site to the decedent's dominant hand, absence of any evidence of struggle at the scene, position of the firearm consistent with the wound pattern (right-hand accessible), documented antecedent history of major depression with recent psychiatric admission, and absence of any alternative history from investigation.

**Trap Logic:** A contact wound at the temple is strongly associated with self-infliction but is not diagnostic. A homicide can be staged to appear self-inflicted, and the pathologist must not assume suicide from the wound pattern alone. The systematic evaluation reasons through: is the wound anatomically accessible for self-infliction, given the decedent's handedness; is the wound range consistent with the position of the recovered firearm; is the wound tract consistent with the position of the decedent at the scene; is there any pattern of struggle or defensive injury; is there scene evidence supporting or contradicting the self-infliction hypothesis. When multiple elements align, the determination is supported; when elements diverge, the alternative manner requires active consideration.

**Certification Anchor:** Range of fire is documented by the physical evidence on the skin — muzzle imprint and stellate tearing for contact, external soot for near-contact, powder tattooing for intermediate, absence of soot and powder for distant. The physical evidence is documented photographically and described in the report so that the range determination can be reconstructed by a reader. Manner determination in firearm cases integrates range, wound site accessibility, wound tract direction, scene evidence, and antecedent history.

## Exit Wounds and Wound Tract Reconstruction

The exit wound is the point at which the projectile leaves the body. Its morphology differs from the entrance wound in ways that support identification of which wound is entrance and which is exit — a determination central to the reconstruction of the direction of fire.

### Exit Wound Morphology

The classic exit wound is characterized by irregular, everted (outward-turned) skin margins with radiating tears, and by the absence of an abrasion rim. The projectile leaves the body with less controlled contact with skin than at entry, and the wound margins tend to be splayed outward by the projectile as it exits. Handgun exit wounds are often smaller than the intervening internal cavity would suggest because the projectile has decelerated and lost energy through the body; rifle exit wounds are often larger and more disruptive because the high-velocity projectile has retained substantial energy. The absence of the abrasion rim is the single most reliable finding distinguishing exit from entrance.

### The Shored Exit Wound and Its Caveat

The shored exit wound is a specific artifact that can confound the entrance-exit determination. When the exit surface of the body is pressed against a firm object at the moment of exit — a wall, the ground, a firm article of clothing — the skin around the exit is supported and produces a marginal abrasion mimicking the abrasion rim of an entrance wound. Shored exit wounds are characteristic of a body found in a specific position at the scene, and the shoring pattern often preserves the outline of the supporting surface. Recognition of shored exits requires attention to the position of the body and to the character of the marginal abrasion. Failure to recognize a shored exit wound has produced published cases in which the entrance-exit determination was reversed, with substantial reconstruction implications.

### The Wound Tract

The wound tract through the body is documented by systematic dissection following the projectile path. The direction of the tract is described in three dimensions: superior-inferior, anterior-posterior, medial-lateral. Structures traversed are documented in order. Projectile fragmentation, if present, is documented with recovery of retained fragments for ballistics analysis. Bone fractures along the tract are documented; the beveling pattern of skull entrance wounds (internal beveling of the calvarium) versus exit (external beveling) is characteristic and supports entrance-exit determination in cranial wounds independent of skin findings. Multiple wound tracts from multiple projectiles are documented individually with each tract reconstructed separately.

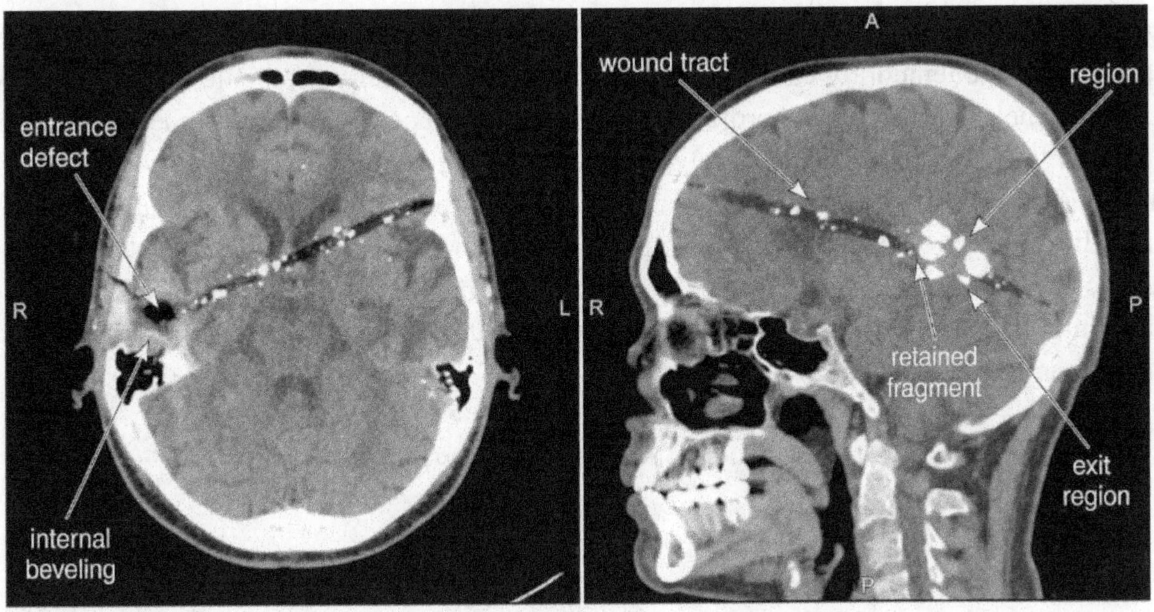


Figure 7.2: Postmortem CT Reconstruction of a Cranial Gunshot Wound Tract

## Shotgun Wounds

Shotgun wounds are distinct from wounds produced by rifled firearms because a shotgun typically discharges multiple projectiles (shot) rather than a single projectile. The wound pattern reflects the spread of the shot column as it travels from the muzzle.

### Contact and Close Shotgun Wounds

At contact and close range, the shot column has not spread substantially and enters the body as a coherent mass. The wound is a single large defect with irregular margins, extensive underlying tissue disruption, and often massive local injury. Wadding — the plastic or paper components that separate powder from shot in the shell — is often carried into the wound at close range and can be recovered during dissection. The character of the wadding may support identification of the shell type. At contact range, similar findings to contact handgun wounds occur — muzzle imprint over bone, stellate tearing from propellant gas expansion, absence of external soot.

### Intermediate and Distant Shotgun Range

As distance increases, the shot column spreads and the wound pattern reflects the spread. Multiple small entrance wounds — termed a shot pattern — appear on the skin, distributed across a region with the pattern size proportional to the distance. Test firing of a candidate shotgun with the same shell type produces a comparison series that permits range estimation from the pattern diameter. Because shot patterns spread predictably with distance, shotgun range estimation is often more precise than handgun range estimation at intermediate distances. Distant shotgun wounds may show highly dispersed shot patterns spread across substantial body regions.

## Rifle and High-Velocity Wounds

Rifle wounds and other high-velocity projectile wounds show characteristic features reflecting the physics of the projectile. The temporary cavity produced by the high-velocity projectile causes extensive tissue disruption at some distance from the projectile path itself. Entrance wounds may appear deceptively small — the projectile enters through a relatively small skin defect — but internal injury is often extensive. Bone injury from rifle wounds is characteristically comminuted and shows features of high-energy transfer. Exit wounds are often large and disrupted, and rifle wound tracts through the trunk may produce injuries whose extent is disproportionate to the entrance wound size. The pathologist reading a rifle wound anticipates internal injury greater than the entrance wound suggests, and systematic examination confirms or refutes the anticipated pattern.

Figure 7.3: Wound Tract Dissection with Probe Placement

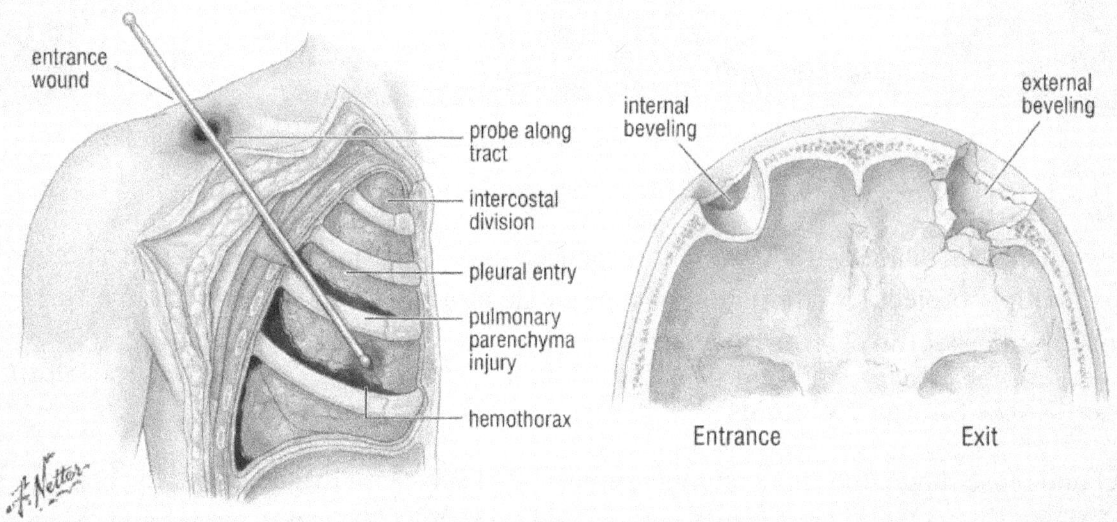


A. Anterior Chest Wall Dissection

B. Cranial Wound Beveling Comparison

## Manner Determination in Firearm Deaths

Firearm death carries the same manner categories as any other traumatic death — natural (rare in firearm death but possible for underlying disease unrelated to the wound), accident, suicide, homicide, and undetermined. The determination integrates the wound pattern with the scene evidence and the antecedent history. The literature on manner determination in firearm death documents that misclassification errors, though uncommon, do occur and typically involve either misclassification of homicide as suicide (when a homicide is staged) or misclassification of suicide as homicide (when scene evidence is misinterpreted).

### Firearm Suicide

Firearm suicide typically involves contact or near-contact range wounds, at sites accessible to the decedent's dominant hand (temple, submental, intraoral, chest), with the firearm recovered at the scene in a position consistent with self-infliction. The most common pattern is single contact or near-contact wound to the head, with the firearm still in the hand or fallen immediately from the hand. Multiple gunshot wounds in suicide are uncommon but documented, particularly when the initial wound was not immediately incapacitating. Wound location, range, tract direction, firearm position, and antecedent history all support the reasoning.

### Firearm Homicide

Firearm homicide typically involves distant-range wounds (though contact wounds occur in homicide when the assailant approaches closely), at sites not chosen by the decedent (back, multiple sites, defensive injuries to the arms), often with multiple wounds. The scene evidence typically documents an assault — the firearm may be absent, a firearm may be present but its position is inconsistent with self-infliction (across the room from the body, in a position inaccessible to the decedent), signs of struggle may be present. Wound distribution, range, and scene reasoning together support the determination.

### Cartridge Identification and the Class of Firearm

The pathologist does not typically identify a specific firearm from a wound, but the wound and any recovered projectile constrain the class and caliber of firearm involved. Retained projectiles are recovered during dissection with care to preserve rifling marks, weighed, and preserved for transfer to the crime laboratory ballistics section. The rifling pattern on the projectile — land and groove impressions — supports comparison with a recovered firearm barrel through microscopic comparison performed by a firearms examiner. Cartridge cases recovered at the scene bear firing pin impressions, breech face marks, and extractor and ejector marks that similarly support comparison with a recovered firearm. Handgun cartridges span calibers from small (.22, .25) through mid-range (.38, 9 mm, .380) to large (.40, .45); rifle cartridges span calibers from small (.22 rimfire, .223) through mid-range (.243, .308) to large (.30-06, .338); shotgun shells are designated by gauge with 12-gauge and 20-gauge dominating civilian and law enforcement use. The pathologist documents the general caliber category when the recovered projectile permits it and defers specific identification to the firearms examiner.

Cartridge and projectile evidence carries chain of custody implications from the moment of recovery. A projectile removed from the body enters the ballistic evidence chain and is documented with the decedent identifier, the recovery location within the body, the date and time of recovery, and the identity of the pathologist recovering it. Preservation in a manner that protects the surface features from damage — typically in a padded container without direct hand contact after removal — protects the rifling comparison possibilities. Handling and packaging follow the office's specific ballistic evidence protocol.

**KEY POINT:** The retained projectile is a piece of ballistic evidence. Its recovery and preservation directly affect the crime laboratory's ability to compare it with a suspect firearm. Careless handling — tool marks from forceps, direct hand contact, packaging that abrades the surface — can foreclose the comparison. The pathologist recovers projectiles with soft-tipped instruments and packages them for transfer with intact chain of custody.

### Wounds Through Intermediate Targets

Projectiles that pass through an intermediate target — a windshield, a door, an article of clothing, another person's body — before striking the decedent may show characteristic modifications of the wound pattern. Projectile deformation from the intermediate target produces an atypical wound that does not match the standard morphology of a direct-fire wound of the same caliber. Deposition of glass fragments, wood splinters, fabric fibers, or bone chips from the intermediate target may be recoverable from the wound tract and can support reconstruction of the shot path. Ricochet projectiles that have struck a surface before entering the body typically show deformation and produce entrance wounds with atypical morphology — often larger and more irregular than a direct-fire wound. Recognition of an atypical entrance wound raises the possibility of an intermediate target or ricochet, and the reconstruction is developed with input from law enforcement scene investigation and, in complex cases, from a shooting reconstruction expert.

### Multiple Gunshot Wounds

Cases with multiple gunshot wounds require documentation of every wound with the same precision as a single-wound case. Each wound is numbered systematically, described for range, tract, and injury, and photographed in overview, mid-range, and close-up. The pattern of wounds — their distribution, the range of each, the direction of each tract — supports reconstruction of the sequence and the positioning at each strike. Sequence determination among multiple wounds is difficult and often not resolvable to reasonable medical certainty. Some inferences are supported: a wound to a lethal site (heart, brainstem, great vessel) that would cause immediate incapacitation is typically among the last wounds in a series if the decedent was still standing during preceding wounds; wounds through clothing that has been displaced by subsequent wounds may support sequencing. In most multiple-wound cases, the pathologist documents each wound completely and defers sequencing to the level of certainty the pattern supports rather than reasoning beyond the evidence.

## Firearm Injury and Survival Time

The interval between firearm injury and death is variable and depends on the site of injury, the extent of tissue damage, and the availability of medical care. Wounds to the brainstem, upper cervical spinal cord, heart, or great vessels typically produce immediate or near-immediate incapacitation and death within minutes. Wounds to the peripheral extremities without major vascular injury may cause no immediate incapacitation and can permit substantial mobility of the decedent for minutes to hours before decompensation from blood loss. Between these extremes lie the majority of firearm wounds, in which decompensation occurs progressively as blood loss and organ injury develop. Estimation of survival time in a firearm death — relevant when the case reconstruction depends on it, as when the decedent moved from the site of the shot to the site of discovery — is done conservatively with reference to the specific injuries and the physical evidence of mobility (blood trails, position of the body relative to the shot site, disturbance of the environment consistent with movement). The estimate is presented as a range consistent with the evidence rather than as a specific time interval.

## Documentation of Clothing in Firearm Cases

Clothing is central evidence in firearm cases and requires disciplined documentation before it is removed from the body. Bullet defects in clothing are photographed in place with a scale in frame. The number, location, and pattern of defects is described. Powder residue on clothing — which persists on fabric more reliably than on skin in some cases — is preserved by careful handling that avoids contamination or displacement. Clothing is removed one item at a time with each item photographed on removal, then preserved in paper packaging (never plastic, which retains moisture and degrades residue) and transferred to the crime laboratory for detailed examination. The pattern of defects on layered clothing may support reconstruction that skin evidence alone cannot: the alignment of defects through multiple layers documents that the layers were in place at the moment of the shot, and the defect character on the outer layer may reveal soot or powder patterns not visible on the underlying skin because the outer garment absorbed the deposition.

Powder residue on the hands of a firearm decedent — evidence that the decedent recently discharged a firearm — is a specific analytical determination performed by the crime laboratory rather than by the pathologist. The pathologist supports the analysis by preserving the hands with paper bags at the scene, avoiding contamination of the hand surfaces during handling and transport, and coordinating with the crime laboratory on the timing and technique of hand sampling. Gunshot residue analysis produces results that are sensitive to sample collection technique and to interpretation; both false positive and false negative results are documented in the literature, and the results are interpreted in context by the firearms examiner.

## Postmortem Imaging in Firearm Cases

Postmortem computed tomography has become an important adjunct to autopsy in firearm cases at offices with the resources to support it. Postmortem CT identifies retained projectile fragments with high sensitivity, documents the wound tract in three dimensions with a fidelity that dissection cannot easily reproduce, identifies bone fragmentation and internal beveling patterns, and preserves the anatomical relationships in a form that can be reviewed after autopsy dissection has disturbed them. The trajectory of a wound through the body — which is central to the reconstruction of the shot direction — can be measured from CT with greater precision than from dissection alone. For complex cases with multiple wounds, cases with retained fragments in critical regions, cases where the anatomical relationships will be central to trial testimony, and cases with religious or family objection to full dissection, postmortem CT substantially strengthens the reconstruction and preserves evidence for later analysis by outside experts.

The role of postmortem CT in firearm case reasoning is a supplement to autopsy rather than a replacement. Findings identifiable only on tissue examination — subtle vital reaction at wound margins, small hemorrhage into tissue planes, microscopic injury to critical structures — require direct examination. The integration of CT and autopsy findings is developed further in Chapter 19.

### The Staged Suicide

A staged suicide — a homicide arranged to appear self-inflicted — is the classic reconstruction failure in firearm case work. Detection depends on systematic analysis of the wound pattern against the physical realities of self-infliction. Contact wounds at the head that would require an anatomically impossible or extremely awkward hand position; multiple wounds inconsistent with a single incapacitating strike; firearm position inconsistent with the fall pattern expected from the wound; defensive injuries suggesting struggle before the fatal wound; scene evidence of struggle inconsistent with a controlled self-inflicted event — each is a signal that requires investigation. No single finding is diagnostic; the reasoning is cumulative.

### SCENE-TO-CERTIFICATION DECISION SYSTEM — Firearm Homicide-Versus-Staged-Suicide Arc

---

**Presenting Death Scenario:** A 51-year-old man is found deceased in his home office by his wife, who reports discovering him after returning from a store errand. The decedent is seated in his office chair, slumped forward across his desk. A single gunshot wound is present at the right temple. A 9 mm semiautomatic pistol is on the floor immediately to the right of the chair, and one spent cartridge case is on the desk in front of the decedent. The wife reports that the decedent had been under financial stress and had recently expressed suicidal ideation to her. The medical examiner's office accepts jurisdiction on the sudden death.

**Autopsy Signature:** External examination documents a single gunshot entrance wound at the right temple, 2 cm anterior to the right external auditory meatus. The entrance wound is a small circular defect with abrasion rim. There is no soot deposition on skin adjacent to the wound and no powder tattooing. The wound tract is documented internally and passes from the right temporal region horizontally through the brain to the left temporal region with a corresponding exit wound. The decedent is right-handed by history. Toxicology is negative apart from a trace of ethanol at 0.03 grams per deciliter. Detailed external examination reveals a small contusion of the right occipital scalp with underlying subgaleal hemorrhage that is not consistent with the exit wound or with any postmortem fall pattern. No defensive injuries are present.

**Cause Determination:** Gunshot wound of the head.

**Manner Determination:** Homicide. The determination rests on the combination of findings: entrance wound range is distant (no soot, no powder tattooing) rather than the contact range typical of self-infliction; the small subgaleal hemorrhage in the occipital region documents blunt injury before the gunshot, consistent with a strike from behind; the position of the recovered firearm on the floor is inconsistent with the pattern expected from a self-inflicted contact wound to the temple; and the scene evidence (single cartridge case on desk) is consistent with a shot fired from a position other than by the decedent himself.

**Trap Logic:** A gunshot wound to the right temple with a recovered firearm and a report of antecedent depression could be certified as suicide without careful evaluation. The trap is to accept the surface pattern of the scene without systematic examination of the physical findings. In this case, the range determination (distant rather than contact), the antemortem blunt injury (occipital contusion inconsistent with a fall pattern), and the physical incompatibility of the firearm position with the wound pattern all point away from suicide. Systematic evaluation of every element — rather than acceptance of the initial impression — is what distinguishes the case.

**Certification Anchor:** Firearm manner determination integrates range of fire, wound site accessibility, wound tract direction, presence or absence of other antemortem injury, firearm position relative to the wound pattern, and antecedent history. Every element is evaluated systematically. A single element out of alignment with the initial impression — an antemortem injury not explained by the shooting, a range inconsistent with self-infliction, a firearm position incompatible with the pattern — requires reasoning through the alternative manner before certification.

## SCENE-TO-CERTIFICATION DECISION SYSTEM — Firearm Determination Arcs

**The Ballistic Framework:** Firearm class — handgun, rifle, shotgun — determines the physics of the projectile and the character of the resulting wound. Handgun wounds deposit energy locally along the tract; rifle wounds produce temporary cavitation and extensive internal injury; shotgun wounds vary with distance from single large defects at close range to spread shot patterns at longer distances. The pathologist reads the wound in the context of the class of firearm involved.

**Range Determination:** Range of fire is documented by physical evidence on the skin: muzzle imprint and stellate tearing for contact, external soot for near-contact, powder tattooing for intermediate, absence of soot and powder for distant. Powder tattooing is not reproducible artifactually and its presence documents intermediate range and living tissue at the moment of the strike.

**Entrance-Exit Distinction:** Entrance wounds have abrasion rims; exit wounds do not, except in shored configurations where a firm supporting surface produces a mimic. Recognition of shored exits requires attention to body position and to the pattern of marginal abrasion. In cranial wounds, internal beveling at entrance versus external beveling at exit supports the distinction independent of skin findings.

**Manner Determination Integration:** Firearm manner rests on integration of range, wound site accessibility for self-infliction, wound tract direction, firearm position relative to the wound pattern, presence or absence of other antemortem injury, defensive injury, scene evidence of struggle, and antecedent history. No single element is diagnostic; the reasoning is cumulative. Systematic evaluation identifies the staged suicide, which is the classic reconstruction failure.

**The Documented Interpretive Reliability:** Published literature on gunshot wound interpretation documents error rates for wound type and range identification that require systematic examination against defined criteria. The pathologist follows the systematic protocol, documents each finding explicitly, and reasons transparently in the report. Testimony reflects the actual reliability of the reasoning; overconfidence about specific ranges or specific firearm identification is not defensible on cross-examination.

## Summary and Key Concepts

Firearm injury is the most consequential category of traumatic death in American forensic caseloads. The forensic pathologist requires working knowledge of firearm mechanics, ammunition, and wound ballistics to interpret gunshot wounds accurately.

Entrance wound morphology reflects the range of fire: contact wounds show muzzle imprint and stellate tearing from propellant gas expansion; near-contact wounds show external soot deposition; intermediate-range wounds show powder tattooing (embedded partially burned powder grains) that is not reproducible artifactually; distant-range wounds show only the projectile defect with abrasion rim.

Exit wounds lack the abrasion rim of entrance wounds and typically show irregular everted margins, though shored exit wounds against firm supporting surfaces can mimic entrance abrasion rims and require careful recognition. Internal beveling at cranial entrance versus external beveling at exit supports the distinction in skull wounds.

Shotgun wounds vary characteristically with range — single large defects at close range, spreading shot patterns at intermediate and distant ranges. Rifle wounds show temporary cavitation with internal injury disproportionate to the entrance wound size. The pathologist reads each firearm class with its characteristic pattern.

Manner determination in firearm death integrates range, wound site accessibility, tract direction, firearm position, other antemortem injury, defensive injury, scene evidence, and antecedent history. The staged suicide — homicide arranged to appear self-inflicted — is detected by systematic evaluation of every element rather than by acceptance of the initial scene impression.

Published literature documents wound-interpretation error rates that require systematic examination against defined criteria. Testimony reflects the actual reliability of the reasoning; overconfidence in specific ranges or specific firearm identification is not defensible on cross-examination.

# CHAPTER 8: ASPHYXIAL DEATHS

**Learning Objectives**

1. Define asphyxia physiologically and describe the mechanisms by which each category of asphyxial death interrupts oxygen delivery to the brain.
2. Distinguish the autopsy findings that support the diagnosis of hanging, ligature strangulation, and manual strangulation, and reason from the pattern of neck injury to the mechanism.
3. Recognize smothering, suffocation, and positional asphyxia and articulate the documentation challenges that accompany each.
4. Distinguish antemortem drowning from postmortem immersion and integrate scene, autopsy, and ancillary evidence to support the determination.
5. Recognize chemical asphyxia — carbon monoxide, cyanide, and hydrogen sulfide — by history, autopsy findings, and confirmatory toxicology.

## The Concept and Categories of Asphyxia

Asphyxia is the physiologic state in which oxygen delivery to the tissues is interrupted to a degree sufficient to cause death. The interruption may occur at any point along the oxygen-delivery pathway: at the atmosphere (oxygen-poor environment), at the airway (obstruction), at the neck (compression of airway and vessels), at the lungs (drowning, aspiration), at the blood (hemoglobin dysfunction from chemical exposure), or at the tissue level (metabolic poisons that prevent oxygen use). The traditional forensic classification groups asphyxial deaths into categories that reflect the mechanism of the interruption, and the autopsy findings that support the diagnosis vary substantially among the categories.

Asphyxial death is a particularly demanding category for forensic reasoning because the autopsy findings are frequently subtle. Unlike blunt force injury or firearm injury, in which the mechanism produces visible destructive changes, asphyxia may produce few or no specific findings on external and internal examination. The pathologist reasons from a constellation of findings — petechial hemorrhages, cervical soft tissue injury, pulmonary edema, cyanosis, and the presence or absence of specific findings for each subcategory — to reach a determination that often depends heavily on scene evidence and antecedent history.

### The Nonspecific Findings

Several findings appear in asphyxial death but are not specific to any single category and are also seen in non-asphyxial deaths. Petechial hemorrhages of the conjunctivae, sclerae, facial skin, and, when severe, the mucous membranes and internal serosal surfaces reflect the rise in venous pressure that accompanies most forms of asphyxia. Their presence supports asphyxia when other findings converge, but petechiae also occur in cardiac arrest of any cause, in coughing or vomiting, and in resuscitation. Congestion and cyanosis of the head and face above the level of neck compression are common in hanging and strangulation but also occur in cardiac and pulmonary disease. Pulmonary edema and congestion are nearly universal in asphyxial death but are also nonspecific. The pathologist reads these findings in the context of the specific subcategory reasoning.

### The Reasoning Discipline

The reasoning discipline for asphyxial death is to identify the specific findings that support the specific subcategory and to integrate them with scene evidence and history. In hanging, the specific finding is the ligature furrow with characteristic morphology, together with the position of the body relative to the suspension point. In manual strangulation, the specific finding is layered cervical soft tissue hemorrhage identified on layered anterior neck dissection. In drowning, the specific finding is the constellation of foam cone at the airways, pulmonary edema with the distinctive character of drowning fluid, and diatom identification in tissue if the drowning medium contained them. In carbon monoxide poisoning, the specific finding is elevated carboxyhemoglobin measured in blood. Each category has its diagnostic anchor, and the case reasoning depends on identifying and documenting the anchor when present.

**KEY POINT:** Asphyxial death is diagnosed by pattern recognition across a constellation of findings, not by any single pathognomonic feature. The pathologist assembles the findings, integrates them with scene evidence, and reasons transparently in the report about which subcategory the pattern supports.

## Hanging and Ligature Strangulation

Hanging and ligature strangulation both involve compression of the neck by a ligature. They are distinguished by the source of the compressive force: in hanging, the ligature is drawn tight by the weight of the body suspended (or partially suspended) from the ligature; in ligature strangulation, the ligature is drawn tight by force applied by another person or by the decedent's own hands. The distinction is central to manner determination because hanging is overwhelmingly a suicide mechanism whereas ligature strangulation is overwhelmingly a homicide mechanism, though exceptions to both occur.

### Hanging: Mechanism and Findings

Hanging causes death by compression of the venous return from the head, with resulting cerebral hypoperfusion; in some cases, additional airway compression contributes; in high-drop hanging (judicial hanging or accidental hanging with substantial drop), cervical spine fracture with cord injury contributes to or dominates the mechanism. The classic finding on the neck is a ligature furrow — a pale, dry, parchment-like depression in the skin at the site of ligature contact. The furrow is typically oriented obliquely on the neck, running from a low anterior position upward to a higher posterior position where the ligature meets the suspension point. The furrow is deepest at the low anterior aspect (where the body weight has drawn the ligature tightest) and shallowest at or near the suspension point (where the ligature was in relatively less tension).

Additional findings support the diagnosis. Congestion of the face and head above the level of ligature contact reflects the venous return interruption. Petechiae of the conjunctivae, sclerae, and facial skin are common. The tongue may be protruded and cyanotic. In complete hanging (full body suspension), the feet do not touch the ground; in incomplete hanging, some portion of the body remains in contact with the ground, and the mechanism reflects partial body weight on the ligature. Incomplete hanging is fully documented as a cause of hanging death — the physiologic mechanism does not require full body weight, only sufficient compression of venous return.

**Ligature Strangulation: Mechanism and Findings**

Ligature strangulation causes death by compression of the neck sufficient to interrupt cerebral perfusion, with the ligature drawn tight by external force (the assailant's hands, in most cases). The findings differ from hanging in specific ways that permit the distinction. The ligature furrow in strangulation is typically oriented horizontally on the neck rather than obliquely, because the ligature is drawn tight from behind or laterally without the vector of gravity that produces the oblique orientation in hanging. The depth of the furrow is more uniform along its length. The location of the furrow tends to be lower on the neck than in hanging. Facial congestion and petechiae are generally more prominent in ligature strangulation than in hanging because the assault typically involves a period of struggle during which venous obstruction is intermittent.

Cervical soft tissue hemorrhage is more prominent in ligature strangulation than in hanging because the applied force is often greater and less well distributed than the passive weight of a hanged body. Layered anterior neck dissection documents hemorrhage in the strap muscles, sternocleidomastoid, and prevertebral tissues. Fracture of the hyoid or thyroid cartilage occurs in a substantial minority of ligature strangulation cases and is more common in adult strangulation than in adolescent strangulation because the hyoid ossifies with age and becomes more fragile. The presence of hyoid or thyroid cartilage fracture is not required for the diagnosis of strangulation and is not by itself diagnostic, but its presence supports the diagnosis when found.

**Figure 8.1: Ligature Furrow Patterns: Hanging Versus Ligature Strangulation**

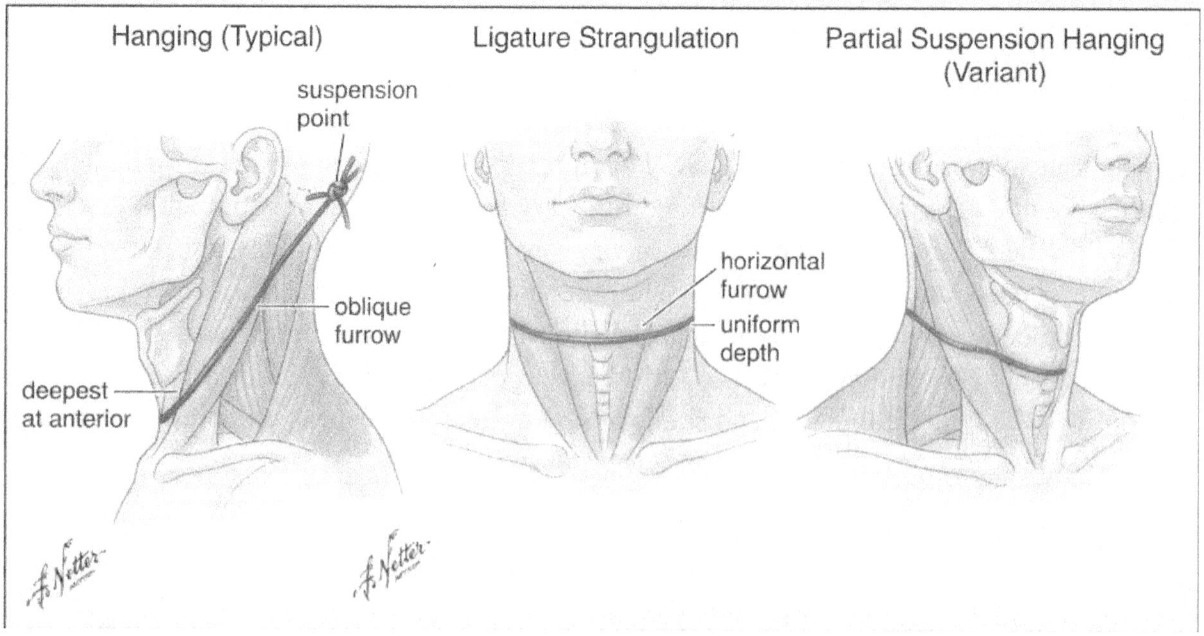

## Manual Strangulation

Manual strangulation is compression of the neck by the assailant's hands (throttling) or forearm (choke hold) without an intervening ligature. It is a mechanism of intimate-partner and physical-assault homicide and, less commonly, of accidental death in restraint contexts. The autopsy findings differ from hanging and ligature strangulation because the compressive surface (a hand) is broader and less uniform than a ligature.

### External Findings

External findings in manual strangulation include contusions and abrasions on the anterior and lateral neck reflecting the pressure and grip of the assailant's hand or hands. Fingertip contusions may be present in a pattern reproducing the hand position (multiple oval contusions along the lateral neck reflecting the fingertips, with a broader palmar contusion opposite them). Fingernail abrasions (crescent-shaped abrasions) may be present where the assailant's fingernails or the decedent's own fingernails (in defensive scratching) contacted the skin. There is no ligature furrow because there is no ligature. Facial congestion, cyanosis, and petechial hemorrhages are typically present and are often more prominent than in hanging or ligature strangulation because the assault typically involves a period of struggle.

**Figure 8.2: Cervical Anatomy in Strangulation:** Points of Injury

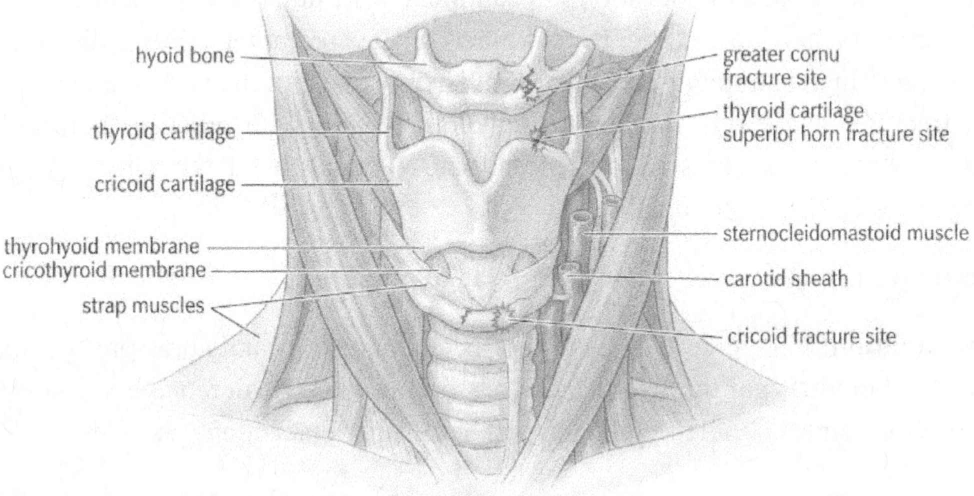


### Internal Findings

The internal examination in manual strangulation is critical. Layered anterior neck dissection — through the skin and subcutaneous tissue, the strap muscles, the sternocleidomastoid, and the prevertebral tissues — documents the pattern of internal hemorrhage. Deep cervical soft tissue hemorrhage is highly characteristic of manual strangulation and is often present even when external findings are minimal. Fracture of the hyoid, thyroid cartilage, or cricoid cartilage occurs in a substantial fraction of manual strangulation cases; the hyoid is the most commonly fractured element in strangulation of adults, particularly older adults with ossified hyoid bone. Hemorrhage into the airway soft tissue, the tongue base, and the periesophageal tissues supports the diagnosis. The pathologist performs the neck dissection carefully to avoid introducing postmortem artifact hemorrhage from vessels manipulated during dissection; standard practice performs the neck dissection after brain removal has drained cranial vasculature.

## SCENE-TO-CERTIFICATION DECISION SYSTEM — Neck Compression Reconstruction Arc

**Presenting Death Scenario:** A 34-year-old woman is found deceased in her apartment by her adult brother, who came to check on her after her failure to answer phone calls for a day. The apartment shows signs of struggle — an overturned chair, disarrayed bedclothes, a broken glass on the kitchen floor. The decedent is on the bedroom floor in a supine position. Her clothing is disarrayed but not removed. There is no ligature at the scene. On external inspection at the scene, contusions are visible on the anterior and lateral neck, and small crescent-shaped abrasions are present on the anterior neck consistent with fingernail contact. The scene is documented photographically before the body is transported to the medical examiner's office. The decedent has a documented history of domestic violence from her estranged husband.

**Autopsy Signature:** External examination confirms multiple contusions on the anterior and lateral neck in a pattern consistent with digital pressure. Crescent-shaped abrasions are present on the anterior neck and on the anterior chest. Facial congestion is prominent with numerous petechial hemorrhages on the conjunctivae, sclerae, facial skin, and the buccal mucosa. Layered anterior neck dissection demonstrates extensive hemorrhage in the strap muscles bilaterally, hemorrhage in the periesophageal and prevertebral tissues, and a fracture of the right greater cornu of the hyoid with adjacent hemorrhage. Fingernail scrapings from the decedent's hands are preserved for DNA analysis. Toxicology is negative apart from a trace of ethanol at 0.02 grams per deciliter.

**Cause Determination:** Asphyxia due to manual strangulation.

**Manner Determination:** Homicide. The pattern of neck contusions and abrasions, the extensive internal cervical soft tissue hemorrhage, the hyoid fracture, the presence of defensive scene evidence, and the antecedent history of domestic violence all support the manner determination.

**Trap Logic:** Manual strangulation frequently presents with minimal external findings, particularly when the assault is brief or occurs against a lightly-pigmented decedent where surface contusion is not immediately apparent. The trap is to rely on external inspection alone and miss the diagnosis when internal findings would have supported it. The countermeasure is systematic layered anterior neck dissection in every case where strangulation is a reasonable differential consideration, including cases where the external neck appears unremarkable. A related trap is postmortem artifact hemorrhage introduced by dissection technique — manipulation of cervical vessels before cranial drainage can produce artifactual hemorrhage that mimics true injury. The countermeasure is standard-technique dissection with brain removal preceding neck dissection.

**Certification Anchor:** Manual strangulation is confirmed by layered anterior neck dissection documenting internal soft tissue hemorrhage, with supporting external findings when present. Hyoid or thyroid cartilage fracture supports the diagnosis when present but is not required. The systematic examination distinguishes strangulation from postmortem artifact and identifies cases where external findings would not otherwise have supported the diagnosis.

## Smothering, Suffocation, and Positional Asphyxia

Smothering, suffocation, and positional asphyxia are asphyxial mechanisms that do not involve neck compression. Each presents a specific set of documentation challenges, and each is a common source of case reasoning difficulty because the autopsy findings are often nonspecific.

### Smothering

Smothering is asphyxia produced by mechanical obstruction of the mouth and nose. The classic mechanism is a soft object (pillow, hand) held over the mouth and nose. The autopsy findings in smothering are frequently minimal or absent. External injury may be limited to small contusions or abrasions of the lips, gingiva, or perioral skin from pressure of the obstructing object; petechial hemorrhages of the conjunctivae and facial skin may be present. Internal findings typically show pulmonary edema and congestion. There is often no diagnostic finding, and smothering is diagnosed from the scene evidence and history when the autopsy is essentially negative and the circumstances support the mechanism. Smothering of an infant — a mechanism that can be difficult or impossible to distinguish from sudden unexpected infant death — is a specific challenge developed in Chapter 12.

### Choking and Airway Obstruction

Choking is asphyxia from obstruction of the airway by a foreign body — food, small objects, aspirated material. The autopsy findings include the obstructing object identified in the airway (typically at the laryngeal inlet or in the trachea), together with pulmonary edema and, in some cases, aspiration of gastric contents. Foreign body identification requires careful examination of the airway before dissection can dislodge the object. Cafe coronary — sudden collapse and death from food impaction in an intoxicated or otherwise impaired decedent — is a specific pattern that may initially suggest cardiac cause and be identified only at autopsy. In children, aspirated objects are a specific concern and the case is documented with attention to what was accessible to the child at the time of collapse.

### Positional Asphyxia

Positional asphyxia is death from a body position that mechanically restricts respiration without any active obstruction of the airway or compression of the neck. Classic scenarios include an intoxicated decedent found wedged between furniture with the chest and abdomen compressed such that adequate ventilation is impossible, a decedent hanging by clothing caught on a fixed object with the body position preventing breathing, or a restrained decedent in a position that mechanically restricts respiration. Positional asphyxia is difficult to document from autopsy findings alone because the autopsy typically shows only nonspecific findings of asphyxia. The diagnosis rests on integration of scene evidence, body position, and the exclusion of alternative causes. Positional asphyxia in restraint contexts — particularly during law enforcement encounters — is a specific case category of substantial contemporary concern, developed further in Chapter 16.

## Drowning

Drowning is asphyxia produced by aspiration of fluid into the lungs. The mechanism is the same in fresh water and salt water drowning — fluid enters the airway, reflex laryngospasm may briefly obstruct further aspiration, and the ultimate cause of death is hypoxia from inadequate pulmonary gas exchange. The chemistry of the drowning medium may modify secondary electrolyte and osmotic effects on the blood, but the primary mechanism and the timeline of death are similar.

### Antemortem Drowning Findings

The classic finding at the airway is the foam cone — a persistent mixture of air, water, mucus, and pulmonary edema fluid that emerges from the mouth and nostrils. The foam cone is highly suggestive of drowning when present but is not specific (it can occur in other causes of severe pulmonary edema) and its absence does not exclude drowning. Pulmonary findings show hyperinflated, boggy lungs with the surfaces overlapping the anterior mediastinum and often bearing rib imprints from the compressed inflation — termed emphysema aquosum. Cut surfaces of the lung show marked pulmonary edema with abundant fluid consistent with the aspirated medium. Water in the sphenoid sinuses and in the stomach documents ingestion of the drowning medium during immersion. Diatoms — microscopic silicaceous algae present in most natural bodies of water — may be identified in tissue samples (bone marrow, liver, kidney) if they entered the vascular system during vital drowning, providing a specific marker of antemortem immersion when the drowning medium contains them.

### Distinction From Postmortem Immersion

A body immersed after death shows some of the findings of drowning — water in the airway, water in the stomach if the body is immersed with the mouth open — but lacks the pulmonary findings characteristic of vital drowning. The lungs of a postmortem-immersed decedent do not show emphysema aquosum and do not contain the abundant edema fluid of vital drowning. Diatoms in tissue require intact circulation to be transported from the airway to distant tissue and are typically absent in postmortem immersion. The scene evidence — the mechanism by which the body entered the water, the position of the body, the state of the clothing and personal effects — also supports the distinction. Integration of the pulmonary findings, diatom analysis where applicable, and the scene reasoning supports the determination of antemortem drowning versus postmortem immersion.

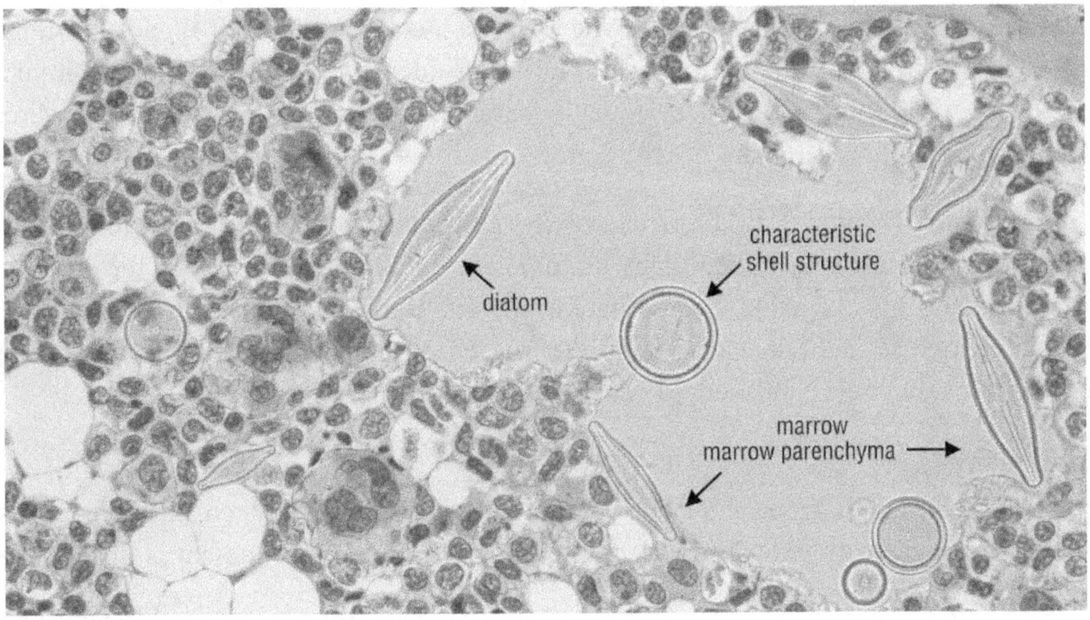


**SCENE-TO-CERTIFICATION DECISION SYSTEM — Drowning-Versus-Postmortem-Immersion Arc**

**Presenting Death Scenario:** A 45-year-old man is found by fishermen floating face-down in a lake, approximately 200 meters from the nearest shore. His personal fishing boat is found beached approximately 500 meters away, unmoored. Water temperature is 18 degrees Celsius. The decedent is wearing casual clothing but no life jacket. He has a documented history of alcohol use and was last seen leaving a bar the previous evening. The scene investigator documents the body position, the location of the boat, the lake conditions, and the water temperature.

**Autopsy Signature:** External examination documents early skin maceration of the hands and feet consistent with immersion for approximately 12 to 24 hours. There is a foam cone visible at the mouth and nostrils. There is no significant external injury. Internal examination shows markedly hyperinflated, boggy lungs with anterior surfaces overlapping the mediastinum and bearing prominent rib imprints. Cut surfaces of the lungs are edematous with abundant pink frothy fluid. Water is present in the sphenoid sinuses and in a moderate amount in the stomach. Diatoms identified on histologic sections of bone marrow and kidney. Toxicology shows blood ethanol of 0.19 grams per deciliter.

**Cause Determination:** Drowning.

**Manner Determination:** Accident. The mechanism is consistent with fall from the boat or entry into the water while intoxicated. The absence of injury of the type consistent with assault, and the intoxication documented by toxicology, support the accident classification.

**Trap Logic:** The trap in cases of body-in-water is to certify drowning based on the finding of a body in water, without confirming vital drowning findings. A body dumped in water after death from another cause — blunt injury, gunshot wound, poisoning — may be recovered from water and superficially appear to be a drowning. The autopsy findings distinguish vital drowning (emphysema aquosum, pulmonary edema of characteristic type, diatoms in tissue when the water contains them) from postmortem immersion (absence of these findings). A related trap is the failure to identify subtle antemortem injury under the postmortem changes of immersion — systematic external examination, radiographic screening, and consideration of the decedent's history are the countermeasures.

**Certification Anchor:** Drowning is confirmed by the constellation of pulmonary findings (emphysema aquosum, characteristic pulmonary edema), by diatom identification in tissue when the drowning medium contains diatoms, and by exclusion of alternative causes. Body-in-water without the vital drowning findings is documented as such; the case reasoning proceeds to identify the alternative cause of death or, where alternatives cannot be established, to certify cause as undetermined.

## Chemical Asphyxia

Chemical asphyxia is death from a substance that interferes with oxygen carriage or use. Carbon monoxide, cyanide, and hydrogen sulfide are the classic agents; the mechanism is different in each and the diagnostic approach reflects the mechanism.

### Carbon Monoxide Poisoning

Carbon monoxide binds to hemoglobin with an affinity approximately 240 times greater than that of oxygen, forming carboxyhemoglobin and preventing oxygen carriage in the blood. Sources include incomplete combustion of any hydrocarbon fuel: house fires (with victims commonly killed by CO poisoning before thermal injury), gasoline engines operating in enclosed spaces (intentional or accidental), poorly vented gas furnaces or water heaters, and vehicle exhaust in enclosed environments. Autopsy findings include the classic cherry-red cyanosis of livor and of internal tissues, reflecting the color of carboxyhemoglobin. Quantitative measurement of blood carboxyhemoglobin confirms the diagnosis; levels above approximately 50 percent in the absence of severe cardiovascular disease are strongly associated with lethal poisoning, and levels above 60 to 70 percent are frequently lethal even in previously healthy individuals. In smoke inhalation cases, the CO poisoning is one component of an integrated smoke inhalation injury that includes thermal injury to the airways and toxic effects of other combustion products.

### Cyanide and Hydrogen Sulfide

Cyanide poisoning interferes with cellular oxygen use by inhibiting cytochrome oxidase in the mitochondrial electron transport chain. Sources include industrial cyanide exposure, combustion of nitrogen-containing polymers (a component of smoke inhalation in many building fires), and intentional poisoning (rare in current American practice but documented). The autopsy findings are limited; cherry-red or bright pink livor may be present but is less consistent than in CO poisoning. Almond odor from the body — a classic teaching finding — is detectable by only a fraction of examiners because ability to detect the odor is genetically determined. Diagnosis rests on quantitative measurement of cyanide in blood. Hydrogen sulfide poisoning occurs in industrial and confined-space contexts (petroleum industry, sewer work, manure pit exposures). The autopsy findings include a characteristic dark or greenish discoloration of tissue at exposure sites and the odor of rotten eggs, though the odor is often not detectable at autopsy hours after exposure. Diagnosis rests on toxicological analysis in cases where the exposure is not documented at the scene.

### Autoerotic Asphyxia

Autoerotic asphyxial death is a distinct pattern in which the decedent has produced partial asphyxia for sexual purposes through hanging, ligature compression, plastic bag occlusion, or chemical exposure (typically volatile hydrocarbons inhaled from a plastic bag), and lost consciousness before releasing the compression or ending the exposure. The pattern is almost exclusively male and predominantly in adolescents and young adults. The scene evidence is characteristic: the decedent is typically found alone in a private location, partially or fully undressed, with sexually explicit material accessible, and with the mechanism arranged in a way that indicates deliberate control (a release mechanism intended to allow the decedent to end the compression at will, which failed or was not activated in time). Prior evidence of similar activity may be present in the environment (wear patterns on the ligature, prior marks on the neck, sexual material curated for the activity).

The manner determination in autoerotic asphyxial death is accident, based on the absence of intent to die. Recognition of the pattern is essential because failure to recognize it produces two common misclassifications: the case may be classified as suicide (with substantial impact on family grief, insurance benefits, and social stigma) or as homicide (with substantial impact on the investigation and on any innocent party who becomes a suspect). The pathologist who recognizes the pattern documents the scene evidence supporting it, communicates the finding with sensitivity to the family, and certifies accident. Family communication in autoerotic asphyxial death is one of the more challenging communications in forensic practice and typically benefits from experienced office staff and, where available, from grief counseling resources for the family.

**CLINICAL PEARL:** The characteristic scene of autoerotic asphyxial death includes a partial or full nudity, arrangement of sexual material, and a release mechanism intended to allow the decedent to end the compression. Recognition of the pattern permits accurate manner determination as accident and avoids the misclassification as suicide. The scene evidence is not shared beyond the case investigators and the family, out of respect for the decedent and family privacy.

### Positional Asphyxia in Custody and Restraint

Positional asphyxia in the context of law enforcement custody or restraint is a specific case category that has received substantial attention in the medicolegal and criminal justice literature over the past several decades. The mechanism proposed is that the prone position, particularly with weight applied to the back or with the arms restrained behind the body, mechanically restricts chest expansion and produces asphyxia when the position is maintained for a sufficient duration. The concept is contested within the specialty; some published analyses have questioned whether positional restriction in the absence of other physiological stressors is sufficient to produce death, and manner determinations in restraint-associated cardiac arrest have shown documented variation among practitioners.

The pathologist encountering a restraint-associated death integrates the autopsy findings (typically nonspecific), the underlying disease of the decedent (cardiovascular disease, obesity, hypertrophy, drug intoxication commonly present), the duration and character of the restraint (documented by body-worn camera footage and by police report), and the timing of decompensation relative to the restraint. The manner determination — accident, homicide, or undetermined — is one of the most difficult in the specialty and is a case category where transparency about reasoning, documentation of all considered alternatives, and openness to peer review substantially strengthen the report. The topic is developed further in Chapter 16.

### Suicide, Homicide, and Accident Patterns in Asphyxial Death

The manner distribution among asphyxial deaths follows category-specific patterns. Hanging is overwhelmingly a suicide mechanism in adult populations; homicidal hanging (in which a hanging is staged after a homicide) is rare and identified by inconsistency between the wound pattern and the physical parameters of the hanging (for example, ligature marks inconsistent with the reported suspension mechanism, or the presence of other antemortem injuries not explained by the hanging). Accidental hanging in children and adolescents occurs from misadventure with cords, blinds, or clothing, and is documented as accident with the scene evidence supporting the mechanism.

Ligature strangulation is overwhelmingly a homicide mechanism. Manual strangulation is essentially always a homicide mechanism because it requires the direct application of force by another person; self-strangulation to death by manual pressure is not achievable in a conscious person. Smothering of infants is a documented homicide mechanism that is extremely difficult to distinguish from sudden unexpected infant death without scene evidence and behavioral context. Drowning distributes across accident (the majority — recreational drowning, accidental fall into water, unattended-child drowning), suicide (documented but less common), and homicide (uncommon, associated with specific scenarios such as immersion of a bound decedent or drowning of an incapacitated person). Chemical asphyxia distributes across suicide (particularly for CO poisoning from vehicle exhaust), accident (CO from faulty appliances, industrial exposures), and homicide (rare).

### Fire Deaths and the Asphyxia Component

Deaths in fires deserve specific attention because the majority of fire fatalities die from asphyxia rather than from thermal injury. The combustion of building materials produces carbon monoxide, cyanide (from combustion of nitrogen-containing polymers such as many synthetic fabrics), and multiple other toxic combustion products. Victims are typically incapacitated by CO and cyanide poisoning within minutes of significant fire exposure and become unable to escape the building or extinguish the fire; thermal injury to the body typically occurs after death from smoke inhalation. The autopsy in a fire death systematically distinguishes antemortem from postmortem thermal injury, quantifies the blood carboxyhemoglobin and cyanide levels, and documents any soot in the airways (indicating antemortem breathing during the fire). Absent soot in the airways in a decedent found in a fire scene raises the specific concern that the decedent was dead before the fire started — a critical distinction for both criminal investigation and insurance investigation. The topic is developed in more detail in the thermal injury discussion of Chapter 9.

### Hyoid and Thyroid Cartilage Fracture Interpretation

The forensic interpretation of hyoid and thyroid cartilage fracture requires understanding of the age-dependent ossification of the structures. The hyoid bone begins as three cartilaginous components (body and paired greater cornua) that gradually ossify and fuse from adolescence through late adulthood. In young adults, the hyoid retains flexibility that permits substantial compression without fracture; the hyoid of an older adult, fully ossified and fused, fractures more readily under similar force. Consequently, hyoid fracture in an adolescent strangulation victim is unusual, whereas hyoid fracture in an elderly strangulation victim is common. The same principle applies to the superior horns of the thyroid cartilage, which ossify progressively with age.

Interpretation of a fractured hyoid must account for perimortem versus postmortem fracture and for the possibility of postmortem artifactual fracture from dissection technique. Perimortem fracture shows adjacent soft tissue hemorrhage; postmortem or artifactual fracture typically does not. The fracture is documented photographically before removal of the hyoid, with the position and orientation of the fracture line recorded. In cases where the fracture will be central to the case reasoning — particularly cases where the diagnosis of strangulation depends on it — the intact hyoid is removed with adjacent soft tissue, fixed, and preserved as evidence with intact chain of custody.

### Bathtub Drowning as a Specific Category

Drowning in a bathtub is a specific case category that warrants attention because it presents both diagnostic and reconstruction challenges. Bathtub drowning may be a natural death (a decedent with a cardiovascular event who was in the tub at the moment of death and drowned in the shallow water); an accident (a decedent who fell in the tub, sustained a head injury, and drowned unable to raise the head above water); a suicide (submersion in the tub as the mechanism, sometimes with additional injury such as wrist incisions); or a homicide (submersion of an incapacitated or resisting victim). The autopsy reasoning must integrate the pulmonary drowning findings with the presence or absence of other injury (particularly head injury from a fall in the tub), with the presence or absence of scene evidence of struggle, and with the antecedent history.

Bathtub drowning of an adult is uncommonly a straightforward accident; the shallow depth of the water and the position of the tub make simple accidental drowning of a competent adult difficult to explain without some contributing factor (intoxication, seizure, cardiac event, mechanical restriction of the head above water). Bathtub drowning of a young child is more commonly accidental, given the depth of water sufficient to submerge a small child's airway and the developmental limitations of the child to escape. Every bathtub drowning is examined with the reasoning of what supports and what contradicts the presumed mechanism, and the report documents both the findings and the reasoning.

### Choking and Complete Airway Obstruction

The specific challenge in choking cases is identification of the obstructing object before airway dissection dislodges it. Standard practice examines the oral cavity, oropharynx, and hypopharynx by direct inspection with a light and by palpation. The larynx and upper trachea are examined in situ, with attention to the position of any foreign object at the laryngeal inlet or at the vocal cords — the classic location of complete airway obstruction. When a foreign body is identified, it is photographed in place before removal, and its character is documented (type of food or object, dimensions, orientation). The airway is inspected below the obstruction for evidence of partial passage or of contents distal to the site of impaction. Aspiration of gastric contents — which produces a different pattern and is not choking in the classic sense — is documented separately when present.

The distinction between antemortem choking and postmortem aspiration is important. Antemortem choking with complete airway obstruction produces distress and vital reaction (petechiae from the effort, mucosal injury at the site of obstruction, occasionally food in the trachea below the obstruction from unsuccessful attempts to clear it). Postmortem regurgitation of gastric contents into the airway is a common finding, particularly in cases with significant postmortem interval or with resuscitation, and does not indicate antemortem aspiration or choking. The distinction depends on the presence of vital reaction at the obstruction site and on the character of the material found (undigested food particles at the larynx supporting antemortem choking, versus gastric acid-modified content in the airway supporting postmortem regurgitation).

### SCENE-TO-CERTIFICATION DECISION SYSTEM — Asphyxia Determination Arcs

**The Category Framework:** Asphyxia comprises neck compression (hanging, ligature strangulation, manual strangulation), airway obstruction (smothering, choking), positional restriction (positional asphyxia), fluid aspiration (drowning), and chemical interference (carbon monoxide, cyanide, hydrogen sulfide). Each category has characteristic findings, and the diagnostic anchor is the pattern of findings specific to the subcategory rather than a single pathognomonic feature.

**Neck Compression Discipline:** Hanging shows an oblique ligature furrow, higher-lying, deepest at the anterior neck. Ligature strangulation shows a horizontal furrow of uniform depth. Manual strangulation shows contusions and abrasions from digital pressure with fingernail crescents and prominent facial congestion. Layered anterior neck dissection is the standard technique for identifying internal soft tissue hemorrhage and cartilage fracture in all three.

**The Subtle-Findings Category:** Smothering and positional asphyxia frequently show minimal or absent specific findings. The diagnosis depends on integration of scene evidence, body position, exclusion of alternative causes, and antecedent history. The pathologist is honest about the limits of autopsy diagnosis in these categories and does not overreach.

**Drowning Confirmation:** Antemortem drowning is confirmed by the pulmonary findings (emphysema aquosum, characteristic edema), by diatom identification when the drowning medium contains them, and by exclusion of alternative causes. Postmortem immersion is distinguished by the absence of these vital findings. Body-in-water is not equivalent to drowning.

**Chemical Asphyxia Confirmation:** Carbon monoxide poisoning is confirmed by quantitative blood carboxyhemoglobin. Cyanide poisoning is confirmed by quantitative cyanide analysis. Hydrogen sulfide poisoning is confirmed by toxicology when the exposure context supports the differential. Autopsy findings in chemical asphyxia are supportive but rarely diagnostic without the confirmatory analytical result.

## Summary and Key Concepts

Asphyxia is the physiologic state of interrupted oxygen delivery to tissue and comprises multiple subcategories, each with characteristic mechanisms and findings. Asphyxial death is a demanding reasoning category because autopsy findings are frequently subtle and the diagnosis depends on pattern recognition across a constellation of findings integrated with scene evidence.

Hanging and ligature strangulation both involve compression of the neck by a ligature, distinguished by the source of the compressive force. The ligature furrow pattern (oblique in hanging, horizontal in ligature strangulation) supports the mechanism determination.

Manual strangulation shows contusion and abrasion patterns from digital pressure with fingernail crescents, together with layered anterior neck soft tissue hemorrhage identified on systematic dissection. Hyoid or thyroid cartilage fracture supports the diagnosis when present but is not required.

Smothering, choking, and positional asphyxia present variable diagnostic challenges. Smothering and positional asphyxia frequently show minimal or absent specific findings; choking is diagnosed by identification of the obstructing object in the airway.

Drowning is confirmed by pulmonary findings (emphysema aquosum, characteristic edema), by diatom identification when the drowning medium contains them, and by exclusion of alternative causes. Postmortem immersion is distinguished by the absence of these vital findings.

Chemical asphyxia — carbon monoxide, cyanide, hydrogen sulfide — is confirmed by quantitative toxicological measurement in each case, with supportive autopsy findings (cherry-red livor in CO poisoning, exposure context in cyanide and hydrogen sulfide) that raise the differential.

# CHAPTER 9: THERMAL, ELECTRICAL, AND CHEMICAL INJURY DEATHS

**Learning Objectives**

1. Distinguish antemortem burn injury from postmortem thermal artifact and reason about the state of the decedent at the onset of fire exposure.
2. Recognize hypothermia and hyperthermia by their autopsy findings and articulate the environmental and physiologic factors that predispose to each.
3. Identify electrical injury by the characteristic entry and exit lesions and reason from the pattern of injury to the mechanism of the electrical event.
4. Recognize chemical burn injury and corrosive ingestion and understand the toxicological correlation required for cause and manner determination.
5. Describe blast injury and its four categories, and recognize radiation injury patterns in the specific contexts where they arise.

## Thermal Injury and Fire Deaths

Thermal injury encompasses burn injury from direct heat exposure, smoke inhalation injury from combustion products, and the systemic effects of severe burn exposure. Fire deaths are among the most common contexts in which forensic pathologists encounter thermal injury, and the reasoning about fire deaths integrates the burn pattern with the smoke inhalation findings, the toxicological confirmation of carboxyhemoglobin and cyanide, and the scene reconstruction of the fire itself.

### Classification of Burn Injury

Burn injury is classified by depth into first-degree (superficial epidermal), second-degree (partial-thickness dermal, with subclassification into superficial partial and deep partial), third-degree (full-thickness with destruction of epidermis and dermis), and fourth-degree (extending into underlying muscle, tendon, or bone). The depth of injury reflects the temperature of exposure and the duration of contact; brief exposure to high temperature and prolonged exposure to moderate temperature both produce full-thickness injury. Extent of burn is quantified as body surface area affected, traditionally by the Rule of Nines (each upper limb 9 percent, each lower limb 18 percent, anterior trunk 18 percent, posterior trunk 18 percent, head and neck 9 percent, perineum 1 percent) with pediatric modifications reflecting the different body proportions of children. Extensive burn injury produces systemic effects — severe fluid loss, hypovolemic shock, systemic inflammatory response — that account for the majority of burn deaths beyond the immediate post-injury period.

In forensic practice, the burn injury classification supports the reasoning about the mechanism and about survival. A partially-preserved decedent from a house fire with predominantly superficial burns on the skin and extensive smoke inhalation likely died from asphyxial mechanism during the fire, with the surface burns representing brief thermal exposure. A decedent with predominantly deep burns and limited smoke inhalation may have died from thermal injury with survival time between fire onset and death long enough for extensive burn injury to develop. Reasoning about these patterns integrates the burn pattern, the toxicological findings for CO and cyanide, and the scene reconstruction of the fire.

**Figure 9.1 Burn Depth Classification and Body Surface Area Estimation**

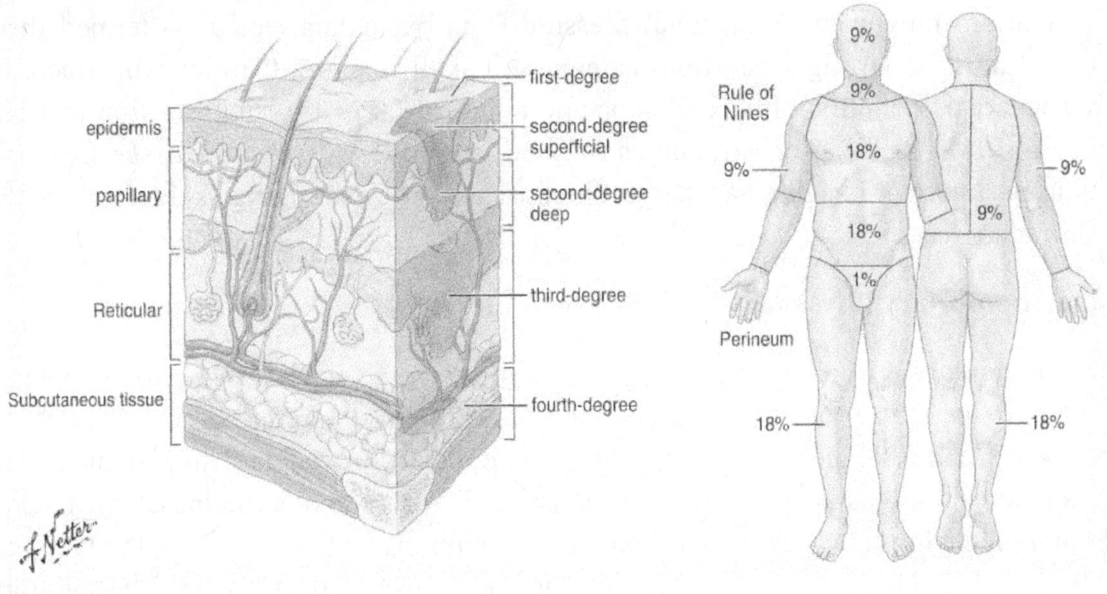


## Antemortem Versus Postmortem Thermal Injury

The distinction between antemortem burn injury and postmortem thermal artifact is central to the forensic reasoning in fire death cases. Antemortem burn injury shows vital reaction — hyperemia and blister formation at the burn margins in survivable exposure, and, in exposures survived for at least minutes, inflammatory infiltrate documented on histology. Postmortem thermal exposure produces charring and destruction of tissue without vital reaction; the burns are limited to the exposed body surfaces and show no evidence of biological response. The distinction supports the reasoning about whether the decedent was alive at the onset of the fire or whether the body was already dead when fire exposure began. The former is consistent with the decedent being killed by the fire (from asphyxia or thermal mechanism); the latter is consistent with the fire being a subsequent event, potentially an attempt to destroy evidence.

## The Airway Examination in Fire Deaths

The airway examination in fire deaths is directed at identifying soot in the airway and evidence of thermal injury to the mucosa. Soot in the trachea and bronchi documents antemortem breathing during smoke exposure. Absent soot in the airway of a decedent found in a fire scene is a specific concern that the decedent was not breathing at the time of the fire — supporting the reconstruction that death occurred before the fire started. Thermal injury to the pharyngeal and laryngeal mucosa documents thermal exposure to the airway and is characteristic of substantial smoke inhalation. Toxicological confirmation of carbon monoxide and cyanide poisoning documents antemortem inhalation of combustion products. These findings integrate to distinguish deaths in fires from deaths preceding fires.

## Fire Death Postmortem Changes

Extensive thermal exposure produces characteristic postmortem changes that must be distinguished from antemortem injury. The pugilistic (boxer) posture — flexion of the elbows, hips, and knees produced by contraction of the flexor muscles under heat exposure — is a postmortem finding of severe thermal exposure and does not indicate any antemortem event. Skull fracture from severe thermal exposure occurs when the calvarium fails under intracranial pressure from expanding steam — termed thermal skull fracture — and must be distinguished from antemortem skull fracture; thermal skull fracture typically shows a characteristic pattern with sutural separation and a lack of the vital reaction that antemortem fracture would show. Charring of extremities may be extensive with loss of tissue that limits injury identification; postmortem imaging can support identification of underlying skeletal injury that surface examination cannot reach.

## Smoke Inhalation Injury Physiology

Smoke inhalation injury is a compound insult: thermal injury to the upper airway from inhaled hot gases, chemical injury to the airway and lung parenchyma from combustion products (organic acids, aldehydes, particulate matter), and systemic toxicity from carbon monoxide and cyanide absorbed into the circulation. The upper airway shows characteristic thermal injury with edema and erythema of the pharyngeal and laryngeal mucosa; the lower airway shows chemical bronchiolitis and pneumonitis; the lung parenchyma shows edema, congestion, and, in survivors of the initial event, delayed acute respiratory distress syndrome. Carbon monoxide binds hemoglobin and interferes with oxygen carriage; cyanide interferes with cellular oxygen use. The combined effect produces incapacitation and death within minutes in significant exposures. Victims of house fires who die from smoke inhalation typically do so before thermal injury of the body itself becomes lethal, which is why absent soot in the airway of a fire scene decedent is a specific concern that death preceded the fire.

## Vehicle Fires and Enclosed-Space Fire Deaths

Vehicle fires present a specific set of case reconstructions. Deaths in vehicle fires occur from collision (with subsequent vehicle fire), from vehicle malfunction with fire onset (electrical short, fuel leak with ignition), from intentional vehicle fire (as a mechanism of concealing a decedent, or as a suicide method), and from carbon monoxide poisoning in a running vehicle in an enclosed space (garage, tunnel). Each pattern has distinctive scene characteristics and integrates with different autopsy reasoning. The pathologist reads a vehicle fire death with attention to the injury pattern from the collision if any (predating the fire), the airway examination for soot documenting antemortem fire exposure, the toxicological confirmation of CO and cyanide, and the position of the decedent in the vehicle relative to the fire origin. Autopsy of a decedent recovered from a running vehicle in a garage (typical scene of carbon monoxide suicide by vehicle exhaust) shows the classic cherry-red cyanosis of CO poisoning and confirmatory toxicological carboxyhemoglobin without significant thermal injury.

**Skin Histology in Burn Interpretation**

Histologic examination of representative burn samples supports the antemortem/postmortem distinction and the depth assessment when the gross appearance is ambiguous. Antemortem burn shows vital reaction — dermal hemorrhage, inflammatory infiltrate if the survival was at least several hours, and edema of the dermis. Postmortem burn shows thermal denaturation of tissue proteins and cellular architecture without vital reaction. The depth of burn is assessed by identifying the deepest layer of involved tissue — epidermal loss for superficial burns, papillary or reticular dermal involvement for partial-thickness burns, full-thickness involvement with destruction of skin appendages for third-degree burns, and involvement of subcutaneous or deeper tissue for fourth-degree burns. Representative samples from multiple body regions are taken in cases where the burn distribution is central to the case reasoning.

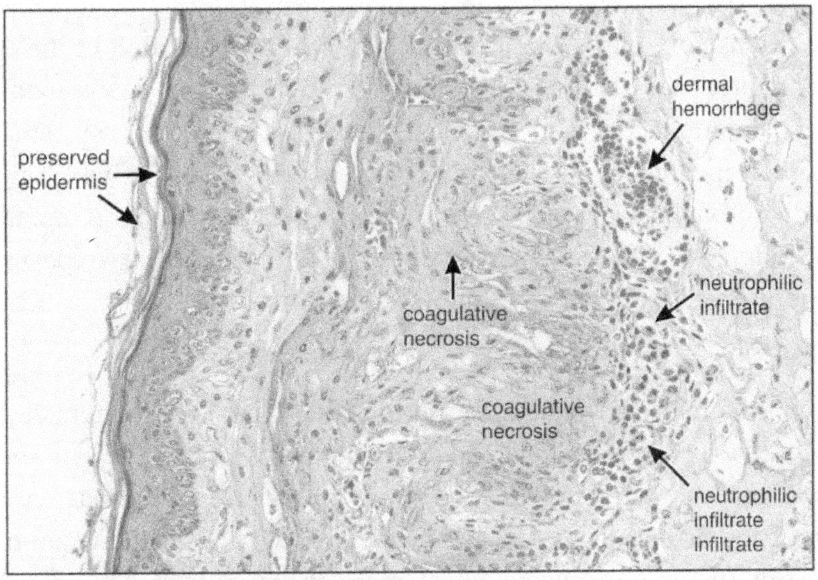


Figure 9.3: Antemortem Skin Burn: Histologic Vital Reaction at Burn Margin

**SCENE-TO-CERTIFICATION DECISION SYSTEM — Antemortem-Versus-Postmortem Fire Injury Arc**

**Presenting Death Scenario:** A single-story residential fire is reported at approximately 3:00 AM. Fire response controls the fire within 45 minutes. A single decedent is recovered from the master bedroom, extensively burned, in a supine position on what remained of the bed. The residence was occupied by a middle-aged man who lived alone. Preliminary fire investigation notes an accelerant pattern consistent with intentional fire setting. Toxicology on postmortem specimens is initiated. The medical examiner's office accepts jurisdiction and the pathologist prepares to examine the body.

**Autopsy Signature:** External examination documents extensive charring of the body with fourth-degree burns involving approximately 85 percent of the body surface. The pugilistic posture is present. Detailed examination of the anterior neck, protected from the fire by the position of the body, identifies a horizontal ligature furrow at mid-neck, approximately 1 cm wide, with parchmentization and adjacent subcutaneous hemorrhage on layered dissection. The oral cavity and airway are largely preserved and show no soot in the trachea and no thermal injury to the mucosa. Toxicology shows carboxyhemoglobin of 3 percent (baseline range for non-fire deaths, indicating no antemortem CO exposure), and cyanide is not detected. Internal examination confirms cervical soft tissue hemorrhage in the strap muscles bilaterally and a fracture of the right greater cornu of the hyoid.

**Cause Determination:** Asphyxia due to ligature strangulation, with postmortem thermal injury.

**Manner Determination:** Homicide. The autopsy establishes that the decedent was strangled before the fire; the accelerant pattern documented by fire investigators is consistent with the fire being set to destroy evidence of the strangulation. The absence of soot in the airway, the near-baseline carboxyhemoglobin, and the identification of the ligature furrow beneath the preserved neck tissue integrate to support this reconstruction.

**Trap Logic:** A body extensively burned in a fire may appear to have died in the fire when the primary cause of death actually preceded the fire. The trap is to certify fire death without documenting the antemortem versus postmortem distinction. The countermeasures are systematic: examination of preserved body regions (typically underneath the body or under protective clothing) for evidence of antemortem injury; airway examination for soot; toxicological documentation of carboxyhemoglobin and cyanide levels. Any single element inconsistent with antemortem fire exposure (absent soot, low carboxyhemoglobin, preserved evidence of antemortem injury) warrants specific evaluation of the alternative reconstruction.

**Certification Anchor:** Antemortem versus postmortem fire injury is distinguished by vital reaction at burn margins, by soot in the airway, by elevated carboxyhemoglobin, and by preserved evidence of prior cause of death. When multiple elements converge on postmortem thermal exposure, the reasoning supports certification of the primary cause of death rather than fire death; when elements converge on antemortem fire exposure, fire and its associated asphyxia or thermal mechanism are the primary cause.

## Hypothermia and Hyperthermia

Environmental temperature extremes cause death through opposite mechanisms: hypothermia through progressive impairment of thermoregulation and cardiac function as body temperature falls, and hyperthermia through breakdown of thermoregulation as body temperature rises.

### Hypothermia

Hypothermic death occurs when body core temperature falls below approximately 28 to 30 degrees Celsius; below this range, cardiac arrhythmia becomes progressively more likely and cardiac arrest often supervenes. Environmental exposure is the classic mechanism; intoxication (particularly ethanol) predisposes by producing peripheral vasodilation, by impairing behavioral responses to cold, and by producing cognitive impairment that prevents recognition of the danger. Elderly decedents, decedents with cardiovascular disease, and decedents with hypothyroidism or other endocrine dysfunction are particularly vulnerable. Homeless populations, decedents intoxicated in outdoor environments, and decedents in inadequately heated residences comprise the major categories in most caseloads.

The autopsy findings in hypothermia are limited but characteristic when present. Skin may show a bright pink or reddish discoloration of livor, particularly over the extremities — a finding termed cold pink livor reflecting the reduced oxygen consumption of cold tissue and the retention of oxyhemoglobin. Gastric mucosal hemorrhages (Wischnewsky lesions) — small punctate hemorrhages of the gastric mucosa — are described in hypothermia and, though not specific, support the diagnosis when found in the appropriate context. Adipose tissue may show a pale yellow character. Paradoxical undressing — the decedent removing clothing before death — is a documented behavior in severe hypothermia and, when reported at the scene, supports the diagnosis. The reasoning integrates the autopsy findings with the environmental context and antecedent history.

**Hyperthermia**

Hyperthermic death occurs when body core temperature rises above approximately 40 degrees Celsius (heat stroke threshold) and thermoregulation fails. Environmental heat exposure is one mechanism; classic heat stroke is common in elderly populations during heat waves, in athletes and workers with prolonged exertion in hot environments, and in decedents left in enclosed vehicles or environments during warm weather. Malignant hyperthermia — a genetic predisposition to hyperthermic crisis triggered by anesthetic agents — is a specific medical cause. Drug-induced hyperthermia occurs with sympathomimetic drugs (cocaine, methamphetamine, MDMA), with certain antipsychotic drug reactions (neuroleptic malignant syndrome), and with serotonin syndrome from serotonergic medication interactions. The autopsy findings are limited but include marked pulmonary edema, cerebral edema, and often significant fluid loss with hemoconcentration. Toxicology supports the diagnosis when drug-related hyperthermia is on the differential.

**Vehicular Hyperthermia in Children**

Death of a child from hyperthermia inside a parked vehicle is a specific case category with substantial contemporary attention. The mechanism reflects the greenhouse effect of a closed vehicle in sunlight, in which cabin temperature can rise substantially above ambient within minutes. Even ambient temperatures in the range of 20 degrees Celsius produce dangerous cabin temperatures with sufficient sunlight exposure, and infants and young children are particularly vulnerable because of their limited ability to escape the environment and their lower body mass with less thermal reserve. The manner determination in these cases depends on the circumstances: unintentional forgetting of the child in the vehicle (a documented mechanism affecting fatigued or distracted caregivers) is typically classified as accident, though the specific determination and any associated criminal charges are made by law enforcement and the prosecutor rather than by the medical examiner. Intentional confinement of a child in a vehicle is a homicide mechanism.

**Stages of Hypothermic Death**

The progression of hypothermic death has been described in three broad stages. In mild hypothermia (core temperature 32 to 35 degrees Celsius), the decedent shows shivering, mild cognitive impairment, and appropriate behavioral responses to cold when able. In moderate hypothermia (28 to 32 degrees Celsius), shivering ceases, cognitive impairment progresses, and paradoxical undressing may occur (the decedent removes clothing before death, thought to reflect the sensation of warmth from failed peripheral thermoregulation). In severe hypothermia (below 28 degrees Celsius), cardiac arrhythmia becomes likely, coma develops, and cardiac arrest supervenes. The final stage often includes the terminal behavior of terminal burrowing, in which the decedent seeks shelter in a small enclosed space (a closet, under furniture, in a corner) before death. Recognition of the terminal burrowing pattern in a decedent found in an unusual location supports hypothermia as the mechanism when the environmental context is consistent.

## Electrical Injury

Electrical death occurs from current passing through the body producing arrhythmia or thermal injury. The pathophysiology depends on the voltage, current, path of the current through the body, and duration of exposure. Low-voltage exposures (household current, 110 to 240 volts) typically produce arrhythmic death from current passing through the chest; the current is often insufficient to produce significant thermal injury. High-voltage exposures (industrial power, transmission lines, thousands to hundreds of thousands of volts) produce both arrhythmic death and extensive thermal injury, with characteristic burns at contact points.

### The Electrical Entry and Exit Mark

The characteristic finding in electrical injury is the electrical entry mark (Joule burn) at the site where current entered the body. The classic entry mark is a small (typically less than 1 cm) area of central pale, dry, blistered skin surrounded by a rim of hyperemia. In high-voltage exposures the mark may be substantially larger with charring and extensive tissue destruction. Exit marks at the site where current left the body have similar morphology, though less consistently identified than entry marks. Both entry and exit marks may be absent when the contact surface was broad (immersion in electrified water, for example) or when the exposure did not produce local tissue heating.

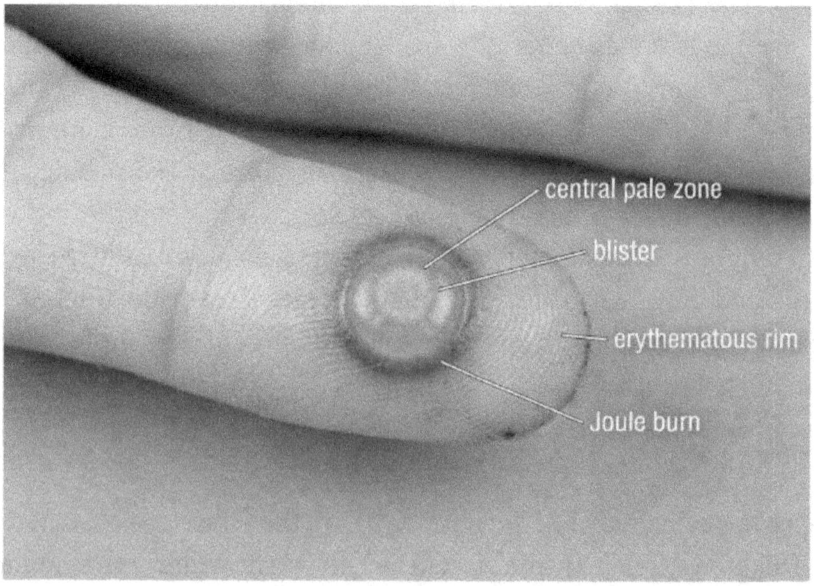


Figure 9.2: Electrical Entry Mark (Joule Burn) at Fingertip

## Reasoning About Electrical Death

Electrical death reasoning integrates the identified entry and exit marks (when present), the scene evidence of the electrical source, the pathophysiologic plausibility of the exposure producing death (low-voltage exposures across the chest are plausibly lethal; low-voltage exposures across a small body region are less likely to be lethal), and the exclusion of alternative causes. The absence of visible electrical marks does not exclude electrical death, particularly in low-voltage exposures through a wet contact surface where local heating is dissipated. Scene evidence documenting the electrical source, the mechanism of contact, and the timing of collapse relative to the exposure supports the diagnosis in cases where the autopsy findings alone would be inconclusive.

## Lightning Injury

Lightning strike produces a specific injury pattern distinct from other electrical injuries. The current involved (thousands to hundreds of thousands of amperes at millions of volts) is far greater than most industrial exposures, but the duration is exceptionally brief (milliseconds), and the current typically flashes over the skin surface rather than passing through the body — termed flashover — which paradoxically produces less internal thermal injury than lower-voltage prolonged contact might. The classic external finding is the Lichtenberg figure — a fern-like, branching pattern of erythema on the skin representing the discharge pattern of the flashover current. The Lichtenberg figure is transient, often disappearing within hours to a day after the exposure, and its documentation is essential when present. Additional findings include tympanic membrane rupture from the pressure wave, keraunoparalysis (transient paralysis of the extremities), and injury from the mechanical effects of the strike (throw of the body, impact from associated debris). Lightning strike is typically an accident but occurs occasionally in unusual homicide reconstructions.

## High-Voltage Versus Low-Voltage Electrical Injury

The distinction between high-voltage and low-voltage electrical injury reflects both the mechanism of death and the case reconstruction. Low-voltage exposures (household 110 to 240 volts) produce arrhythmic death from current across the chest, typically with minimal thermal injury; entry marks are small and can be subtle. High-voltage exposures (thousands of volts and up) produce both arrhythmic death and substantial thermal injury; entry marks are frequently extensive and easily identifiable. High-voltage exposures may throw the decedent by muscle contraction, producing associated blunt injury from the fall. Industrial and utility contexts (power lines, high-voltage equipment) are the classic settings for high-voltage exposure; occupational safety documentation is central to the case reconstruction. Low-voltage exposures typically occur in residential contexts (defective appliances, damaged electrical cords, contact with energized wiring during repair or renovation work); the scene reconstruction integrates the exposure mechanism with the physiologic plausibility.

**SCENE-TO-CERTIFICATION DECISION SYSTEM — Electrical Death Reconstruction Arc**

**Presenting Death Scenario:** A 28-year-old electrician is found deceased in the crawl space beneath a residence where he was working alone on rewiring. The homeowner returned to find him unresponsive and called emergency services. The crawl space contained exposed wiring, some of it energized. The circuit breaker was in the on position when responders arrived. Emergency personnel de-energized the circuit before extraction and transport.

**Autopsy Signature:** External examination documents two electrical entry marks: one on the volar surface of the right index finger (approximately 6 mm diameter, characteristic Joule burn morphology) and one on the volar surface of the left thumb (similar morphology). No exit mark is visible on external inspection. There is no other significant external injury. Internal examination shows no significant natural disease. The heart is of normal size and weight; the coronary arteries are widely patent. Histology of the myocardium shows no acute or chronic pathology. Toxicology is negative.

**Cause Determination:** Electrocution. The autopsy findings integrate: characteristic electrical entry marks on both hands consistent with the reported mechanism (contact with energized wiring during rewiring work), scene evidence of an energized circuit consistent with the exposure, and exclusion of alternative causes on complete autopsy and toxicology.

**Manner Determination:** Accident. The occupational context, the physical evidence of contact with energized wiring during work, and the absence of any evidence of intent to injure or of third-party involvement support the accident classification.

**Trap Logic:** Electrical death may present without visible entry or exit marks, particularly when the contact was broad or through a wet surface. The trap in the other direction is to attribute a death to electrocution based on scene context without confirming that the physiologic mechanism is plausible — for example, contact with low-voltage current through a small skin area far from the chest would not typically be lethal in a healthy young decedent. The reasoning integrates the marks (when present), the scene evidence of the electrical source, the plausibility of the exposure producing death, and the exclusion of alternative causes.

**Certification Anchor:** Electrical death is confirmed by the constellation of electrical entry mark (when present), scene evidence of the electrical source and exposure mechanism, physiologic plausibility of the exposure producing arrhythmic death, and exclusion of alternative causes. Absent visible marks do not exclude the diagnosis but shift greater reasoning weight to the scene and to the exclusion.

## Chemical Burns and Corrosive Injury

Chemical injury occurs from exposure to corrosive substances — acids, alkalis, and reactive chemicals. Acids produce coagulative necrosis with a characteristic dry, discolored appearance of the affected tissue. Alkalis produce liquefactive necrosis with a softer, more edematous appearance and typically penetrate more deeply into tissue than acids of similar concentration. Concentrated hydrofluoric acid is a specific concern because it penetrates deeply, produces systemic effects (hypocalcemia, cardiotoxicity), and can be lethal from relatively small skin exposures.

### Corrosive Ingestion

Corrosive ingestion — accidental in children who access household products, intentional in adult suicide, and in some assault cases — produces characteristic injury to the oral cavity, esophagus, and stomach. The oral cavity shows burns of the lips, tongue, and pharyngeal mucosa. The esophagus is severely affected in ingestions of concentrated corrosive with characteristic ulceration or perforation; the stomach shows chemical injury with characteristic mucosal appearance depending on the agent. Systemic effects include shock from fluid loss, chemical pneumonitis from aspirated fumes, and specific chemical toxicity depending on the agent. Toxicological confirmation of the specific chemical involved supports the case reasoning.

### Common Corrosive Agents and Their Patterns

Specific corrosive agents produce recognizable patterns of injury. Sodium hydroxide and potassium hydroxide (lye) — present in drain cleaners and some industrial cleaning products — are strong alkalis that produce deep liquefactive necrosis with characteristic soft, edematous appearance. Sulfuric acid — present in some drain cleaners and in industrial applications — is a strong acid that produces coagulative necrosis with a characteristic dark, dry appearance from the dehydrating effect on tissue. Hydrochloric acid — sometimes accessed as swimming pool acid or from industrial sources — produces similar coagulative necrosis with tissue discoloration. Bleach (sodium hypochlorite) at household concentrations produces mucosal irritation and mild burn; concentrated industrial bleach can produce more severe injury. Ammonia produces mucosal injury and pulmonary irritation. Recognition of the specific agent by the character of the injury supports the case reconstruction; toxicological analysis of gastric contents identifies the agent when the history is unclear.

### Systemic Toxicity of Chemical Exposures

Beyond local burn injury, many corrosive and reactive chemicals produce systemic effects that contribute to or dominate the mechanism of death. Hydrofluoric acid produces hypocalcemia from fluoride binding of calcium, with cardiotoxicity and arrhythmic death from even small skin exposures. Methylene chloride — present in some paint strippers — is metabolized to carbon monoxide, producing delayed CO poisoning after apparent recovery from acute exposure. Organophosphate pesticide exposure produces cholinergic toxicity with characteristic constellation of miosis, hypersalivation, bronchorrhea, and neuromuscular effects. Each of these categories requires specific toxicological confirmation, and the pattern of exposure documented at scene supports the case reasoning.

## Blast Injury

Blast injury results from explosive detonation. Its categories are conventionally described as primary (direct effect of the pressure wave on air-filled organs — lungs, tympanic membranes, bowel), secondary (injury from fragments propelled by the explosion — shrapnel, secondary projectiles), tertiary (injury from the body being thrown or the environment collapsing on the body), and quaternary (thermal injury, chemical injury, and other blast-related exposures).

### Primary Blast Injury Physiology

The primary blast injury is produced by the pressure wave from the explosion — a supersonic wave of compressed gas that propagates outward from the detonation point. Air-filled organs are particularly vulnerable because the abrupt compression and decompression of the gas within them produces shear injury at tissue interfaces. The lung shows characteristic pulmonary hemorrhage — subpleural hemorrhage, contusion, and, in severe cases, rupture with pneumothorax. The tympanic membrane is highly sensitive to the pressure wave and ruptures at relatively low overpressure exposures; its rupture is a marker of significant blast exposure and is documented in every blast case. The bowel shows characteristic mucosal hemorrhage from the pressure wave with, in some cases, transmural rupture. The pattern of primary blast injury reflects the magnitude of the pressure wave and the position of the decedent relative to the detonation.

### Blast Injury Documentation

Documentation of blast injury requires attention to each injury category. Primary blast injury is documented by examination of the lungs (characteristic pulmonary hemorrhage and rupture), of the tympanic membranes (rupture from pressure wave exposure), and of hollow organs (bowel injury from pressure wave). Secondary blast injury is documented as ballistic-style injury from shrapnel and fragments, with recovery of retained foreign material for later analysis. Tertiary blast injury is documented as blunt force injury from the body being thrown or crushed. Quaternary effects include burns, chemical exposure, and inhalation injury. Blast injury frequently occurs in mass casualty events, and the individual case documentation supports the aggregate reconstruction of the event.

### Blast Reconstruction and Mass Casualty Response

The reconstruction of a blast event depends on integration of individual case findings across multiple decedents. Fragment analysis from multiple decedents documents the character of the explosive device — the fragmentation pattern reveals whether the device contained added shrapnel and, if so, what materials. Body position of decedents relative to the detonation point supports mapping of the blast wave propagation. In mass casualty events — whether accidental (industrial explosion, gas main rupture) or intentional (bombing) — the forensic pathology contribution is one element of a multidisciplinary reconstruction that includes fire investigation, structural engineering, ballistics, and law enforcement investigation. The individual autopsy case documentation is calibrated to serve this aggregate purpose.

## Radiation Injury

Radiation injury results from acute high-dose or chronic exposure to ionizing radiation. In forensic practice, radiation injury is uncommon and typically arises in specific contexts — nuclear or radiological incidents, medical radiation over-exposure, industrial radiation source exposure, and, historically, weapons exposure. Acute radiation syndrome from high-dose whole-body exposure produces characteristic hematopoietic, gastrointestinal, and neurovascular effects depending on dose.

### Acute Radiation Syndrome

Acute radiation syndrome from whole-body ionizing radiation exposure follows a dose-dependent progression. At doses in the range of 1 to 2 gray, the hematopoietic effects dominate — progressive bone marrow suppression with resulting cytopenia over days to weeks after exposure; survival is typical with supportive care. At doses of 4 to 6 gray, the hematopoietic effects are more severe and are accompanied by gastrointestinal injury with mucosal denudation and secondary infection; survival requires advanced medical management. At doses above approximately 8 to 10 gray, neurovascular effects appear with cerebral and cardiovascular collapse within hours; death typically occurs within days regardless of intervention. Beyond approximately 20 gray, immediate neurologic decompensation and death within hours are the pattern. Radiation exposures below the acute threshold may produce chronic effects including malignancy years to decades later, but these do not present as acute forensic cases.

### Autopsy in Radiation Deaths

Autopsy in a radiation death requires coordination with radiation safety authorities because the body may itself be a radiation source depending on the exposure. Standard practice for suspected radiation deaths includes coordination with a health physicist or radiation safety officer before autopsy, appropriate radiological screening of the body, and use of personal protective equipment specific to the radiation type. Postmortem findings in acute radiation death include marrow depletion, gastrointestinal mucosal denudation, and characteristic organ pathology; chronic radiation exposure produces different patterns including tissue-specific injury and secondary malignancy in survivors. The forensic pathologist consults with radiation medicine specialists in cases where the pattern of radiation exposure is central to the case reasoning.

### SCENE-TO-CERTIFICATION DECISION SYSTEM — Thermal, Electrical, Chemical Determination Arcs

---

**Fire Death Discipline:** Fire death reasoning distinguishes antemortem thermal exposure (with vital reaction, soot in airway, elevated carboxyhemoglobin) from postmortem thermal exposure (without vital reaction, without soot, without CO). This distinction is central to identifying deaths that preceded the fire and cases where fire was used to destroy evidence.

**Environmental Temperature Extremes:** Hypothermia is diagnosed by cold pink livor, gastric mucosal hemorrhages, and integration with environmental exposure and antecedent history. Hyperthermia is diagnosed by marked pulmonary and cerebral edema and integration with exposure or drug context. Neither has a single pathognomonic finding; both depend on pattern integration.

**Electrical Injury Reasoning:** Electrical death is confirmed by electrical entry marks (when present), by scene evidence of the electrical source and mechanism of contact, by physiologic plausibility of the exposure producing lethal arrhythmia, and by exclusion of alternative causes. Absent marks do not exclude the diagnosis but shift greater reasoning weight to scene and exclusion.

**Chemical and Corrosive Injury:** Chemical burn injury produces characteristic tissue patterns (coagulative necrosis with acids, liquefactive necrosis with alkalis). Corrosive ingestion produces characteristic upper gastrointestinal injury patterns. Toxicological confirmation of the specific agent supports the reasoning.

**Blast and Radiation:** Blast injury is documented across the four categories — primary (pressure wave), secondary (fragments), tertiary (body throw), quaternary (thermal, chemical, other exposures). Radiation death requires coordination with radiation safety authorities and typically consultation with radiation medicine specialists for the specific pattern of exposure and organ effects.

## Summary and Key Concepts

Thermal injury is classified by depth and extent and integrated with smoke inhalation and toxicological findings to reason about the mechanism of fire death. Distinction between antemortem and postmortem thermal injury is central: vital reaction at burn margins, soot in the airway, and elevated carboxyhemoglobin all support antemortem fire exposure.

Hypothermia and hyperthermia are diagnosed by pattern recognition across characteristic autopsy findings integrated with environmental context and antecedent history. Neither has a single pathognomonic finding, and the reasoning depends on the integration.

Electrical death is diagnosed by identification of electrical entry marks (Joule burns) at contact sites, integrated with scene evidence of the electrical source and mechanism. Absent visible marks do not exclude the diagnosis when scene evidence and physiologic plausibility support it.

Chemical burn injury produces characteristic tissue patterns for acids (coagulative necrosis) and alkalis (liquefactive necrosis). Corrosive ingestion produces upper gastrointestinal injury with specific patterns depending on the agent. Toxicological confirmation supports the case reasoning.

Blast injury is documented across the four categories — primary, secondary, tertiary, quaternary — with attention to each category during examination. Radiation death requires coordination with radiation safety authorities and specialist consultation for the pattern of exposure.

# CHAPTER 10: SUDDEN CARDIAC DEATH

**Learning Objectives**

1. Define sudden cardiac death in forensic practice and articulate the epidemiological patterns that distinguish it across age groups.
2. Recognize and quantify coronary atherosclerotic disease at autopsy and reason about its role in sudden cardiac death cases.
3. Distinguish the major cardiomyopathies — hypertrophic, dilated, arrhythmogenic — by autopsy morphology and histology and articulate their forensic significance.
4. Recognize valvular heart disease, congenital heart disease, and other structural causes of sudden death, and integrate the findings with the case reasoning.
5. Apply the molecular autopsy approach in cases of sudden death with structurally normal heart and articulate the family screening implications.

## Defining Sudden Cardiac Death in Forensic Practice

Sudden cardiac death is defined variably in the epidemiology literature but converges on the concept of natural death from a cardiac cause occurring within one hour of the onset of symptoms in a person who was known to be alive within the preceding 24 hours. The forensic pathology working definition modifies this to include unwitnessed deaths where the decedent was known to be alive within 24 hours and where the postmortem findings are consistent with a cardiac mechanism. The forensic significance is that sudden cardiac death represents the single largest category of unexpected death that enters the medicolegal system, dominates the natural-death caseload of most offices, and requires systematic examination to distinguish natural death from the alternative causes with which it may be confused.

The epidemiology of sudden cardiac death differs across age groups in ways that shape the pretest reasoning at autopsy. In decedents over 40 years of age, atherosclerotic coronary artery disease dominates the etiology; the decedent typically has a severe underlying coronary disease with evidence of an acute or subacute event superimposed. In decedents between adolescence and 40 years, structural cardiomyopathies (hypertrophic cardiomyopathy in particular), congenital heart disease (including anomalous coronary artery origin), valvular disease, and inherited arrhythmia syndromes account for a larger fraction of cases. In decedents under 20 years, structurally normal hearts with inherited arrhythmia syndromes as the presumed mechanism become the dominant category, along with commotio cordis, myocarditis, and rare congenital lesions. The autopsy approach adapts to these pretest distributions.

The forensic pathologist encounters sudden cardiac death in a wide range of scenes and contexts. The classic scene is a witnessed collapse in a middle-aged decedent with cardiovascular risk factors, but sudden cardiac death also presents as an unwitnessed death in a residence, as a sudden death during athletic exertion, as an unexpected death of a decedent under medical care for other conditions, and as death during interaction with law enforcement or in custody. Each context has specific reconstruction implications developed elsewhere in this book. This chapter develops the autopsy findings and their interpretation.

### The Reasoning Framework

The reasoning framework for sudden cardiac death is to identify structural disease of sufficient severity to explain sudden death; when structural disease is present and adequate, the case is certified as natural cardiac death from the identified process. When structural disease is present but not adequate to explain sudden death, additional workup pursues either an alternative primary cause or an arrhythmogenic mechanism on the background of the identified disease. When no structural disease is identified, the case enters the differential of sudden arrhythmic death syndrome, and molecular autopsy for inherited arrhythmia syndromes becomes the standard next step. The pathologist walks this reasoning explicitly in the autopsy report so the determination is reconstructible from the record.

**KEY POINT:** The presence of coronary artery disease at autopsy in a middle-aged or elderly decedent does not automatically establish it as the cause of death. The reasoning must satisfy the question: is this disease of sufficient severity to plausibly produce sudden death without an alternative mechanism? A 30 percent coronary stenosis in a 45-year-old is present but does not by itself explain a sudden death, and the reasoning must pursue the alternative causes.

## Coronary Artery Disease

Atherosclerotic coronary artery disease is the dominant cause of sudden cardiac death in adults and requires systematic evaluation at autopsy. The pathologist assesses the extent, distribution, and character of coronary lesions and integrates the findings with any evidence of an acute or subacute event superimposed on the underlying disease.

### Coronary Artery Examination Technique

The coronary arteries are examined by serial 3 mm sectioning perpendicular to the long axis of each artery, from the origin at the aortic root through the major branches. The left main, left anterior descending, circumflex, and right coronary arteries are each examined systematically. Each significant stenosis is documented for location, percent luminal narrowing (assessed from cross-sectional inspection), and character (fibroatheromatous, calcified, thrombotic, dissected). Grossly significant stenosis — typically 75 percent or greater luminal narrowing — is quantified precisely; lesser lesions are documented but do not typically drive the reasoning about sudden death.

The alternative technique of removing the heart with the coronary arteries perfused and formalin-fixed before sectioning is used in some offices, particularly for cases where subtle coronary findings may be central to the reasoning. The perfusion-fixation technique produces cleaner cross-sections and can identify small thrombi more readily than fresh sectioning, but requires equipment and time that most routine autopsies do not accommodate. For the majority of adult coronary cases, systematic fresh 3 mm sectioning is adequate.

Histologic examination of representative coronary sections supports the assessment of atherosclerotic plaque character. Stable fibrous plaques with intact fibrous caps and small lipid cores are the substrate of chronic ischemia rather than the substrate of sudden death. Vulnerable plaques with thin fibrous caps, large lipid cores, and inflammatory infiltrate at the shoulder region are the substrate of acute events — plaque rupture, thrombosis, and acute occlusion. The identification of a vulnerable plaque at the site of an acute event supports the reasoning that the sudden death was mediated by the acute coronary event.

**Acute Coronary Events and Their Recognition**

The classic acute coronary event underlying sudden death is atherosclerotic plaque rupture with subsequent thrombus formation on the exposed plaque and acute coronary occlusion. The thrombus is identified during sectioning as a red or mixed red-white intraluminal mass adherent to the vessel wall at the site of plaque disruption. Histology confirms the thrombus and identifies the underlying plaque. Coronary artery dissection — the tear of the intima with propagation of blood into the media — is a less common but well-documented cause of acute coronary occlusion, particularly in younger adults and in the peripartum period. Coronary spasm as a contributor to sudden death is difficult to document at autopsy because the spasm resolves after death; the diagnosis rests on clinical history and on the exclusion of alternative causes.

Myocardial infarction is the tissue-level counterpart of acute coronary occlusion. Acute infarction is not visible grossly for the first several hours after the event and is identified histologically. Contraction band necrosis and hypereosinophilia of myocytes appear within hours, followed by neutrophilic infiltrate, myocyte necrosis, and eventually granulation tissue and scarring. In sudden death cases where the decedent died within minutes of the acute event, no infarction may be identifiable histologically; the death is arrhythmic on the substrate of the acute coronary occlusion rather than mediated by frank infarction. Documentation of chronic ischemic disease — old scars, myocardial fibrosis, chronic ischemic changes — supports the substrate for arrhythmia even when acute infarction is not identified.

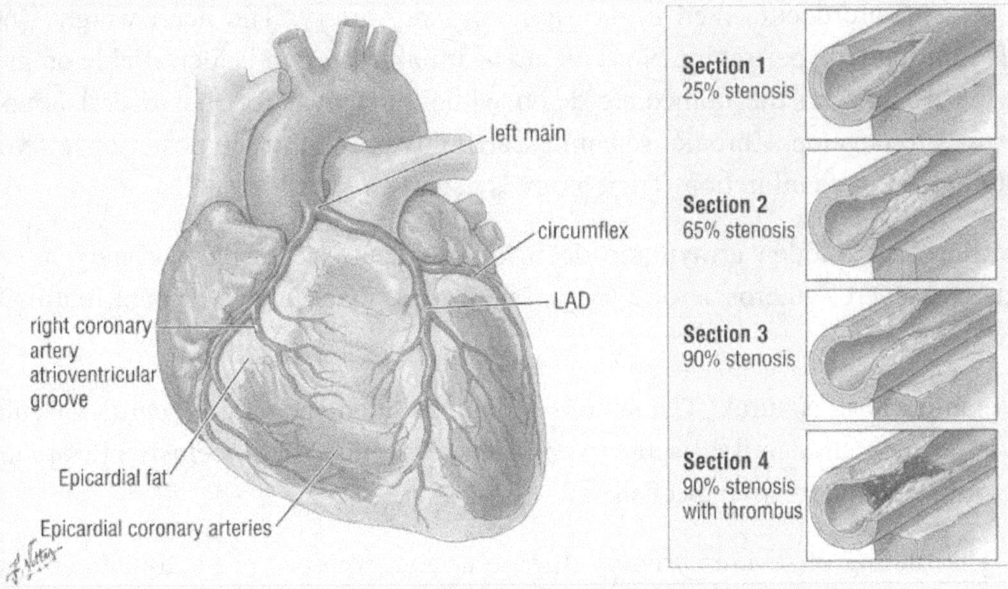


**Figure 10.1: Systematic Coronary Artery Sectioning Approach**

### The Reasoning About Adequacy of Coronary Disease

The reasoning about whether identified coronary disease is adequate to explain sudden death integrates several factors. Severity of stenosis is the first consideration — severe stenosis (75 percent or greater) in one or more major coronary arteries with acute superimposed event (thrombus, plaque rupture) is adequate. Severe stenosis without acute event supports a substrate for arrhythmia but does not by itself establish acute cause; the reasoning must consider what triggered the event. Chronic remote infarction with left ventricular dysfunction supports vulnerability to arrhythmia and can be adequate cause even without acute change. Coronary anomalies (anomalous origin from the wrong sinus, coronary arising from pulmonary artery) can produce sudden death without significant atherosclerotic disease and are documented as separate categories.

### SCENE-TO-CERTIFICATION DECISION SYSTEM — Coronary Artery Sudden Death Arc

---

**Presenting Death Scenario:** A 57-year-old man collapses while shoveling snow in his driveway. Neighbors witness the collapse and initiate CPR immediately. Emergency response arrives within 6 minutes and provides advanced resuscitation without return of spontaneous circulation. Death is pronounced at the scene approximately 30 minutes after collapse. The decedent has a documented history of hypertension, hyperlipidemia, and cigarette smoking, with no prior diagnosis of coronary disease. He had not seen a physician in the preceding two years. The medical examiner's office accepts jurisdiction on the sudden death.

**Autopsy Signature:** External examination documents resuscitation-related sternal contusion and bilateral costochondral rib fractures without other significant findings. Internal examination shows severe atherosclerotic coronary artery disease. The proximal left anterior descending artery shows 95 percent stenosis with an acute occlusive thrombus overlying a ruptured atherosclerotic plaque. Additional severe stenoses (80 percent) are documented in the right coronary artery. The heart weighs 460 grams with concentric left ventricular hypertrophy. No acute myocardial infarction is identifiable on gross inspection or histology, consistent with the immediate death without survival for the several hours required for histologic changes to develop. Chronic ischemic scarring is present in the posterior left ventricular wall consistent with prior remote infarction. Toxicology is negative.

**Cause Determination:** Sudden arrhythmic death due to acute occlusive coronary artery thrombosis superimposed on severe atherosclerotic coronary artery disease, with contributing hypertensive cardiovascular disease.

**Manner Determination:** Natural. The autopsy findings identify natural cardiovascular disease of sufficient severity, with an identified acute event (plaque rupture with occlusive thrombus), to explain sudden death without an alternative mechanism.

**Trap Logic:** The finding of severe coronary disease at autopsy does not automatically establish acute cause when no acute event is identified; the reasoning must document why the disease produced sudden death at this particular time. In this case, the acute occlusive thrombus over a ruptured plaque provides the identified acute event. Without this finding, the reasoning would proceed differently — the severe chronic disease would support the substrate but would require reasoning about the trigger (exertion-related, arrhythmogenic on scar). The trap is to assume sudden death is coronary because coronary disease is common, without documenting the reasoning that ties the death to the disease. The countermeasure is systematic documentation of the acute event or of the substrate-and-trigger reasoning.

**Certification Anchor:** Sudden death from coronary artery disease is certified when severe atherosclerotic disease is identified with an acute event superimposed (occlusive thrombus over ruptured plaque, coronary dissection, or acute occlusion), or when severe chronic disease with substrate for arrhythmia (chronic infarction, severe hypertrophy) is documented with reasoning about the trigger. The reasoning is stated in the autopsy report so the determination is reconstructible.

## Cardiomyopathies

The cardiomyopathies are structural diseases of the myocardium producing dysfunction independent of coronary disease, valvular disease, or hypertension. Three principal categories — hypertrophic, dilated, and arrhythmogenic — account for the vast majority of cardiomyopathy-related sudden deaths encountered in forensic practice.

### Hypertrophic Cardiomyopathy

Hypertrophic cardiomyopathy is the most common inherited cardiovascular disease and is the leading cause of sudden cardiac death in young athletes and in decedents under 35 years of age in most series. It is characterized by asymmetric or diffuse ventricular hypertrophy with disorganized myocyte architecture (myocyte disarray) on histology. The gross findings include heart weight elevated for body habitus (often 400 to 600 grams or more in an adult of average size), septal thickness greater than 15 mm (with variability by measurement site), and, in the classic obstructive form, asymmetric septal hypertrophy with anterior mitral valve leaflet contact producing dynamic outflow obstruction. Histology shows characteristic myocyte disarray with disorganized myofibril orientation, myocyte hypertrophy, and interstitial fibrosis; these findings are the pathognomonic microscopic features.

The forensic significance of hypertrophic cardiomyopathy extends beyond the individual case because it is genetic. Identification of hypertrophic cardiomyopathy in a decedent triggers recommendation for cardiological evaluation of first-degree relatives, who carry a 50 percent risk of inheriting the causative variant. Family screening has substantial implications for identification of at-risk relatives before their own sudden death, and this family communication is one of the more important interventions the forensic pathology office can facilitate. Molecular autopsy can confirm the specific causative variant when tissue is preserved, supporting focused family screening.

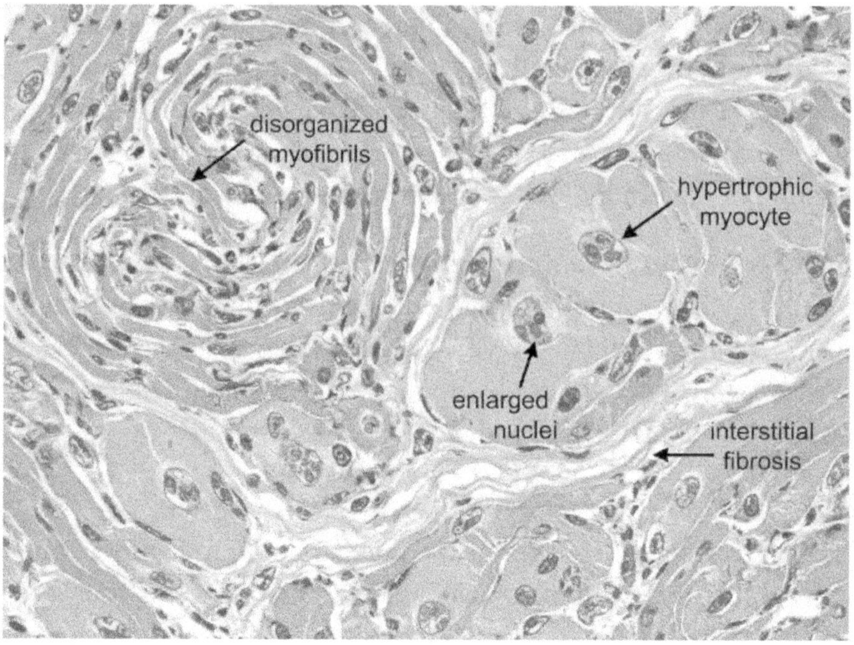


### Dilated Cardiomyopathy

Dilated cardiomyopathy is characterized by four-chamber dilation with impaired systolic function and, at autopsy, cardiomegaly with dilated ventricles and relatively thin ventricular walls. Multiple etiologies converge on the dilated cardiomyopathy phenotype: idiopathic (many cases with genetic contribution), post-viral (following myocarditis with progressive remodeling), toxic (chronic alcohol exposure being the classic pattern), peripartum, and drug-induced (chemotherapy agents including anthracyclines being the classic causes). The autopsy identifies the dilated phenotype and, where possible, the underlying etiology. Sudden death in dilated cardiomyopathy is arrhythmic, occurring on the substrate of chamber dilation, myocardial fibrosis, and electrical remodeling.

### Arrhythmogenic Cardiomyopathy

Arrhythmogenic cardiomyopathy — previously termed arrhythmogenic right ventricular cardiomyopathy (ARVC) and now recognized to affect left ventricle in some variants — is characterized by fibrofatty replacement of the ventricular myocardium, particularly of the right ventricular free wall. The gross findings include right ventricular dilation, thinning of the right ventricular wall with visible fatty infiltration through the epicardium, and, when the left ventricle is involved, similar findings in the left ventricular wall. Histology confirms the fibrofatty replacement of myocardium. The disease is genetic in most cases, with mutations in desmosomal proteins accounting for the majority of identified variants. Sudden death, often during exertion, is a characteristic presentation, and the disease has particular importance in young athletes where it must be considered in cases of sudden death during exercise.

## Valvular and Congenital Heart Disease

Valvular heart disease and congenital heart disease account for a smaller but important fraction of sudden cardiac deaths and require systematic examination for identification.

### Aortic Stenosis

Aortic stenosis is a documented cause of sudden death, particularly in the elderly with degenerative calcific stenosis and in adults with congenital bicuspid aortic valve. The forensic identification of hemodynamically severe aortic stenosis requires assessment of the valve morphology (leaflet number, thickness, calcification, mobility) at autopsy. Severe stenosis is characterized by heavily calcified, thickened, immobile leaflets; the annular circumference and orifice area cannot be reliably measured at postmortem but qualitative assessment is possible. In cases of sudden death with severe aortic stenosis identified, the reasoning integrates the valve findings with the clinical history and with the exclusion of alternative causes.

### Mitral Valve Prolapse

Mitral valve prolapse — characterized by myxomatous degeneration of the leaflets with billowing into the left atrium during systole — has been documented as a cause of sudden death in a subset of patients, particularly those with bileaflet involvement and characteristic tricuspid regurgitation on echocardiography during life. The forensic significance is that mitral valve prolapse is prevalent (2 to 3 percent of the general population) but sudden death from it is rare; the reasoning must integrate the finding with other supporting evidence and typically requires exclusion of alternative causes before the mitral prolapse is accepted as the primary cause.

### Anomalous Coronary Artery Origin

Anomalous origin of a coronary artery from the opposite sinus of Valsalva — particularly left coronary from the right sinus or right coronary from the left sinus — is a specific congenital abnormality that can produce sudden death during exercise. The mechanism reflects the anomalous artery's course between the aorta and pulmonary artery, where it is compressed during exercise-induced increases in cardiac output. The finding is easily missed at autopsy if not specifically looked for; the entering fellow trains to examine the coronary origins as a standard part of every cardiac examination and to document the anatomical relationships. Anomalous coronary origin is a leading cause of sudden death in young athletes and is a diagnosis that changes the manner determination from unexplained sudden death to natural cardiac death with a specific structural cause.

### Aortic Dissection as Sudden Cardiac Death

Acute aortic dissection is a category of sudden cardiac-adjacent death that requires specific attention. The tear in the aortic intima propagates within the media, producing a false lumen that may extend proximally into the coronary ostia or into the pericardial sac (producing hemopericardium and cardiac tamponade) or distally along the aorta. Sudden death from aortic dissection typically occurs from tamponade, coronary compromise, or exsanguination. The pretest reasoning is important: aortic dissection is associated with hypertension, with connective tissue disease (Marfan syndrome, Ehlers-Danlos vascular type, Loeys-Dietz syndrome), with bicuspid aortic valve, and with cocaine use. The autopsy identifies the intimal tear typically in the ascending aorta or in the descending thoracic aorta, follows the dissection plane through the aortic media, and documents the extent of proximal and distal propagation. Hemopericardium with tamponade is the classic acute lethal complication and is documented by measurement of pericardial blood at autopsy.

### Myocarditis

Myocarditis is a category of myocardial inflammation that can produce sudden death, particularly in young decedents. The classic viral myocarditides — coxsackievirus, adenovirus, parvovirus B19 — are established causes, and, since 2020, SARS-CoV-2 has entered the differential in populations exposed to significant viral disease. Non-viral causes include autoimmune myocarditis (particularly giant cell myocarditis with characteristic multinucleated giant cells on histology), drug-induced myocarditis (with specific patterns for immune checkpoint inhibitor myocarditis and other agents), and eosinophilic myocarditis. The autopsy findings include cardiomegaly, ventricular dilation, and myocardial pallor with focal or diffuse hemorrhage. Histology confirms the diagnosis with lymphocytic (or other characteristic cellular) infiltrate with associated myocyte necrosis — the Dallas criteria for pathological diagnosis of myocarditis. Sudden death in myocarditis is arrhythmic on the substrate of the inflamed myocardium and may occur early in the course of disease when clinical presentation has been subtle or absent.

**Figure 10.3**
Severe Coronary Artery Stenosis with Occlusive Thrombus

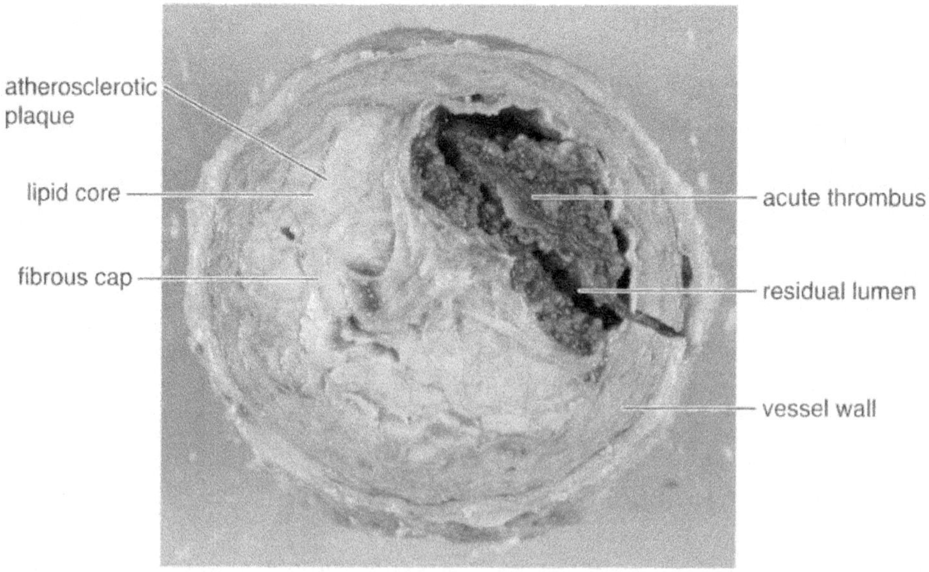

### Left Ventricular Hypertrophy as Independent Substrate

Left ventricular hypertrophy from hypertension or from other causes is an independent substrate for arrhythmic sudden death, even in the absence of coronary disease or of cardiomyopathy per se. Hypertensive heart disease with concentric left ventricular hypertrophy is common in decedents with poorly controlled hypertension, and the hypertrophied myocardium is electrically vulnerable to arrhythmia particularly during physiologic stress. The autopsy identifies the hypertrophy by increased ventricular wall thickness and by increased heart weight for body habitus, integrated with the antecedent history and with the exclusion of other structural causes. Sudden death in hypertensive heart disease is typically certified as sudden arrhythmic death due to hypertensive cardiovascular disease when the pattern is present.

## Inherited Arrhythmia Syndromes

The inherited arrhythmia syndromes — long QT syndrome, catecholaminergic polymorphic ventricular tachycardia, Brugada syndrome, short QT syndrome, and related conditions — produce sudden death in decedents with structurally normal hearts on gross and microscopic examination. The autopsy in these cases is negative for structural disease, and the diagnosis is established by molecular autopsy for the causative variant.

### The Structurally Normal Heart

The decedent with sudden death and structurally normal heart on complete autopsy presents a specific diagnostic challenge. The category is termed sudden arrhythmic death syndrome (SADS) in the epidemiology literature. Molecular autopsy for the panel of inherited arrhythmia syndrome genes — KCNQ1, KCNH2, SCN5A, RYR2, CASQ2, and others depending on the specific panel — identifies a causative variant in approximately 30 percent of SADS cases in published series. The identification has immediate implications for surviving relatives, who may carry the same variant and benefit from cardiological evaluation and preventive treatment. Molecular autopsy has become standard of care in SADS cases at offices with the resources to support it, and family notification with recommendation for cardiological evaluation of first-degree relatives is a standard practice regardless of whether molecular studies are available.

**SCENE-TO-CERTIFICATION DECISION SYSTEM — Structurally Normal Heart / Molecular Autopsy Arc**

---

**Presenting Death Scenario:** A 17-year-old girl is found deceased in bed by her mother in the morning. There is no evidence of injury and no signs of struggle at the scene. She had no known medical history. She had participated in high school swimming and had passed a pre-participation physical examination six months earlier. The mother reports that her daughter had recently had two episodes of syncope — attributed at the time to dehydration — and had complained of a racing heartbeat during swimming practice on multiple occasions. The medical examiner's office accepts jurisdiction on the sudden death of a young person.

**Autopsy Signature:** External examination is unremarkable. Internal examination shows a structurally normal heart of appropriate size for body habitus (250 grams; ventricular wall thicknesses normal; valves morphologically normal; coronary arteries widely patent without atherosclerotic or anomalous origin findings). Histology of the myocardium shows no fibrosis, no myocyte disarray, no infiltrative disease, and no evidence of myocarditis. The lungs, brain, and other organs are unremarkable. Toxicology is negative. Peripheral blood and tissue (myocardium, spleen, liver) are retained frozen for molecular studies. The pathologist initiates molecular autopsy for the inherited arrhythmia syndrome panel and, given the history of exertion-related symptoms and swimming (a documented trigger), specifically requests screening for long QT syndrome including the type 1 variant most associated with swimming-related triggering.

**Cause Determination:** Sudden arrhythmic death syndrome, pending molecular autopsy results. The determination will be updated to include the specific inherited arrhythmia syndrome if a causative variant is identified.

**Manner Determination:** Natural. The autopsy findings and history support natural sudden arrhythmic death; no alternative mechanism is identified.

**Trap Logic:** The structurally normal heart at autopsy does not exclude cardiac cause; it identifies the case as sudden arrhythmic death syndrome pending molecular workup. The trap is to close the case as "sudden death, cause undetermined" without initiating molecular autopsy or family notification. The countermeasure is systematic identification of SADS cases at intake, retention of appropriate specimens for molecular analysis, and communication with family regarding the recommendation for cardiological evaluation of first-degree relatives regardless of molecular results. In this case, the antecedent history of exertion-related symptoms and swimming is a specific pointer to long QT syndrome type 1, and the molecular panel is specifically requested to include this variant.

**Certification Anchor:** Sudden arrhythmic death syndrome in a young decedent with structurally normal heart triggers molecular autopsy and family notification. The retention of appropriate specimens (frozen tissue and blood) at the primary autopsy is essential; failure to preserve specimens forecloses the molecular workup and the family screening opportunity that follows. Family members of SADS decedents warrant cardiological evaluation regardless of the molecular result.

## The Autopsy Approach to Sudden Cardiac Death

The autopsy approach to sudden cardiac death integrates systematic cardiac examination with appropriate ancillary studies and, in cases of structurally normal heart, molecular autopsy and family notification. The approach is calibrated to the pretest probability determined by age, history, and scene.

### Standard Cardiac Examination

Standard cardiac examination includes heart weight, chamber examination with wall thickness measurements, valve examination with leaflet assessment, coronary artery origin examination for anomalous origin, systematic 3 mm sectioning of the coronary arteries, and multiple representative histologic sections from anterior wall, posterior wall, septum, papillary muscles, and the four chambers. Conduction system examination — sinoatrial node, atrioventricular node, His bundle and bundle branches — is not routinely performed but is available for cases where inherited arrhythmia is on the differential and the conduction system findings may support the diagnosis.

### Documentation for Family and Genetic Counseling

Documentation of the cardiac findings in sudden death cases carries implications beyond the immediate case reasoning. Family members of decedents with identified inherited cardiovascular disease benefit from communication of the finding and recommendation for cardiological evaluation. The medical examiner's office is often the first source of this information to the family, and the communication is calibrated to family circumstances — often mediated through the death investigator or through office administrative staff and integrated with grief counseling resources where available. The autopsy report is retained as a medical record that family members may need to share with their own physicians during genetic evaluation.

### Sudden Death From Pulmonary Embolism

Pulmonary embolism accounts for a significant fraction of sudden deaths certified as natural cause and warrants systematic consideration in every case of unexpected death without immediately obvious cardiac findings. The pretest reasoning identifies risk factors: recent immobilization (postoperative state, prolonged travel, hospitalization), malignancy, hormonal exposure (oral contraceptives, hormone replacement), pregnancy and the postpartum period, obesity, prior venous thromboembolic disease, and inherited thrombophilias. Autopsy identifies pulmonary embolism by careful bilateral pulmonary artery examination — the main pulmonary arteries and their branches are opened and inspected before extensive dissection disturbs any thromboemboli. Saddle emboli lodged at the pulmonary artery bifurcation, main branch emboli, and multiple smaller emboli scattered through the segmental branches each have specific reconstruction implications. Confirmation of the source (deep vein thrombosis in the lower extremities, or less commonly in the pelvic or upper extremity venous system) supports the diagnosis. Sudden death from massive pulmonary embolism reflects acute right heart failure and cardiac arrest; the decedent may have symptoms in the preceding hours (dyspnea, chest pain, syncope) or may collapse abruptly without warning.

### Conduction System Disorders

The cardiac conduction system — sinoatrial node, atrioventricular node, His bundle, bundle branches, Purkinje network — mediates the electrical activation sequence of the heart. Disorders of the conduction system can produce sudden death through complete heart block with escape failure, through tachyarrhythmia from re-entry circuits, or through accessory pathway conduction (as in Wolff-Parkinson-White syndrome). The conduction system is not routinely examined in most forensic autopsies because its histological examination requires specialized technique and interpretation, but consultation with a cardiac conduction pathologist is available when the case reasoning depends on identifying a conduction system abnormality. Structural conduction system disease may accompany other cardiovascular disease (aortic stenosis with calcification extending into the conduction system, cardiomyopathy with fibrosis involving the bundle branches) or may be primary (idiopathic bundle branch fibrosis in older decedents, Lenegre disease).

### Sudden Death in Young Athletes

Sudden death of a young athlete during or shortly after competition or training is a specific category of substantial public and forensic attention. Published series identify hypertrophic cardiomyopathy as the leading structural cause, followed by anomalous coronary artery origin, myocarditis, arrhythmogenic cardiomyopathy, and commotio cordis (sudden arrhythmic death from precordial impact during a specific vulnerable phase of the cardiac cycle, most classically from a projectile such as a baseball). Substantial fractions of athletic sudden deaths have structurally normal hearts on complete autopsy and enter the sudden arrhythmic death syndrome category with molecular autopsy indicated. The pretest reasoning in an athletic sudden death case includes attention to the specific circumstances (which sport, what phase of activity, any recent symptoms), the exclusion of drug or supplement use (some sports supplements and performance-enhancing drugs have documented cardiotoxicity), and the family history of premature cardiac death. The autopsy applies systematic examination of every category and, where the heart is structurally normal, initiates molecular autopsy and family notification.

**CLINICAL PEARL:** Sudden death in a young athlete requires a systematic cardiac evaluation focused on the categories with the highest pretest probability in that population: hypertrophic cardiomyopathy (detailed septal and free wall measurement, myocyte disarray on histology), anomalous coronary origin (specific examination of the coronary origins from the sinuses of Valsalva), arrhythmogenic cardiomyopathy (systematic examination of the right ventricular free wall), myocarditis (representative myocardial histology), and, when heart is structurally normal, molecular autopsy for inherited arrhythmia syndromes. Family notification with recommendation for cardiological evaluation of first-degree relatives is standard practice.

### Communicating Sudden Cardiac Death Findings to Families

The communication of sudden cardiac death findings to families is one of the more consequential communications the forensic pathology office produces. Families of decedents with sudden cardiac death frequently seek understanding of what happened, whether it could have been prevented, and — in cases of inherited disease — whether other family members are at risk. The pathologist supports the communication through the autopsy report (written for a family audience as well as a professional audience where feasible), through direct conversation with the family in some offices, and through documentation of the genetic implications where applicable. Family notification of the recommendation for cardiological evaluation of first-degree relatives in cases of hypertrophic cardiomyopathy, arrhythmogenic cardiomyopathy, dilated cardiomyopathy with genetic basis, and sudden arrhythmic death syndrome is a professional obligation that the office typically integrates with the return of the autopsy report to the family. The communication may occur through a variety of channels — the pathologist directly, the death investigator, office administrative staff — depending on the office structure and the family circumstances.

**SCENE-TO-CERTIFICATION DECISION SYSTEM — Sudden Cardiac Death Determination Arcs**

**The Age-Stratified Framework:** Sudden cardiac death etiology varies with age. Coronary atherosclerotic disease dominates over 40; structural cardiomyopathies, congenital disease, and inherited arrhythmia syndromes dominate under 40. The autopsy approach adapts to the pretest distribution of the age group.

**The Coronary Disease Reasoning:** Severe coronary artery disease at autopsy supports natural cardiac death when accompanied by an acute event (thrombus, plaque rupture) or by substrate-and-trigger reasoning (severe chronic disease, remote infarction, exertion or physiologic stress). The reasoning is documented in the report; the finding alone does not automatically establish acute cause.

**The Cardiomyopathies:** Hypertrophic cardiomyopathy (with characteristic myocyte disarray on histology), dilated cardiomyopathy (with the four-chamber dilated phenotype), and arrhythmogenic cardiomyopathy (with fibrofatty replacement of the ventricular wall) are the principal categories. All have genetic bases with family screening implications.

**Structural Causes Beyond Coronary:** Aortic stenosis, mitral valve prolapse (in specific subsets), anomalous coronary artery origin, and other congenital lesions account for a subset of sudden deaths. Systematic examination identifies these findings when present; anomalous coronary origin is a specific finding that is easily missed without deliberate looking.

**The Structurally Normal Heart:** Sudden death with structurally normal heart on complete autopsy is sudden arrhythmic death syndrome, and the standard workup is molecular autopsy for inherited arrhythmia syndrome variants together with family notification and recommendation for cardiological evaluation of first-degree relatives. Retention of appropriate specimens at the primary autopsy is essential.

## Summary and Key Concepts

Sudden cardiac death is the leading category of unexpected natural death entering the medicolegal system and requires systematic examination to distinguish from alternative causes. The epidemiology varies substantially by age group, with coronary atherosclerotic disease dominating over 40 and structural, congenital, and inherited electrical causes dominating in younger decedents.

Coronary artery disease is evaluated by systematic 3 mm sectioning with documentation of stenosis severity, plaque character, and any acute event (thrombus, plaque rupture, dissection). The reasoning about adequacy of coronary disease as cause of sudden death integrates the severity of disease with the presence or absence of an acute event.

The cardiomyopathies — hypertrophic, dilated, arrhythmogenic — are principal categories of structural heart disease producing sudden death and each has genetic bases with family screening implications.

Hypertrophic cardiomyopathy is the leading cause of sudden death in young athletes and requires specific attention in the pretest reasoning for this population.

Valvular disease (aortic stenosis, mitral valve prolapse in specific subsets) and congenital heart disease (anomalous coronary artery origin, in particular) account for a subset of sudden deaths. Anomalous coronary origin is a specific finding easily missed without deliberate examination of the coronary origins and is a leading cause of sudden death in young athletes.

Sudden death with structurally normal heart is sudden arrhythmic death syndrome. Molecular autopsy for inherited arrhythmia syndrome variants identifies a causative variant in approximately 30 percent of cases, and family notification with recommendation for cardiological evaluation of first-degree relatives is standard practice regardless of molecular results. Retention of appropriate specimens at the primary autopsy is essential to preserve the molecular workup opportunity.

# CHAPTER 11: SUDDEN DEATH FROM NEUROLOGICAL, PULMONARY, AND OTHER NATURAL CAUSES

**Learning Objectives**

1. Recognize the neurological causes of sudden natural death and reason from the autopsy findings to the specific mechanism.
2. Distinguish pulmonary embolism, asthma, and other pulmonary causes of sudden death by autopsy findings and clinical integration.
3. Identify gastrointestinal, renal, and hepatic causes of sudden death, particularly those that may not be immediately apparent on external examination.
4. Recognize endocrine emergencies (diabetic ketoacidosis, adrenal crisis) and metabolic causes of sudden death from postmortem findings and ancillary testing.
5. Apply systematic reasoning to the case of natural sudden death without an identified cause — the undetermined natural death — and articulate when the classification is appropriate.

## Neurological Causes of Sudden Death

Neurological causes account for a significant fraction of natural sudden deaths after cardiac cause has been excluded. The mechanisms range from acute vascular events (intracranial hemorrhage from ruptured aneurysm or from spontaneous intracerebral hemorrhage), through seizure-related death, to less common causes including brain herniation from mass effect and complications of chronic neurologic disease. The autopsy approach to suspected neurological sudden death combines careful gross examination of the brain with formalin fixation for detailed sectioning and, when indicated, neuropathology consultation.

The pretest reasoning for neurological sudden death considers age, antecedent history, and scene evidence. Ruptured berry aneurysm producing subarachnoid hemorrhage is a classic cause in decedents from the third through sixth decades and is often associated with a scene report of sudden severe headache, abrupt collapse, and rapid unresponsiveness. Spontaneous intracerebral hemorrhage is more common in older decedents with hypertension. Seizure-related death spans the age spectrum but has particular importance in decedents with known epilepsy, where sudden unexpected death in epilepsy (SUDEP) is a recognized category. Meningitis and other infectious causes require history of preceding febrile illness or immunocompromise for the pretest reasoning to identify them.

### Ruptured Berry Aneurysm and Subarachnoid Hemorrhage

The ruptured berry aneurysm at a branch point of the circle of Willis producing subarachnoid hemorrhage is the classic scene of neurological sudden death. The scene is typically of a previously well decedent who complained of sudden severe headache before collapsing, or who was found dead without warning.

Autopsy identifies extensive subarachnoid blood over the base of the brain and, on careful dissection, the site of the ruptured aneurysm. The circle of Willis anatomy — the anterior cerebral, middle cerebral, and posterior cerebral arteries connected by anterior and posterior communicating arteries — has predictable sites for aneurysm formation. The anterior communicating artery is the single most common site, followed by the posterior communicating artery, the middle cerebral bifurcation, and the basilar tip. Multiple aneurysms are documented in a substantial minority of aneurysm cases and may or may not include the ruptured lesion at the time of death.

The examination technique matters. The brain is removed with the arachnoid intact so the subarachnoid blood is preserved for photographic documentation. The base of the brain is inspected before the vessels are disturbed. The circle of Willis is dissected carefully to identify the aneurysm; small aneurysms can be missed if the dissection is rushed. Fixation of the brain before final examination supports detailed identification when the initial gross inspection is inconclusive. Photographs of the base of the brain with the arachnoid intact document the extent and distribution of the subarachnoid blood — findings that support the reconstruction of which aneurysm ruptured when multiple are present.

**Figure 11.1:** Circle of Willis Anatomy and Common Sites of Berry Aneurysm Formation

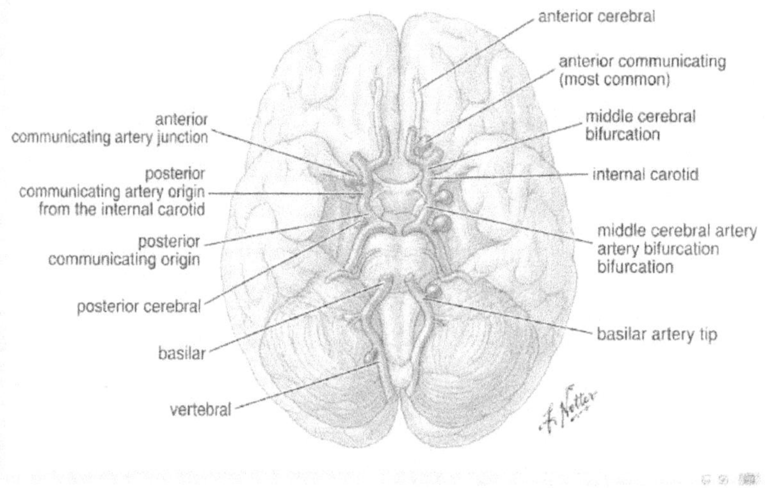


## Spontaneous Intracerebral Hemorrhage

Spontaneous intracerebral hemorrhage — hemorrhage into the brain parenchyma without prior trauma — is the classic hypertensive stroke, producing sudden collapse and death in decedents with poorly controlled hypertension. The bleeding typically originates from small perforating arteries with hypertensive vascular changes, and the classic sites are the basal ganglia, thalamus, pons, and cerebellum. The autopsy identifies the location of the hematoma, its extent, any extension into the ventricular system (which worsens the prognosis substantially), and any mass effect. Hypertensive vascular changes on histology (arteriolar hyalinosis, Charcot-Bouchard microaneurysms) confirm the pathogenetic setting. Alternative causes of intracerebral hemorrhage include amyloid angiopathy in elderly decedents (cortical hemorrhage location, cerebral amyloid on histology), arteriovenous malformation (identified by careful dissection through the hemorrhage), and hemorrhagic transformation of ischemic stroke.

## Seizure-Related Death and SUDEP

Sudden unexpected death in epilepsy (SUDEP) is a documented category of sudden death in decedents with known epilepsy. The mechanism is incompletely understood but is thought to involve postictal cardiac arrhythmia, apnea, or a combination of the two. The autopsy findings are typically nonspecific: the decedent has a documented history of epilepsy (often uncontrolled), often prone in bed on the pillow (a pattern suggesting the death occurred during or after a seizure), and the autopsy shows no structural cause of death. Toxicology may show low or absent antiepileptic drug levels supporting nonadherence as a contributing factor. The manner is natural; the certification typically states sudden unexpected death in epilepsy or sudden death associated with epilepsy. Family notification and communication about SUDEP risk for other family members with epilepsy is often integrated with the case closure.

Deaths during acute seizure activity differ. Aspiration of gastric contents during seizure with subsequent asphyxial mechanism, drowning during seizure in the bathtub or in water, and traumatic death during seizure (falls, particularly from height) are documented mechanisms. Each is certified with reference to the specific mechanism and its interaction with the underlying epilepsy. Status epilepticus — prolonged seizure activity — has its own metabolic and cardiovascular consequences and can produce sudden death independent of SUDEP mechanism.

## Ischemic Stroke and Cerebral Herniation

Massive ischemic stroke with cerebral herniation can produce sudden death, particularly in decedents with large territory infarcts from proximal arterial occlusion (internal carotid or proximal middle cerebral artery). The mechanism reflects the expanding cerebral edema after infarction, with mass effect producing herniation of brain tissue across dural reflections (uncal herniation across the tentorium, tonsillar herniation through the foramen magnum) with brainstem compression and death. The autopsy identifies the ischemic territory (with characteristic pallor and softening in early cases, or with cystic encephalomalacia in remote cases), the herniation pattern (with characteristic notching of the uncus, tonsils, and mesial temporal lobe against dural edges), and the vascular source of the infarction (embolic source from cardiac disease, thrombotic occlusion of atherosclerotic vessel). Reasoning about the vascular source integrates the pattern of infarction with the coronary and cerebrovascular findings and with the antecedent history.

## Chronic Neurological Disease as Substrate

Decedents with chronic neurological disease including neurodegenerative disorders (Alzheimer, Parkinson, multiple system atrophy), chronic epilepsy, and remote traumatic brain injury may present with sudden death that reflects the substrate of the chronic disease rather than an acute event. Autopsy findings show the chronic disease features — cortical atrophy, characteristic proteinopathy on histology, remote traumatic scarring — and the sudden death is reasoned as complications of the underlying disease. Sudden aspiration in an advanced Parkinson decedent with severe dysphagia, sudden death in a decedent with advanced dementia and multiple comorbidities, and sudden death after minor injury in a decedent with remote traumatic brain injury each represent this category. The certification reflects the interaction of the chronic disease with the immediate mechanism.

**SCENE-TO-CERTIFICATION DECISION SYSTEM — Neurological Sudden Death Reasoning Arc**

---

**Presenting Death Scenario:** A 42-year-old woman collapses at her workplace shortly after complaining of a sudden severe headache to a coworker. Emergency response arrives within 8 minutes and finds her unresponsive. She is transported to the emergency department where she is pronounced dead approximately 30 minutes after collapse despite advanced resuscitation. She has no known medical history apart from occasional migraine headaches. The medical examiner's office accepts jurisdiction on the sudden death. Her family reports that her mother died suddenly at age 45 from a brain hemorrhage.

**Autopsy Signature:** External examination documents resuscitation-related sternal contusion. Internal examination shows an unremarkable heart, lungs, and abdominal organs. Cranial examination shows extensive subarachnoid hemorrhage over the base of the brain, extending into the ventricular system through the third ventricle. The brain is fixed for one week before detailed sectioning. Careful dissection of the circle of Willis identifies a 6 mm saccular aneurysm at the anterior communicating artery with a visible rupture site through the wall. No additional aneurysms are identified. Toxicology is negative.

**Cause Determination:** Ruptured saccular aneurysm of the anterior communicating artery with subarachnoid hemorrhage.

**Manner Determination:** Natural.

**Trap Logic:** Subarachnoid hemorrhage may be traumatic or spontaneous. In a decedent with recent head trauma, the reasoning must distinguish traumatic subarachnoid hemorrhage (typically over the convexity, often unilateral, associated with cortical contusion) from spontaneous aneurysmal hemorrhage (typically over the base of the brain, often diffuse, associated with an identified aneurysm). In this case, the absence of trauma history and the classic pattern of basal subarachnoid blood with an identified anterior communicating aneurysm supports the spontaneous mechanism. A related trap is failure to identify the ruptured aneurysm when the initial gross inspection is negative; brain fixation and careful dissection are essential in these cases.

**Certification Anchor:** Ruptured berry aneurysm producing subarachnoid hemorrhage is confirmed by careful dissection of the circle of Willis after brain fixation, with photographic documentation of the aneurysm and its rupture site. Family history of sudden death from brain hemorrhage in a first-degree relative supports the recommendation for cardiological and neurological screening of surviving family members for familial aneurysm predisposition.

## Pulmonary Causes of Sudden Death

Pulmonary causes of sudden natural death include pulmonary embolism (developed briefly in Chapter 10 and expanded here), acute asthma with severe bronchospasm, alveolar hemorrhage syndromes, and less common causes including pulmonary hypertension crisis and pulmonary infection.

### Pulmonary Embolism: Detailed Reasoning

Pulmonary embolism accounts for a substantial fraction of sudden deaths certified as natural. The pretest reasoning identifies risk factors: recent immobilization (postoperative state, prolonged travel, hospitalization), malignancy with active or recent treatment, hormonal exposure (oral contraceptives, hormone replacement therapy), pregnancy and the postpartum period, obesity, prior venous thromboembolic disease, and inherited thrombophilias (factor V Leiden, prothrombin gene variant, protein C or S deficiency, antithrombin deficiency). The autopsy approach identifies pulmonary embolism by careful bilateral pulmonary artery examination performed before extensive dissection disturbs thromboemboli. The main pulmonary arteries and their major branches are opened systematically, and any thromboembolus is documented for location, size, and the character of the thrombus (fresh, organizing, remote).

Saddle emboli lodged at the pulmonary artery bifurcation are the classic massive pulmonary embolism with sudden death; the mechanism is acute right heart failure from the abrupt obstruction of pulmonary blood flow. Multiple smaller emboli scattered through the pulmonary vasculature can also produce cardiovascular collapse. The source is typically deep vein thrombosis in the lower extremities, and examination of the deep veins of the legs — the popliteal, femoral, and iliac veins — typically identifies the source thrombus. When the source thrombus has embolized completely, the source vein may be difficult to identify. Peripheral pulmonary emboli from chronic recurrent embolism without a single massive event are documented in cases with organizing thrombi and pulmonary hypertensive changes.

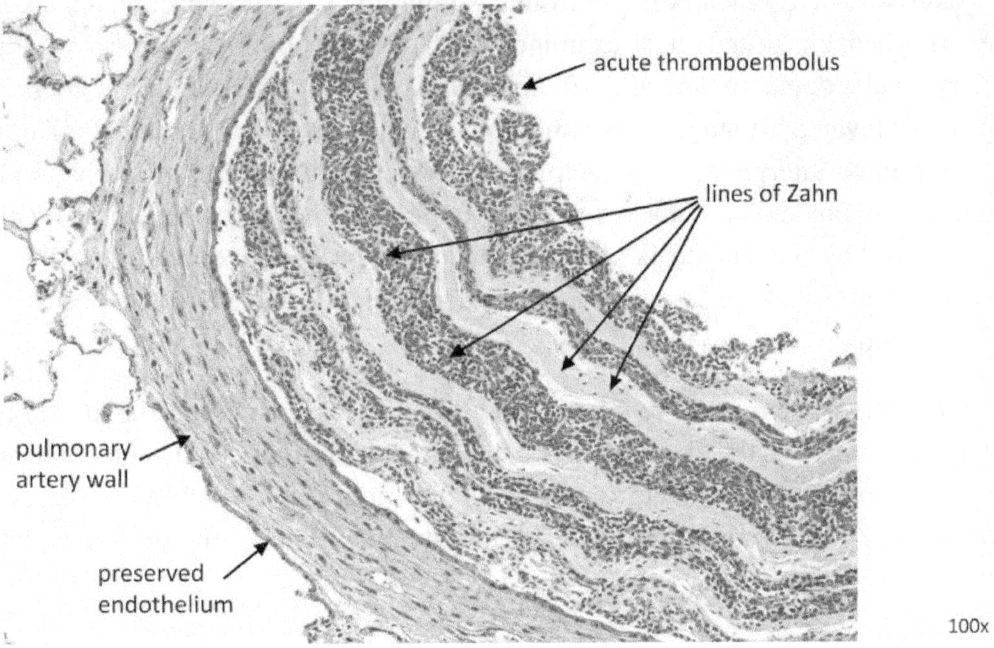

### Acute Asthma Death

Acute asthma exacerbation with sudden death occurs in decedents with known asthma, particularly those with poorly controlled disease, nonadherence to controller medications, prior severe exacerbations, and specific risk factors including allergen exposure, respiratory infection, and beta-agonist overuse. The autopsy findings include hyperinflated lungs (with the surfaces overlapping the anterior mediastinum), extensive mucus plugging of the airways with tenacious mucous material occluding bronchi and bronchioles, and eosinophilic inflammation on histology of the airway walls. The diagnosis integrates the antecedent history of asthma, the scene evidence (medications present, the pattern of preceding illness), the autopsy findings, and the exclusion of alternative causes.

### Alveolar Hemorrhage and Other Pulmonary Emergencies

Diffuse alveolar hemorrhage is a category of pulmonary emergency with characteristic findings of extensive intra-alveolar red blood cells and hemosiderin. Causes include autoimmune disease (Goodpasture syndrome, ANCA-associated vasculitis, systemic lupus with pulmonary hemorrhage), coagulopathy, and drug reactions. The autopsy documents the pulmonary findings and integrates with clinical history to identify the specific etiology when possible. Pulmonary hypertension crisis — acute right heart failure in decedents with severe chronic pulmonary hypertension — produces sudden death with autopsy findings including right ventricular hypertrophy, dilated pulmonary arteries, and, on histology, characteristic plexiform lesions of severe pulmonary hypertension.

### Fatal Asthma and Anaphylaxis

The distinction between sudden death from asthma exacerbation and sudden death from anaphylaxis is important because the two conditions overlap in some features but reflect different mechanisms. Anaphylaxis is a systemic immunological reaction with airway involvement (laryngeal edema, bronchospasm), cardiovascular collapse from vasodilation and third-spacing, and skin findings (urticaria, angioedema) when the decedent is examined shortly after collapse. Autopsy findings in anaphylaxis include laryngeal edema (a specific finding when present), pulmonary hyperinflation with mucus plugging, and elevated tryptase in postmortem serum (a marker of mast cell degranulation, though postmortem tryptase interpretation is complicated by potential postmortem elevation from tissue release). The setting of anaphylaxis — known allergen exposure, food or medication ingestion shortly before collapse — supports the diagnosis. Anaphylaxis from bee stings, food ingestion (peanuts, tree nuts, shellfish being common), or medication (particularly antibiotic and NSAID exposures) is a specific pattern requiring recognition.

**EVIDENCE:** Postmortem tryptase measurement in suspected anaphylaxis has documented limitations. Elevated tryptase supports the diagnosis when the clinical setting is consistent, but tryptase can be elevated postmortem for reasons other than antemortem anaphylaxis, and normal tryptase does not exclude anaphylaxis when the setting supports it. The measurement is one line of evidence within an integrated diagnosis.

## Gastrointestinal, Renal, and Hepatic Causes

### Gastrointestinal Hemorrhage

Massive gastrointestinal hemorrhage can produce sudden death, most classically from ruptured esophageal varices in decedents with cirrhotic portal hypertension. The scene evidence often includes vomited blood (hematemesis) or melena. Autopsy identifies large amounts of intraluminal blood in the stomach, small intestine, and colon; the source is identified by systematic examination of the esophagogastroduodenal mucosa and, when varices are present, of the esophageal submucosal veins. Alternative sources include peptic ulcer disease with erosion into a major artery (posterior duodenal ulcer eroding into the gastroduodenal artery), Mallory-Weiss tears at the gastroesophageal junction (typically producing survivable hemorrhage but occasionally massive), aortoenteric fistula (rare, associated with aortic prosthetic grafts), and colonic sources including diverticular hemorrhage and colon cancer with erosion into a vessel.

### Bowel Ischemia and Perforation

Acute bowel ischemia from mesenteric artery occlusion (thrombotic or embolic) can produce sudden death particularly in elderly decedents with atherosclerotic disease or in decedents with atrial fibrillation and thromboembolism. The autopsy identifies the ischemic bowel segment with characteristic dusky discoloration, hemorrhagic infarction of the mucosa, and, in advanced cases, perforation with peritonitis and sepsis. Bowel perforation from other causes (peptic ulcer, diverticular perforation, foreign body, tumor perforation) similarly can produce sudden death from sepsis. The reasoning integrates the autopsy findings with the antecedent history and with the exclusion of alternative causes.

### Renal and Hepatic Causes

Renal causes of sudden death are less common but include acute renal failure with severe hyperkalemia (potassium-mediated cardiac arrhythmia), acute urinary tract obstruction with associated sepsis, and complications of chronic kidney disease including dialysis-related sudden death and uremic pericarditis with tamponade. Hepatic causes include acute liver failure from viral hepatitis or from acetaminophen or other hepatotoxic exposure, hepatic encephalopathy with cerebral edema, and complications of cirrhosis including hepatorenal syndrome and hepatic hemorrhage from spontaneous rupture of a hepatocellular carcinoma. Each has specific autopsy findings that support the diagnosis, and the toxicological workup identifies exogenous hepatotoxins when present.

### Abdominal Aortic Aneurysm Rupture

Abdominal aortic aneurysm rupture is a specific vascular emergency with characteristic autopsy findings. The aneurysm typically arises in the infrarenal aorta, with progressive dilation over years to decades. Rupture produces catastrophic hemorrhage into the retroperitoneum with rapid cardiovascular collapse. The classic autopsy finding is a large retroperitoneal hematoma centered around the ruptured aneurysm, with the intact rupture site or its remnant identifiable on careful dissection. In some cases, the rupture is contained by the surrounding retroperitoneal structures (contained rupture) and the decedent survives for hours or days before the containment fails; in others, the rupture extends into the peritoneal cavity with rapid exsanguination. The pretest reasoning identifies risk factors: age (typically over 65), male sex, hypertension, smoking history, family history of aneurysm, and connective tissue disease. Sudden death of an elderly decedent with these risk factors and with a scene of collapse without obvious cause warrants systematic examination of the aorta before certification of an alternative cause.

### Cerebral Venous Thrombosis

Cerebral venous sinus thrombosis is a less common but important cause of sudden neurological death, particularly in younger decedents. Risk factors include hormonal exposure (oral contraceptives, pregnancy, postpartum period), inherited thrombophilia, dehydration, and infection. The autopsy identifies the thrombosis in the dural venous sinuses (typically superior sagittal sinus, transverse sinus, or straight sinus) and may show venous infarction of the underlying cerebral cortex with hemorrhagic transformation. Identification requires deliberate examination of the dural sinuses at autopsy — they are readily missed if not specifically examined. Histology confirms the thrombosis and its age (fresh, organizing, remote). The reasoning integrates the finding with the antecedent history to identify the specific etiology when possible.

### Hemorrhagic Complications of Anticoagulation

Decedents on therapeutic anticoagulation (warfarin, direct oral anticoagulants, therapeutic heparin) are at elevated risk of sudden death from spontaneous hemorrhage, particularly intracerebral, retroperitoneal, and gastrointestinal. The autopsy identifies the site of hemorrhage and integrates with the toxicological confirmation of the anticoagulant level. Supratherapeutic anticoagulation (INR substantially above 3.0 for warfarin, or elevated levels of direct oral anticoagulants) supports the reasoning that the therapy was a contributing factor; therapeutic levels support the reasoning that the underlying vascular pathology dominated. The certification typically reflects the interaction: hemorrhage in an anticoagulated decedent with underlying vascular disease is certified with reference to both the hemorrhage and the contributing anticoagulation.

## Endocrine and Metabolic Causes

### Diabetic Ketoacidosis

Diabetic ketoacidosis (DKA) can produce sudden death particularly in decedents with type 1 diabetes and in decedents with new-onset diabetes who have not been diagnosed. The autopsy findings are limited: the vitreous humor glucose is elevated (typically markedly, above 500 mg/dL), the vitreous acetone or beta-hydroxybutyrate is elevated indicating ketosis, and the general findings of dehydration and metabolic derangement may be present. Postmortem serum glucose is unreliable because of postmortem glycolysis and glycogenolysis; vitreous glucose is the specimen of choice. Diagnosis rests on the vitreous chemistry integrated with the clinical history when available. New-onset DKA in a decedent without known diabetes is a specific reconstruction that emerges from the autopsy chemistry.

### Adrenal Crisis and Other Endocrine Emergencies

Adrenal crisis — acute cortisol deficiency in the setting of Addison disease or other causes of adrenal insufficiency — produces cardiovascular collapse with sudden death. The autopsy findings include adrenal gland pathology (atrophy in autoimmune Addison, hemorrhage in acute adrenal hemorrhage, replacement by metastatic disease or tuberculosis in specific cases). Postmortem cortisol measurement is not reliable, and the diagnosis rests on the adrenal findings integrated with clinical history. Thyroid storm — acute severe thyrotoxicosis — is a rare cause of sudden death with hyperthyroid findings on organ examination and a history of hyperthyroidism. Pheochromocytoma crisis can produce sudden hypertensive death with the tumor identified at autopsy.

### Electrolyte and Metabolic Derangement

Severe hyperkalemia (often from renal failure, from potassium-sparing diuretic reactions, or from rhabdomyolysis) produces cardiac arrhythmia and sudden death. Postmortem potassium is not reliable because of postmortem release from cells, and antemortem hyperkalemia is inferred from the clinical setting and vitreous potassium in appropriate cases (though vitreous rises with postmortem interval as noted in Chapter 3). Severe hyponatremia, hypernatremia, and other electrolyte disorders can cause sudden death when severe. Metabolic disorders including inherited enzymopathies (in pediatric decedents particularly) present with specific autopsy findings and require metabolic autopsy workup to establish the diagnosis.

## Infectious Disease Sudden Death

Infectious causes of sudden death include meningitis (particularly bacterial meningitis with rapid progression in previously healthy decedents), sepsis with septic shock, invasive infections including epiglottitis and severe streptococcal or staphylococcal infection with toxic shock, and specific infections including influenza and, since 2020, SARS-CoV-2 with associated pulmonary and multiorgan involvement. The autopsy identifies the infectious cause through gross examination, histology, microbiologic culture (with recognition of postmortem contamination limits), and molecular studies. The reasoning integrates the autopsy findings with the antecedent history of preceding febrile illness.

### Meningitis

Bacterial meningitis in a previously healthy decedent can produce sudden death, particularly the classic Neisseria meningitidis (meningococcal) infection with rapid progression from apparent health to fatal septic shock within hours. Autopsy findings include purulent exudate over the meninges, cerebral edema, and the specific findings of septic shock including Waterhouse-Friderichsen syndrome (bilateral adrenal hemorrhage). Cerebrospinal fluid culture confirms the organism when postmortem contamination has not compromised the specimen. The public health implications of meningococcal infection are substantial — identification of the case triggers contact tracing and prophylaxis of exposed individuals — and the medical examiner's office coordinates with public health authorities to initiate the response.

### Sepsis and Systemic Infection

Sepsis with septic shock can produce sudden death, particularly in immunocompromised decedents or in decedents with severe underlying comorbidity. The autopsy findings include the primary site of infection (pneumonia, urinary tract infection, skin and soft tissue infection, intra-abdominal source), the systemic effects of sepsis (multiorgan dysfunction, disseminated intravascular coagulation with microthrombi in small vessels), and evidence of shock. Postmortem cultures require interpretation against contamination but can identify the responsible organism when appropriate specimens are collected. Toxic shock syndrome from staphylococcal or streptococcal toxin production produces characteristic diffuse erythroderma and multiorgan involvement in the appropriate clinical context.

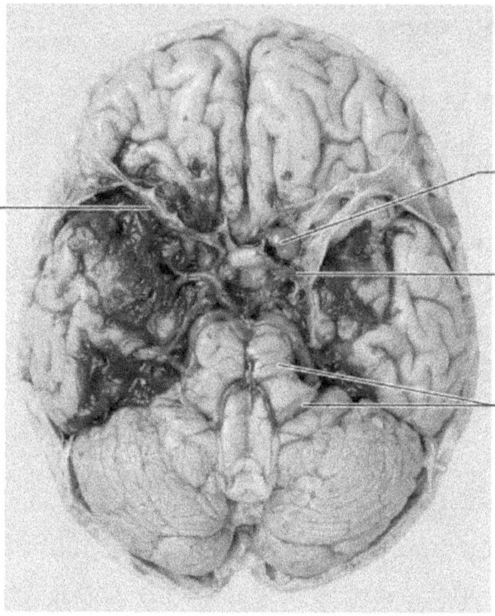


## The Undetermined Natural Death

In a subset of sudden natural death cases, complete autopsy with appropriate ancillary studies fails to identify a specific cause. The case is certified with cause undetermined or, when the reasoning supports it, with the presumptive natural mechanism (sudden cardiac death, presumed arrhythmic; sudden death associated with epilepsy). The determination of undetermined is a professional determination, not a professional failure, and the systematic use of the category preserves the credibility of specific determinations in cases where they are made.

### When Undetermined Is Appropriate

Undetermined cause of death is appropriate when the autopsy is complete (including all indicated ancillary studies), no cause of death has been identified to reasonable medical certainty, and no specific alternative can be reasoned as the presumptive cause. It is not appropriate when the pathologist has not completed the workup that would identify the cause — for example, when molecular autopsy would identify an inherited arrhythmia syndrome but has not been performed, or when appropriate toxicological analysis has not been completed. The reasoning in the report documents what was examined, what was excluded, and why the determination is undetermined.

## SCENE-TO-CERTIFICATION DECISION SYSTEM — Undetermined Natural Death Arc

**Presenting Death Scenario:** A 61-year-old man is found deceased in his residence by a neighbor. He had a documented history of hypertension, coronary artery disease with prior stent placement, and type 2 diabetes. He lived alone. The last confirmed contact was 24 hours before discovery. The scene shows no evidence of injury, no signs of struggle, and no evidence of scene alteration. Medications are present in the residence consistent with his history. The medical examiner's office accepts jurisdiction on the unwitnessed death of a person with known cardiovascular disease.

**Autopsy Signature:** External examination is unremarkable apart from early postmortem changes. Internal examination shows moderate coronary artery disease with a widely patent prior coronary stent, no acute coronary event, no significant myocardial pathology, and no acute or chronic ischemic changes to the heart. Vitreous glucose is 720 mg/dL. Vitreous ketones are positive at moderate levels. There is no other significant pathology on gross or histologic examination. Toxicology is negative apart from levels of the decedent's prescribed medications consistent with therapeutic use.

**Cause Determination:** Diabetic ketoacidosis, on the substrate of type 2 diabetes and cardiovascular disease. The vitreous chemistry supports the diagnosis: vitreous glucose above 500 mg/dL with ketosis on vitreous ketone measurement is highly supportive of DKA as the acute mechanism, even in a decedent without prior DKA history.

**Manner Determination:** Natural.

**Trap Logic:** The finding of coronary artery disease at autopsy could support a presumptive cardiac cause of death, but the moderate severity of the disease and the absence of acute event do not support this as the sudden mechanism. Without vitreous chemistry, this case could have been certified as "probable cardiac death" or "undetermined natural death" and the actual mechanism of DKA missed. The trap is failure to obtain vitreous chemistry in every sudden death of a decedent with known diabetes; the ancillary study is inexpensive, easily performed, and identifies an important category of cause that gross and microscopic examination alone cannot establish. A related trap is overinterpretation of moderate coronary disease as adequate to explain sudden death — the reasoning about adequacy must be systematic, not by default assumption.

**Certification Anchor:** Undetermined natural death is a professional determination reserved for cases where complete workup has failed to identify a cause to reasonable medical certainty. Systematic vitreous chemistry (glucose, ketones, urea, electrolytes) in decedents with known diabetes or with clinical presentations suggestive of metabolic derangement identifies DKA and other metabolic causes that gross and microscopic examination miss. When the appropriate workup identifies a cause, undetermined is no longer the correct classification.

**SCENE-TO-CERTIFICATION DECISION SYSTEM — Natural Sudden Death Determination Arcs**

**Neurological Sudden Death:** Neurological causes include ruptured berry aneurysm with subarachnoid hemorrhage (classic anterior communicating site), spontaneous intracerebral hemorrhage (typically hypertensive, in basal ganglia or brainstem), seizure-related death including SUDEP, and less common causes. Brain fixation and careful dissection are essential in cases with subtle findings.

**Pulmonary Sudden Death:** Pulmonary embolism is systematically identified by bilateral pulmonary artery examination before extensive dissection. Acute asthma death, alveolar hemorrhage syndromes, and pulmonary hypertension crisis are additional categories requiring specific attention and integration with clinical history.

**Gastrointestinal, Renal, Hepatic Causes:** Massive gastrointestinal hemorrhage from esophageal varices or peptic ulcer disease, bowel ischemia from mesenteric artery occlusion, and hepatic emergencies including acute liver failure and hepatocellular carcinoma rupture require systematic examination and integration with clinical setting.

**Endocrine and Metabolic Causes:** Diabetic ketoacidosis is confirmed by vitreous chemistry (glucose above 500 mg/dL with ketosis). Adrenal crisis, thyroid storm, pheochromocytoma crisis, and severe electrolyte derangement each have specific autopsy findings and require the appropriate ancillary workup for identification.

**Infectious and Undetermined Cases:** Infectious causes including meningitis and sepsis are identified by autopsy findings integrated with microbiology and clinical history. Undetermined natural death is the appropriate classification when complete workup fails to identify a cause; the classification preserves credibility for cases where cause is specifically determined.

## Summary and Key Concepts

Neurological causes of sudden death include ruptured berry aneurysm with subarachnoid hemorrhage, spontaneous intracerebral hemorrhage (typically hypertensive), seizure-related death including sudden unexpected death in epilepsy, and infectious causes including bacterial meningitis. Brain fixation and careful dissection support the identification of subtle findings.

Pulmonary embolism is a major cause of sudden natural death and requires systematic bilateral pulmonary artery examination for identification. Acute asthma with severe bronchospasm, diffuse alveolar hemorrhage syndromes, and pulmonary hypertension crisis account for additional pulmonary sudden deaths.

Gastrointestinal, renal, and hepatic causes include massive gastrointestinal hemorrhage (from esophageal varices, peptic ulcer disease, or other sources), acute bowel ischemia from mesenteric artery occlusion, acute liver failure, and specific renal complications. Systematic examination identifies these findings.

Endocrine and metabolic emergencies including diabetic ketoacidosis (confirmed by vitreous chemistry), adrenal crisis, and severe electrolyte derangement produce sudden death and require specific ancillary workup for identification. Postmortem serum chemistry is unreliable for glucose and potassium; vitreous humor is the specimen of choice for glucose, ketones, and specific electrolytes.

Infectious causes including bacterial meningitis, sepsis, and specific severe infections require integration of autopsy findings with clinical history and microbiologic workup. Public health implications of certain infections (meningococcal disease) trigger coordination with public health authorities.

Undetermined natural death is the appropriate classification when complete workup has failed to identify a specific cause. Systematic use of the category — rather than default certification with a presumptive cause — preserves credibility for cases where cause is specifically established.

# CHAPTER 12: PEDIATRIC FORENSIC PATHOLOGY: SUID, SIDS, AND THE SUDDEN INFANT DEATH INVESTIGATION

**Learning Objectives**

1. Define the sudden unexpected infant death (SUID) framework and articulate its differences from the older SIDS-centric approach to infant death investigation.
2. Perform a comprehensive pediatric autopsy according to standard protocol, including full-body skeletal survey and metabolic autopsy specimens.
3. Apply the diagnostic criteria for sudden infant death syndrome (SIDS) and articulate why the diagnosis has become one of exclusion in modern practice.
4. Recognize the pattern of unsafe sleep environment and reason about accidental suffocation as a mechanism of infant death.
5. Distinguish sudden infant death syndrome, accidental suffocation, and homicidal suffocation, and articulate the traps documented in the peer-reviewed literature.

## The Sudden Unexpected Infant Death Framework

The investigation of sudden infant death has evolved substantially over the past several decades, reflecting improved understanding of the mechanisms and better documentation of the scene circumstances that produce infant death. The older approach centered on sudden infant death syndrome (SIDS) as a diagnostic category of exclusion, applied to any sudden death of an infant under one year with a negative complete investigation. The modern approach centers on sudden unexpected infant death (SUID) as an umbrella term encompassing all sudden deaths of infants regardless of eventual specific diagnosis, with SIDS reserved for the subset that meets specific criteria after complete investigation.

The framework shift matters because it changed the epidemiology and the investigation. Under the SUID framework, deaths that would previously have been reflexively labeled SIDS are now systematically investigated with scene reconstruction, doll reenactment, complete pediatric autopsy, and specific consideration of accidental suffocation from unsafe sleep environment as a distinct mechanism. The consequence has been a substantial reduction in cases certified as SIDS and a corresponding increase in cases certified as accidental suffocation, undetermined, or specific identified causes. The framework has also increased the recognition of the substantial fraction of infant deaths that reflect unsafe sleep environments, with implications for public health messaging about safe sleep practices.

The forensic pathology fellow entering pediatric death investigation must understand both the technical protocol and the epidemiological framework. Every SUID case is a demanding investigation because the diagnostic categories overlap substantially at the case level, because the scene evidence is often critical and rapidly deteriorating, and because the manner determination has substantial implications for the family, for surviving siblings (whose subsequent risk is affected by the mechanism identified), and for any subsequent legal proceedings. The pathologist approaches every case with systematic protocol and honest reasoning about what the evidence supports.

### The Scale of the Problem

Sudden unexpected infant death accounts for approximately 3,500 deaths annually in the United States. Rates have declined substantially since the Back to Sleep campaign of the 1990s (now Safe to Sleep) but remain a leading cause of infant death beyond the first month of life. Rates vary substantially by race and socioeconomic status, with higher rates in Black and American Indian infants and in populations with lower socioeconomic resources; these disparities reflect a combination of environmental exposures, healthcare access, and systemic factors that the individual case investigation does not resolve but that the aggregate data has consistently documented.

**KEY POINT:** SUID is the umbrella category; SIDS is a specific diagnostic subset. Under the modern framework, SIDS is a diagnosis of exclusion requiring complete pediatric autopsy, complete scene investigation, and specific consideration of alternative causes. The framework shift has substantially reduced the fraction of SUID cases certified as SIDS.

## The Pediatric Autopsy Protocol

The pediatric autopsy in SUID cases follows a standardized protocol that differs from the adult autopsy in specific elements. The protocol is designed to identify the range of causes that can produce sudden infant death and to preserve the evidence needed to certify the case to reasonable medical certainty.

### Documentation and Photographic Standards

Photographic documentation in pediatric cases exceeds the standard adult protocol substantially. Every body region is photographed at overview and close-up, with attention to skin surfaces where subtle injury might be present. Fingernail scrapings are collected before any handling of the hands. The mouth is examined carefully for evidence of intraoral injury including frenulum injury (a specific finding in some abuse patterns). The genitourinary and anal regions are photographed and examined systematically. Body weight, length, and head circumference are measured and recorded. Overall body proportions and appearance are documented as evidence of nutritional state.

Radiographic skeletal survey is performed on every pediatric case where abuse is a differential consideration — which is essentially every SUID case. The survey includes multiple views of the skull, spine, chest, pelvis, and long bones. The survey identifies occult fractures characteristic of abuse: metaphyseal corner fractures of the long bones (highly specific for infant abuse when identified), rib fractures at various sites and stages of healing (posterior rib fractures being particularly specific for abuse), and complex skull fractures inconsistent with the reported mechanism. The skeletal survey is read by a pediatric radiologist when possible; findings are integrated with the autopsy examination and with the case history.

## External Examination in Detail

The external examination of an infant proceeds with attention to every surface and every body region. Skin color and any discoloration — lividity, contusion, jaundice, cyanosis — is documented. Any lesion, mark, or abnormality is described with location, dimension, and character; the description does not conclude about mechanism at this stage but preserves the observation for later reasoning. The fontanelles are palpated for tension. The oral cavity is inspected carefully for injury of the lips, gingiva, tongue, palate, and frenula. The ears are inspected for otoscopic findings and for external injury. The eyes are examined for hemorrhage of the conjunctivae and sclerae, and — in cases where abusive head trauma is a differential — for retinal hemorrhages on postmortem ophthalmologic examination. Retinal examination requires eye removal or ophthalmologic consultation and is not a routine element of every autopsy; its indication is developed in Chapter 13.

Figure 12.1: Pediatric Skeletal Survey: Standard Radiographic Views

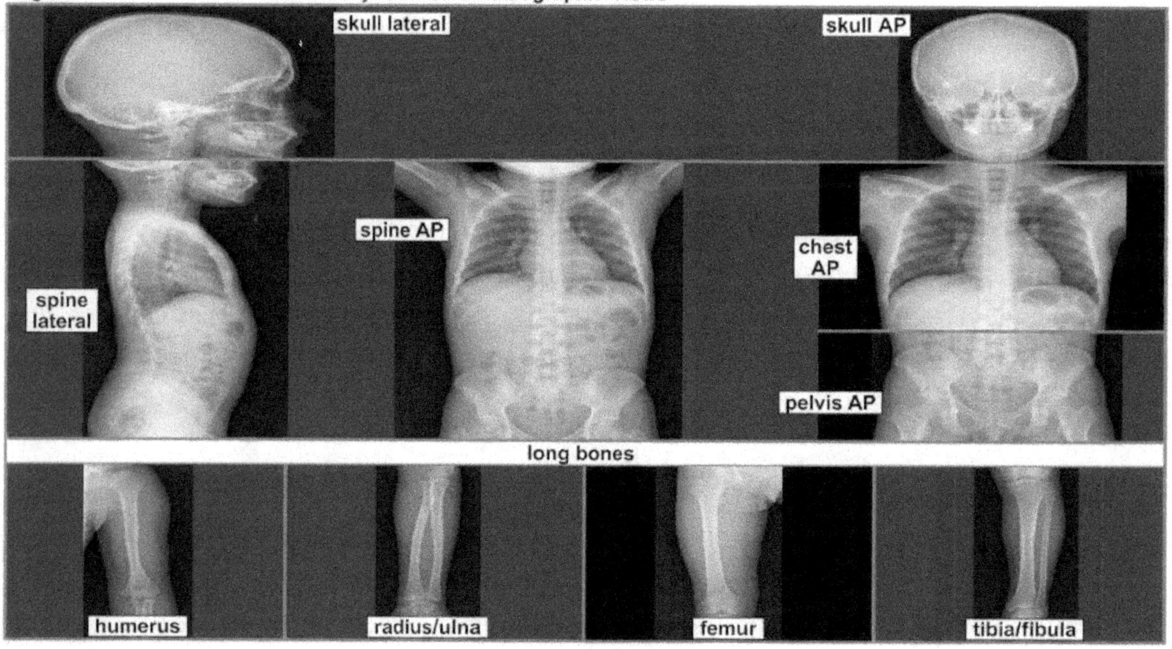


## Internal Examination

The internal examination proceeds through standard evisceration with attention to elements specific to the pediatric setting. Organ weights are recorded and compared to published pediatric reference ranges; small variations from expected weights can be diagnostically important. The heart is examined for structural abnormalities including congenital lesions (aortic coarctation, hypoplastic left heart, anomalous coronary origin, cardiomyopathy). The lungs are examined for evidence of pneumonia, aspiration, and other pathology. The gastrointestinal tract is examined for evidence of aspiration, feeding abnormalities, or specific pathology. The genitourinary system is examined including specific attention to any findings suggesting sexual assault. Brain examination follows the standard approach with formalin fixation for detailed later examination in most SUID cases.

The cervical spine and craniocervical junction warrant specific attention. Ligamentous injury at the atlanto-occipital joint from severe shaking or from mechanical injury is a documented finding in some pediatric cases and requires careful dissection to identify. The neck soft tissue is examined layered for evidence of compression or other injury. The eyes may be preserved with the extraocular tissue for postmortem retinal examination if the case reasoning requires it.

### Specimen Collection

Specimen collection in pediatric autopsy is broader than adult autopsy. Standard collection includes blood (peripheral and central), vitreous humor, urine when available, gastric contents, and bile. Tissues for histology follow the standard pattern. Additional collection for pediatric cases includes: blood spot for metabolic panel (the same specimen used for newborn metabolic screening, applied postmortem for identification of inborn errors of metabolism that can produce sudden infant death); frozen tissue (myocardium, spleen, liver) for molecular studies including inherited arrhythmia syndromes and metabolic disorders; representative sections of every organ for histology; and cerebrospinal fluid when appropriate. The collection is comprehensive because subsequent case questions may not be predictable at the time of autopsy, and the specimens support later molecular and metabolic workup as the case develops.

## Sudden Infant Death Syndrome and Its Diagnostic Criteria

Sudden infant death syndrome (SIDS) is defined as the sudden death of an infant under one year of age that remains unexplained after a thorough case investigation, including a complete autopsy, examination of the death scene, and review of the clinical history. The diagnostic criteria have become more stringent over time; the current framework applies SIDS only when the complete investigation has excluded specific alternative causes.

### The Current Diagnostic Criteria

The San Diego definition of SIDS, adopted in modified form by most American medical examiner offices, requires: complete autopsy including radiographic skeletal survey, complete death scene investigation with doll reenactment, review of medical and social history, exclusion of alternative causes (accidental suffocation, natural disease adequate to explain death, metabolic disease, homicide), and consistency of the case with the epidemiological profile of SIDS (age typically 2 to 4 months, unwitnessed death during sleep, absence of struggle at the scene). Cases meeting all criteria are classified as SIDS. Cases with any positive finding — a natural disease adequate to explain death, evidence of accidental suffocation, positive metabolic screening — are classified with the identified cause.

### SIDS as a Diagnosis of Exclusion

The category of SIDS has narrowed substantially since the systematic implementation of the SUID framework. Deaths that would previously have been reflexively labeled SIDS are now investigated for accidental suffocation in unsafe sleep environments (bed-sharing with adults, prone sleep position, soft bedding, blankets that could occlude the airway), for inflicted injury (through skeletal survey, retinal examination, and layered examination), and for specific natural disease (through metabolic and molecular workup). The result is that many cases previously certified as SIDS are now certified as "accidental suffocation in an unsafe sleep environment" or "undetermined" rather than as SIDS specifically. The change reflects better investigation, not a change in the underlying epidemiology.

The reasoning discipline is important. A case that meets the SIDS criteria after complete investigation is certified as SIDS; the diagnosis is not a euphemism for undetermined but a specific classification with epidemiological meaning. A case that has some findings suggesting accidental suffocation but where the reconstruction is uncertain may be certified as undetermined; the certification reflects the honest assessment that the mechanism cannot be established. Cases with definite evidence of homicidal mechanism are certified as homicide regardless of the difficulty of demonstrating specific injury. The pathologist reasons through the differential and certifies to the level of certainty the evidence supports.

## Unsafe Sleep and Accidental Suffocation

Accidental suffocation in an unsafe sleep environment has emerged as the most commonly identified specific mechanism in SUID cases in recent years. The mechanism involves mechanical obstruction of the infant airway by soft objects (pillows, blankets, mattress edges, adult bodies during co-sleeping) with resulting asphyxia. The pattern is documented in scene evidence — the position of the infant relative to the airway obstruction — and integrates with the autopsy findings, which are typically nonspecific.

### Risk Factors for Unsafe Sleep Death

The identified risk factors for accidental suffocation in unsafe sleep environments include: bed-sharing with an adult (particularly with a caregiver who is intoxicated, obese, or exhausted); prone or side sleep position (particularly with an inexperienced sleeper); soft bedding including pillows, comforters, blankets, and bumper pads in the sleep environment; sleeping on a couch, chair, or adult bed rather than a crib meeting safe sleep standards; overheating from excessive clothing or bedding; and premature birth (with associated increased vulnerability). The Safe to Sleep campaign has systematically addressed each risk factor with public health messaging, with substantial documented reductions in rates over the campaign period but with persistent risk in populations where the messaging has been less effectively received or where the sleep environment is constrained by resource limitations.

### Scene Documentation for Suspected Accidental Suffocation

Scene documentation is central to the identification of accidental suffocation. The scene investigator documents the sleep surface, the presence of soft bedding, the position of the infant when found, the presence of other individuals in the sleep environment, and the position of the infant relative to any potentially obstructing objects. Doll reenactment — in which the caregiver demonstrates with a doll where the infant was placed to sleep, where the infant was found, and what interventions were attempted — is standard practice in most jurisdictions and captures the scene reconstruction in a form that supports later reasoning about the mechanism. The pathologist reviews the scene documentation before autopsy and integrates it with the autopsy findings for the case determination.

## SCENE-TO-CERTIFICATION DECISION SYSTEM — SUID Investigation Arc

**Presenting Death Scenario:** A 3-month-old infant is found unresponsive by his mother in the morning. The infant had been placed to sleep the previous night in the parents' bed, on his back, alongside his mother. The mother reports that when she went to sleep, the infant was between her and her husband. Emergency response is initiated but resuscitation is unsuccessful. The scene is documented photographically. The bed shows adult pillows and a comforter. The infant was found in a prone position with his face partially against the comforter. The medical examiner's office accepts jurisdiction. Doll reenactment with the parents documents the initial and found positions of the infant.

**Autopsy Signature:** External examination is unremarkable apart from small crescentic marks on the face consistent with contact against firm surface (possibly the mattress or the comforter). Full-body radiographic skeletal survey is negative for occult fracture. Internal examination shows congestion of the head and upper chest, mild pulmonary edema, and no significant structural pathology. Postmortem retinal examination is negative for hemorrhage. Metabolic panel from blood spot is unremarkable. Toxicology is negative. The vitreous chemistry is unremarkable. Histology shows no evidence of infection, no structural cardiac abnormality, and no other significant findings. Frozen tissue is retained for molecular studies for inherited arrhythmia syndromes.

**Cause Determination:** Sudden unexpected infant death in an unsafe sleep environment. The determination reflects: the unsafe sleep environment documented at scene (adult bed, bed-sharing, soft bedding), the position of the infant when found (prone, face against soft bedding), the mild external findings consistent with contact with soft bedding, the complete autopsy without alternative cause, and the absence of any evidence supporting inflicted injury.

**Manner Determination:** Undetermined — with reasoning that the case is most consistent with accidental suffocation in an unsafe sleep environment. Some offices would certify this specific case as accident with the specific mechanism of accidental suffocation. The determination reflects office practice; the reasoning is documented in the report so the determination is transparent.

**Trap Logic:** The trap in SUID cases is either overreach (certifying SIDS or a specific accidental suffocation without adequate investigation) or underreach (certifying homicide without adequate evidence of inflicted injury). Both errors have substantial consequences for the family. The systematic approach: complete pediatric autopsy protocol with skeletal survey and metabolic panel; complete scene investigation with doll reenactment; retinal examination if abusive head trauma is a differential; molecular workup for inherited arrhythmia syndromes when the heart is structurally normal; and reasoning through the differential with reference to specific findings. When the mechanism cannot be established to reasonable medical certainty, undetermined is the appropriate certification.

**Certification Anchor:** SUID cases are worked with a comprehensive protocol and certified with attention to the specific mechanism when identified. SIDS is reserved for cases meeting the specific diagnostic criteria after complete investigation. Accidental suffocation in an unsafe sleep environment is certified when scene evidence supports the mechanism and autopsy findings are consistent. Undetermined is appropriate when the mechanism cannot be established. Homicide requires evidence of inflicted injury or of homicidal intent.

## Distinguishing SIDS From Homicidal Suffocation

The distinction between SIDS, accidental suffocation, and homicidal suffocation is one of the most demanding reasoning problems in forensic pathology. The three categories overlap substantially at the autopsy level — all three may show minimal or absent specific findings on complete autopsy — and the distinction depends heavily on scene evidence, on behavioral history, and on the pattern of findings across a case series when multiple infant deaths occur in the same family.

### Findings Suggestive of Inflicted Suffocation

Specific findings that raise concern for inflicted suffocation include: injury to the face, particularly around the nose and mouth (contusions, abrasions, frenulum injury); petechial hemorrhages of the face and conjunctivae (though these occur in both accidental and inflicted suffocation and are not specific); retinal hemorrhages (which have specific significance in the context of pediatric death and are developed in Chapter 13); intraoral injury from forced pressure; pattern of skeletal injury on skeletal survey; and family history of multiple unexplained infant deaths (which raises the possibility of Munchausen syndrome by proxy or of intentional harm to multiple children). Each of these findings requires careful documentation and reasoning.

### Frenulum Injury and Intraoral Findings

Frenulum injury — tearing of the frenulum of the upper lip, or of the lingual frenulum, from forced pressure applied to the mouth — is a documented finding in inflicted suffocation and in inflicted force-feeding. The finding is best identified by careful eversion of the upper lip during external examination, revealing the frenulum insertion into the alveolar mucosa. Fresh frenulum tear shows characteristic hemorrhage and disruption of the connective tissue; healing frenulum injury may show fibrosis or residual disruption. The finding is not pathognomonic — frenulum injury can occur from accidental mechanism (an infant striking the mouth against a firm surface, or from forceful pacifier removal) — but its presence in a case with other concerning findings supports the reasoning about inflicted mechanism. Intraoral injury more broadly — contusions of the alveolar mucosa, hemorrhage in the palatal soft tissue, injury to the tongue — is documented systematically in every pediatric autopsy where inflicted injury is a differential.

### Retinal Hemorrhage as a Pediatric Finding

Retinal hemorrhages have specific and contested significance in pediatric forensic pathology. In infant deaths with suspected abusive head trauma, the finding of extensive multilayered retinal hemorrhages — particularly hemorrhages extending into the peripheral retina and involving multiple layers of the retina — has been associated with mechanisms involving repetitive acceleration-deceleration forces ("shaken baby syndrome", in the older terminology, or abusive head trauma with rotational injury). The finding is not fully specific and can occur in birth (in the days after delivery), in specific hematologic conditions, and in accidental head trauma with sufficient mechanism. In sudden death cases without known head trauma, retinal hemorrhages may be sparse and limited to the posterior pole, or may be absent. Postmortem retinal examination is performed by ophthalmology consultation or by eye removal for later examination and is indicated in cases where abusive head trauma is a differential; the finding is documented photographically and integrated with other reasoning.

**EVIDENCE:** The interpretation of retinal hemorrhage in pediatric forensic pathology is a documented area of controversy in the peer-reviewed literature. Extensive multilayered retinal hemorrhage with a specific distribution supports mechanisms involving acceleration-deceleration forces but is not fully specific. Sparse or absent retinal hemorrhage does not exclude inflicted injury when other findings support it. Interpretation is developed with reference to ophthalmology consultation and to the specific pattern of hemorrhage identified.

### The Doll Reenactment Protocol

The doll reenactment is a specific investigation technique used in SUID cases to reconstruct the sleep environment and the sequence of events. The caregiver is asked to demonstrate, using a doll of appropriate size and weight, where the infant was placed to sleep, in what position, with what bedding, and what the caregiver did upon discovering the infant. The reenactment is documented photographically and by narrative account, and captures information that is often not fully expressed in verbal interview. The reenactment can reveal unsafe sleep practices that the caregiver has not initially disclosed (bed-sharing, prone position, soft bedding), and it captures the discovery position that supports reconstruction of the mechanism. Reenactment is delivered with sensitivity to the caregiver's grief and is not intended as an interrogation; the framing is that the investigation needs to understand the sequence of events to determine what happened. Trained scene investigators perform the reenactment; the pathologist reviews the documentation as part of the case file.

### The Multi-Death Family

Two or more unexplained infant deaths in the same family require specific investigation. The classical dictum that "one SIDS is a tragedy, two SIDS is suspicious, three SIDS is homicide until proven otherwise" reflects the epidemiological rarity of recurrent SIDS and the documented pattern of Munchausen syndrome by proxy and of intentional suffocation of multiple children. The forensic pathology approach to a second unexplained infant death in a family is to conduct the standard SUID protocol on the current case, to obtain complete records on the previous case, and to work with law enforcement, child protective services, and the pediatric medical team to develop the specific reasoning. Molecular workup for shared inherited disorders is standard because some inherited conditions do produce recurrent infant death and must be excluded. The case reasoning is developed with substantially higher scrutiny than the single-death case.

## Munchausen Syndrome by Proxy and Fabricated or Induced Illness

Munchausen syndrome by proxy (now more commonly termed fabricated or induced illness in a child) is a documented pattern in which a caregiver intentionally causes or exaggerates illness in a child in order to obtain medical attention, emotional gratification, or other secondary gain. The behavior in its extreme form includes suffocation of the child to produce apneic episodes that require emergency medical attention, and, in some documented cases, has escalated to fatal suffocation. Recognition of the pattern depends on features that emerge across multiple presentations rather than on a single case: unexplained recurrent illness in a child, illness that improves when the caregiver is separated from the child, discrepancies between the caregiver's reported history and the medical findings, and, in some cases, prior death of a sibling with similar unexplained illness. The pattern is one context in which recurrent infant death in a family raises specific concern. Recognition and investigation require multidisciplinary involvement including pediatric abuse specialists, mental health evaluation, and law enforcement, and the forensic pathology contribution is one element of the aggregate reasoning.

**CAUTION:** The multi-death family requires careful reasoning with attention to both the specific findings and to the epidemiological pattern. Overreach to homicide in the absence of specific evidence, and underreach to natural cause without excluding inflicted mechanism, are both documented errors. Consultation with peer forensic pathologists, with child abuse pediatricians, and with pediatric geneticists supports the reasoning.

Figure 12.2: Metaphyseal Corner Fracture: Highly Specific Finding of Infant Abuse

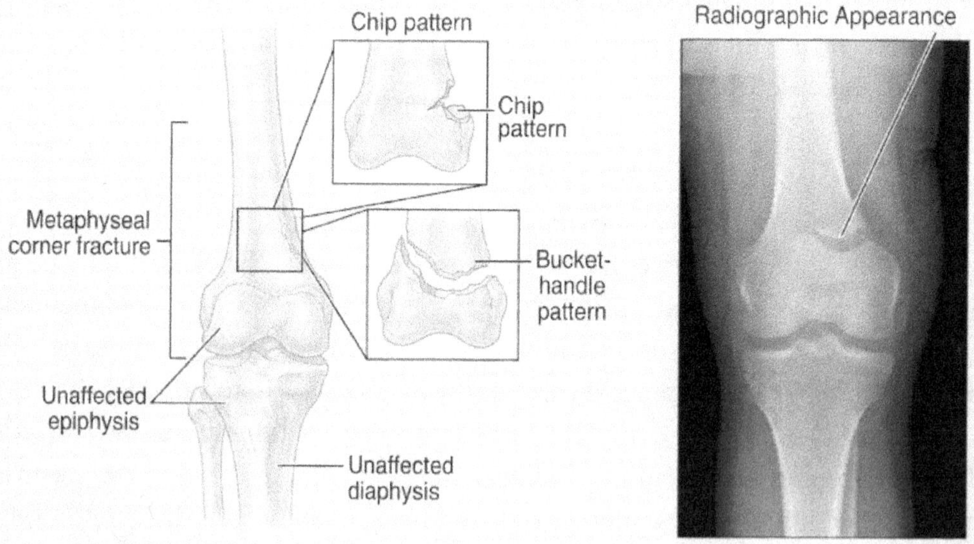

## The Metabolic Autopsy

The metabolic autopsy identifies inborn errors of metabolism that can produce sudden infant death. The category is important because these disorders are treatable in surviving relatives and because the diagnosis has implications for family reproductive counseling. The panel of disorders considered includes: fatty acid oxidation defects (particularly medium-chain acyl-CoA dehydrogenase deficiency, MCADD), organic acidemias, urea cycle disorders, and specific inborn errors of carbohydrate metabolism (galactosemia, glycogen storage disorders).

### Specimen Collection and Analysis

The metabolic autopsy specimens include blood spot collected on newborn screening filter paper and preserved for later analysis (the same specimen and processing used for prospective newborn metabolic screening); vitreous humor for glucose, ketones, and electrolytes; frozen liver and skeletal muscle tissue for enzyme assay if a specific disorder is suspected; and, when the resources are available, dried blood spot for acylcarnitine profile and amino acid analysis. The acylcarnitine profile identifies fatty acid oxidation defects with high sensitivity. Positive metabolic screening triggers confirmatory testing and family evaluation.

### The Molecular Autopsy in Pediatric Cases

The molecular autopsy in pediatric SUID cases parallels the molecular autopsy in adult sudden cardiac death but includes broader gene panels reflecting the inherited disorders that can produce infant death. Panels include inherited arrhythmia syndrome genes (with particular attention to variants that present in infancy), inherited cardiomyopathy genes, and metabolic disorder genes not captured by the biochemical panel. Positive molecular results identify a specific etiology, support family screening, and inform reproductive counseling for the parents. Retention of appropriate specimens (frozen blood and tissue) at the primary autopsy is essential; failure to preserve the specimens forecloses this workup.

### Categories Identified by the Metabolic and Molecular Workup

The panel of disorders that the metabolic and molecular workup identifies is broad and reflects both inborn errors of metabolism and inherited electrical and structural cardiac disorders. Fatty acid oxidation defects (medium-chain acyl-CoA dehydrogenase deficiency being the most common) present classically with hypoglycemic crisis and sudden death during fasting or during viral illness; positive acylcarnitine profile identifies the diagnosis. Long-chain fatty acid oxidation defects (VLCAD, LCHAD, trifunctional protein deficiency) present with cardiac and skeletal muscle involvement and can present with sudden death from arrhythmia. Organic acidemias (methylmalonic acidemia, propionic acidemia, isovaleric acidemia) present with acidosis and can produce sudden death in the setting of catabolic stress. Urea cycle disorders (particularly ornithine transcarbamylase deficiency, which is X-linked and predominantly affects male infants) present with hyperammonemic crisis. Inherited arrhythmia syndromes with infancy-onset presentations include severe forms of long QT syndrome (particularly LQT8, or Timothy syndrome), catecholaminergic polymorphic ventricular tachycardia, and severe Brugada syndrome variants. Each category has specific implications for family screening and for reproductive counseling.

## The Aged-Up Pediatric SUID Case: Sudden Death in the Older Child

Sudden death in children older than one year but before adolescence is a smaller epidemiological category than infant death but presents its own investigation challenges. The differential broadens to include specific structural cardiac disease (hypertrophic cardiomyopathy, anomalous coronary origin, arrhythmogenic cardiomyopathy), inherited arrhythmia syndromes, complications of chronic pediatric illness, and specific infections (myocarditis, sepsis, meningitis). Sudden death in a school-age or older child triggers investigation for these categories with the standard pediatric autopsy protocol plus specific attention to the age-appropriate differentials. The autopsy in a child aged 1 to adolescence differs from the infant autopsy in the range of expected findings but preserves the systematic approach: complete external and internal examination, skeletal survey if abuse is a consideration (with less specificity for abuse-specific findings than in the infant age range), metabolic and molecular workup as appropriate, and reasoning about the specific cause and manner determinations.

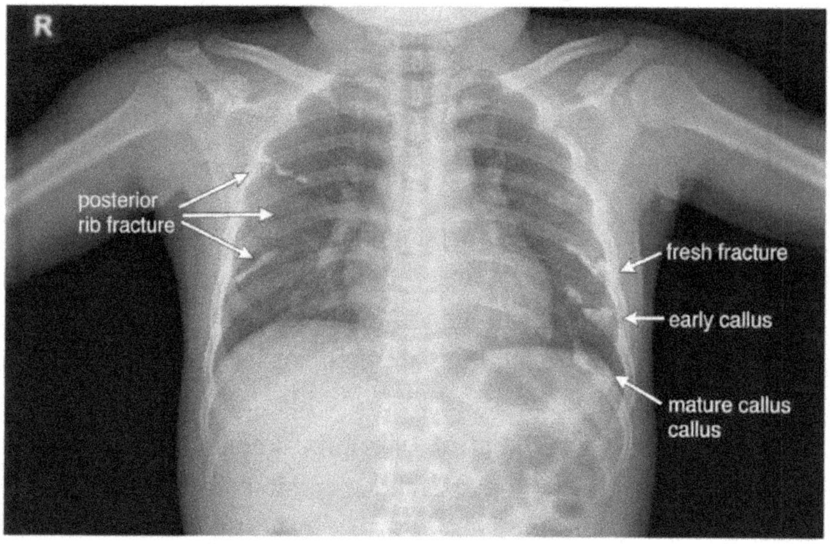


**Figure 12.3:** Healing Rib Fractures in Multiple Stages: Radiographic Appearance of Chronic Infant Abuse

## SCENE-TO-CERTIFICATION DECISION SYSTEM — SIDS-Versus-Suspected-Inflicted-Suffocation Arc

**Presenting Death Scenario:** A 5-month-old infant is brought unresponsive to the emergency department by her mother, who reports that she found the infant not breathing in her crib after a nap. Resuscitation is unsuccessful. The infant is transported to the medical examiner's office. Records review documents that the same mother had a previous infant die at 4 months of age two years earlier; that death was certified as SIDS after complete investigation at the time. No third-party witnesses to either death exist. The scene investigation of the current death documents a proper crib with tight-fitting sheet and no additional bedding; the reported sleep environment was appropriate.

**Autopsy Signature:** External examination is unremarkable apart from facial congestion and small petechial hemorrhages of the conjunctivae. Full-body radiographic skeletal survey shows no acute or healing fractures. Internal examination shows nonspecific findings of asphyxia (congestion, pulmonary edema, mild petechial hemorrhages on serosal surfaces) without structural abnormality. Postmortem retinal examination is unremarkable. Complete histology shows no acute or chronic pathology. Metabolic panel from blood spot is unremarkable. Toxicology is negative. Molecular workup for inherited arrhythmia syndrome variants and for shared inherited disorders that could have produced both infant deaths is initiated on frozen specimens.

**Cause Determination:** Cause of death is undetermined pending completion of molecular workup. The determination cannot be made to reasonable medical certainty from the current findings; the case is closed with cause undetermined and updated if molecular results identify a specific inherited etiology accounting for both this death and the previous infant death.

**Manner Determination:** Undetermined pending investigation. The classical dictum regarding recurrent SIDS in a family ("one tragedy, two suspicious, three homicide until proven otherwise") is a heuristic reflecting the epidemiological rarity of recurrent SIDS, but it is not a determinative rule. Two SIDS in one family may reflect a shared inherited disorder (which the molecular workup may identify), may reflect recurrent unsafe sleep exposure, may reflect intentional harm, or may reflect two independent cases with the same negative-workup outcome. The manner determination requires evidence beyond the epidemiological unlikelihood.

**Trap Logic:** The trap in this case is either premature certification of homicide based on the epidemiological pattern without specific evidence, or premature certification of SIDS/undetermined without pursuing the specific molecular workup that could identify a shared inherited disorder. The countermeasures are systematic: complete pediatric autopsy protocol for the current death; complete records review of the previous death; molecular workup for shared inherited disorders; consultation with law enforcement, child protective services, pediatric abuse specialists, and pediatric genetics; and integration of all findings with transparent reasoning documented in the report. The case is worked with substantially higher scrutiny than a single-death case but is not automatically certified as homicide without specific evidence.

**Certification Anchor:** Recurrent unexplained infant death in a family requires substantially higher scrutiny than the single-death case but does not automatically certify as homicide. Specific evidence of inflicted injury (facial injury, retinal hemorrhage in appropriate context, skeletal injury, corroborating scene evidence) supports homicide. Positive molecular workup identifying a shared inherited disorder supports natural cause for both deaths. Absent both, the case may be certified as undetermined, and the reasoning is documented transparently in the report.

### Communicating the SUID Investigation With Families

The communication of the SUID investigation and its findings with the family is one of the more consequential communications the office produces. Families lose an infant unexpectedly and often in circumstances that raise their own questions of guilt and self-blame. The office's communication is calibrated to family circumstances, is typically mediated through the death investigator or through office administrative staff, and is often integrated with grief counseling resources and with support from organizations focused on infant death loss. When the case identifies accidental suffocation in an unsafe sleep environment, communication with the family addresses safe sleep practices for surviving and future siblings; the communication is delivered with sensitivity and without blame while accurately reflecting the mechanism identified. When the case identifies an inherited disorder, communication addresses genetic implications and recommends evaluation for surviving relatives. When the case is certified as SIDS or as undetermined, communication addresses the honest limits of the investigation and the meaning of the classification for the family.

**SCENE-TO-CERTIFICATION DECISION SYSTEM — Sudden Infant Death Determination Arcs**

**The SUID Framework:** SUID is the umbrella category for all sudden unexpected infant deaths; SIDS is a specific diagnostic subset requiring complete investigation and exclusion of alternative causes. The framework shift over recent decades has substantially reduced the fraction of cases certified as SIDS in favor of specific mechanisms including accidental suffocation and undetermined.

**The Comprehensive Protocol:** The pediatric autopsy protocol includes complete photographic documentation, full-body radiographic skeletal survey, complete external and internal examination, metabolic autopsy specimens (blood spot, vitreous, frozen tissue), and molecular autopsy specimens. Retinal examination is added when abusive head trauma is a differential. The protocol is systematic and comprehensive because the diagnostic differential is broad.

**SIDS Diagnostic Criteria:** The current SIDS diagnostic criteria (San Diego definition) require complete autopsy including skeletal survey, complete scene investigation with doll reenactment, review of medical and social history, exclusion of alternative causes, and consistency with the epidemiological profile of SIDS. Cases meeting all criteria are certified as SIDS; cases with positive findings are certified with the identified cause.

**Unsafe Sleep and Accidental Suffocation:** Accidental suffocation in unsafe sleep environments has emerged as the most commonly identified specific mechanism in SUID cases in recent years. Scene documentation — sleep surface, soft bedding, position of the infant when found, presence of other individuals — is central to identification. The Safe to Sleep messaging addresses the identified risk factors.

**The Differential Reasoning:** Distinguishing SIDS from accidental suffocation from homicidal suffocation depends on scene evidence, on behavioral history, and on the pattern of findings across a case series. Specific findings suggestive of inflicted mechanism (facial injury, retinal hemorrhage in appropriate context, skeletal injury, multiple unexplained infant deaths in the family) require careful documentation and consultation. Overreach and underreach both have substantial family consequences.

## Summary and Key Concepts

The sudden unexpected infant death (SUID) framework has largely replaced the SIDS-centric approach to infant death investigation. SUID is the umbrella category for all sudden unexpected infant deaths; SIDS is a specific diagnostic subset requiring complete investigation.

The pediatric autopsy protocol includes complete photographic documentation, full-body radiographic skeletal survey, complete external and internal examination, metabolic autopsy specimens, and molecular autopsy specimens. The protocol is systematic and comprehensive because the differential diagnosis for sudden infant death is broad.

The current SIDS diagnostic criteria require complete autopsy including skeletal survey, complete scene investigation, review of history, exclusion of alternative causes, and consistency with the epidemiological profile of SIDS. Cases meeting all criteria are certified as SIDS.

Accidental suffocation in unsafe sleep environments has emerged as the most commonly identified specific mechanism in SUID cases. Scene documentation of the sleep environment, position of the infant, and other individuals present is central to the identification. Doll reenactment supports the reconstruction.

The distinction between SIDS, accidental suffocation, and homicidal suffocation is demanding because the categories overlap at the autopsy level. Specific findings suggestive of inflicted mechanism require careful documentation. Multi-death families require substantially higher scrutiny and typically consultation.

The metabolic autopsy and molecular autopsy identify inborn errors of metabolism and inherited disorders that can produce sudden infant death. Positive findings have implications for surviving family members and for future reproductive decisions. Specimen retention at the primary autopsy is essential to preserve the workup opportunity.

# CHAPTER 13: ABUSIVE HEAD TRAUMA, CHILD PHYSICAL ABUSE, AND NEGLECT FATALITIES

**Learning Objectives**

1. Recognize the constellation of findings that characterizes abusive head trauma and distinguish it from accidental head injury in children.
2. Identify skeletal injuries characteristic of infant and child abuse, including metaphyseal corner fractures and posterior rib fractures at multiple stages of healing.
3. Interpret blunt abdominal and thoracic injury in children in the context of the reported mechanism and reason about consistency between injury pattern and history.
4. Recognize the constellation of findings in neglect fatalities including malnutrition, dehydration, and complications of untreated medical conditions.
5. Reason systematically about the age-discrepancy question — the mismatch between injury age and reported history — and integrate the reasoning with the multidisciplinary child abuse investigation team.

## Abusive Head Trauma

Abusive head trauma is the leading cause of fatal child abuse in infants and young children and one of the most contested areas of forensic pathology. The category encompasses inflicted head injury from multiple mechanisms — shaking with or without impact, direct impact injury, and combinations of the two — and the reconstruction of specific mechanism from the constellation of findings is a demanding reasoning problem. The older terminology of "shaken baby syndrome" has been substantially replaced by "abusive head trauma" in the peer-reviewed literature and in professional society position statements, reflecting the understanding that the injury pattern reflects inflicted mechanism without specifying which mechanism produced it in an individual case.

The classic triad of abusive head trauma includes subdural hemorrhage, retinal hemorrhage, and encephalopathy with cerebral edema. The triad was described in the older literature as diagnostic of shaking mechanism, and this diagnostic reliability has been substantially challenged in the peer-reviewed literature over the past two decades. The current understanding is that the triad is a pattern of findings highly associated with inflicted head injury but not fully specific; the specific mechanism producing the triad in an individual case is inferred from the pattern of findings integrated with the reported history. The pathologist reasons from the findings to the mechanism with attention to the documented interpretive limits of individual findings.

## Subdural Hemorrhage in Infants

Subdural hemorrhage in an infant or young child raises the differential of abusive head trauma, accidental head injury, birth-related hemorrhage (in the days after delivery), specific medical conditions (coagulopathy, benign external hydrocephalus with expanded subarachnoid space, some metabolic disorders), and less commonly other causes. The reasoning about which mechanism produced the hemorrhage integrates the clinical history, the pattern of the hemorrhage, the presence or absence of associated findings, and the age of the child. Acute subdural hemorrhage from abusive head trauma is typically bilateral, often thin-film in appearance rather than dense mass-effect producing collections, and is commonly associated with the other findings of the triad. Subdural hemorrhage from accidental impact is typically unilateral, associated with the site of impact, and shows a mechanism consistent with the history.

Chronic subdural hemorrhage — organized subdural collections with a developed membrane — has a different differential. In infants, chronic subdural collections may reflect a prior inflicted event with subsequent survival, may reflect benign external hydrocephalus (a self-limited condition of infant subarachnoid space expansion with vulnerability to bridging vein tear from minor mechanism), or may reflect other specific medical conditions. The distinction requires careful integration of imaging findings, clinical history, and, where available, prior imaging documenting the subdural collection's evolution. The distinction has substantial implications for the reasoning about mechanism and manner in the sudden death case.

## Retinal Hemorrhage: Extended Discussion

Retinal hemorrhage in pediatric death cases has been extensively studied and the interpretive framework has evolved substantially. Extensive multilayered retinal hemorrhages with peripheral retinal involvement have been strongly associated with abusive head trauma mechanisms, particularly mechanisms involving repetitive angular acceleration-deceleration forces. The finding is not fully specific: severe accidental head trauma at forces well beyond routine household mechanisms, specific hematologic conditions, birth trauma in the days after delivery, and cardiopulmonary resuscitation (rarely, in prolonged CPR with severe pulmonary and cardiac disease) can produce retinal hemorrhage patterns overlapping with abusive head trauma. The pathologist consults with ophthalmology for detailed retinal examination when the case reasoning requires it, and the interpretation is calibrated to the specific pattern of hemorrhage identified.

Postmortem retinal examination is performed either by ophthalmology consultation with in-situ examination of the eyes at the time of autopsy or by eye removal with formalin fixation and later examination by ophthalmology or by specialist pathology. Photographic documentation of the retinal findings supports later review. The findings are described by distribution (posterior pole only, extension to mid-periphery, extension to peripheral retina), by layer involvement (superficial only, or multilayered including deep retinal and preretinal), and by density. The findings are integrated with the other elements of the constellation.

Figure 13.1: Retinal Hemorrhage Distribution Patterns in Pediatric Head Trauma

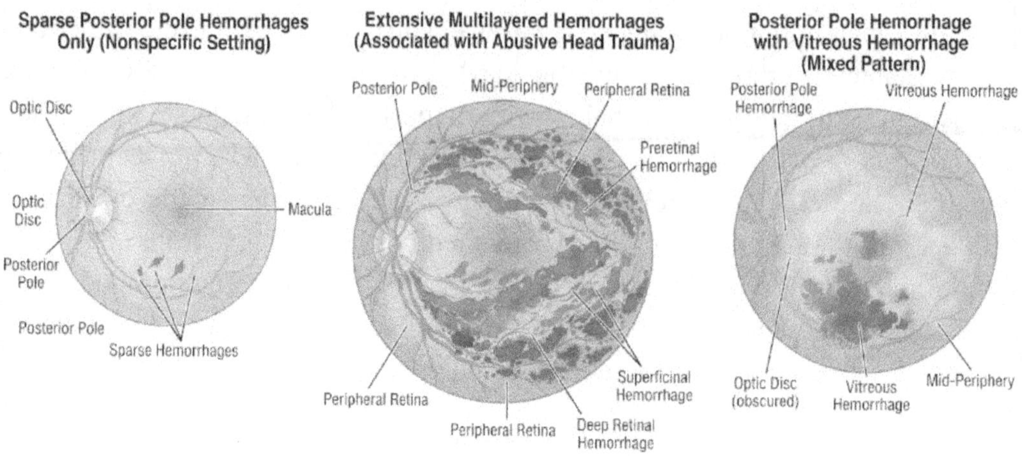


## The Reasoning About Mechanism

The reasoning about which specific mechanism produced abusive head trauma in a given case is contested in the peer-reviewed literature. The older interpretation that the triad was specifically diagnostic of shaking mechanism has been substantially challenged by biomechanical studies suggesting that shaking alone may not produce the forces required for the observed injuries, and that impact against a firm surface (with the impact obscured on external examination by a soft contact surface such as a mattress) may be involved in many cases. The current professional standard, reflected in position statements from the American Academy of Pediatrics, the National Association of Medical Examiners, and other professional bodies, is that the constellation of findings supports inflicted mechanism without necessarily specifying which specific mechanism produced the injuries. The pathologist documents the findings and reasons about inflicted versus non-inflicted mechanism; specific mechanism identification within the inflicted category is not typically the pathologist's reasoning task.

## SCENE-TO-CERTIFICATION DECISION SYSTEM — Abusive-Head-Trauma-Versus-Accidental Arc

**Presenting Death Scenario:** A 4-month-old infant is brought to the emergency department by his father in cardiac arrest. The father reports that the infant fell from the couch to the carpeted floor — an approximate 60 cm fall — and became immediately unresponsive. Resuscitation is unsuccessful. The infant is transported to the medical examiner's office. History review documents that the infant had no prior medical concerns and that the family reports no other recent illness or injury.

**Autopsy Signature:** External examination documents resuscitation-related sternal contusion and mild facial cyanosis. Full-body radiographic skeletal survey identifies four posterior rib fractures at various stages of healing (fresh, early callus, mature callus), a metaphyseal corner fracture of the right distal tibia (fresh), and a healing fracture of the left ulnar shaft with mature callus. Internal examination shows bilateral acute subdural hemorrhage (thin-film distribution), extensive cerebral edema, and cortical contusions. Postmortem ophthalmologic examination identifies extensive multilayered retinal hemorrhages extending to the peripheral retina bilaterally. Toxicology is negative. Metabolic panel is unremarkable. Molecular studies for inherited disorders are unremarkable.

**Cause Determination:** Abusive head trauma with associated skeletal injuries of variable ages. The constellation of findings — bilateral acute subdural hemorrhage with cerebral edema; extensive multilayered retinal hemorrhages extending to the peripheral retina; skeletal injuries in multiple different stages of healing (indicating repeated injury over time rather than a single event); metaphyseal corner fracture (highly specific for infant abuse); and severity of the head injury inconsistent with the reported mechanism (a 60 cm fall from a couch onto carpeted floor produces documented injury patterns that do not include this constellation) — all support inflicted mechanism.

**Manner Determination:** Homicide. The autopsy findings identify inflicted injury as the mechanism; the reported history of accidental fall is inconsistent with the injury pattern; and the skeletal findings document prior injury events not attributed to the reported mechanism, supporting a pattern of ongoing abuse rather than a single accidental event.

**Trap Logic:** The reported history of a household mechanism (fall from couch, fall from bed, rolling off a changing table) is one of the classic patterns given in inflicted infant injury cases. The trap is to accept the reported history and reason from it to the injury pattern; the correct approach is to examine the injury pattern independently and reason to what mechanism could have produced it. Biomechanical studies of routine household falls in infants document injury patterns typically limited (small linear skull fractures, unilateral small subdural hemorrhages, small contusion) rather than the constellation of bilateral subdural hemorrhage, extensive multilayered retinal hemorrhage, and cerebral edema. When the injury pattern is inconsistent with the reported mechanism, the reasoning identifies the inconsistency and pursues the alternative mechanism. A related trap is failure to obtain the complete skeletal survey and retinal examination, which are essential for the case reasoning.

**Certification Anchor:** Abusive head trauma is supported by the constellation of findings integrated with the reported history. When the injury pattern is inconsistent with the reported mechanism and includes findings characteristic of inflicted injury (skeletal injuries in multiple stages of healing, metaphyseal corner fracture, extensive multilayered retinal hemorrhage), the reasoning supports inflicted mechanism. The systematic protocol including skeletal survey and retinal examination is essential.

## Non-Accidental Skeletal Injury

Skeletal injuries in infants and young children have specific patterns that support the reasoning about inflicted versus accidental mechanism. The full-body radiographic skeletal survey identifies the pattern; the specific findings are interpreted with reference to their published specificity for inflicted injury.

### Metaphyseal Corner Fractures

The metaphyseal corner fracture — sometimes termed the classic metaphyseal lesion or bucket-handle fracture — is a small chip-like fracture at the metaphysis of a long bone, produced by shearing forces applied at the metaphyseal region during pulling, twisting, or shaking of the extremity. The finding is highly specific for infant abuse mechanism, with limited alternative explanations (some birth injury in the days after delivery, rare specific medical conditions). The mechanism involves force applied to the extremity such that the metaphysis fails at its junction with the epiphyseal region rather than the diaphysis. Recognition of the finding on skeletal survey requires attention to the metaphyseal region on multiple views; the fracture may be subtle and easily missed without deliberate examination. Pediatric radiologist interpretation is standard for skeletal survey in these cases.

### Rib Fractures

Rib fractures in infants and young children are highly specific for inflicted injury, particularly posterior rib fractures at the costovertebral junction. The mechanism involves compression of the chest wall during grasping or shaking of the infant, with the ribs bending anteriorly against the transverse processes of the vertebrae. Anterior compression of the chest (as from cardiopulmonary resuscitation) can produce anterior rib fractures at the costochondral junctions, but posterior rib fractures at the costovertebral junction are not typically produced by CPR. Multiple rib fractures at various stages of healing document repeated injury events. Careful skeletal survey identification requires oblique views to demonstrate the posterior rib fractures, which are frequently occult on standard anteroposterior projection.

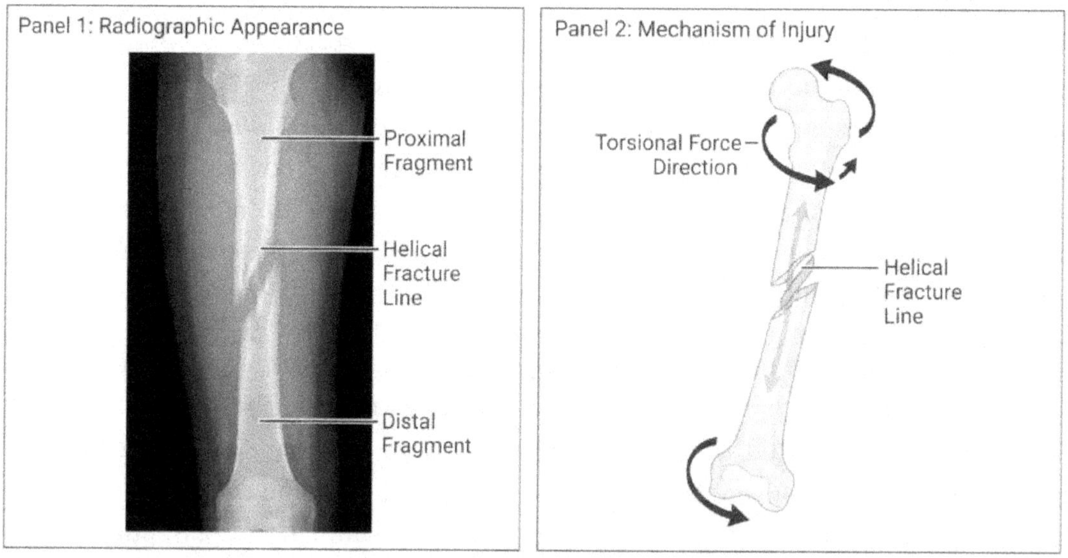


Figure 13.2: Spiral Fracture of a Long Bone: Mechanism and Radiographic Appearance

### Other Skeletal Findings

Additional skeletal findings that raise concern for inflicted injury in infants and young children include: complex skull fractures with multiple fracture lines or crossing suture lines (single simple linear parietal fractures from documented mechanism are more consistent with accidental injury); spiral fractures of long bones (particularly in pre-ambulatory infants who cannot generate torsional forces themselves); vertebral compression fractures; scapular fractures (uncommon in accidental mechanism); sternal fractures; and any fracture in a location not typically produced by accidental mechanism in the child's developmental stage. The pattern of injuries at various stages of healing is a specific finding of ongoing abuse, and the identification of prior injury not previously known to the medical system is a specific concern requiring documentation and integration with the case reasoning.

### The Skeletal Survey Protocol

The standard skeletal survey in suspected infant and child abuse includes multiple projections designed to identify occult and subtle fractures. Standard views include the skull in anteroposterior and lateral projections, the cervical spine in lateral projection, the thoracolumbar spine in lateral projection, the chest in anteroposterior and both oblique projections (to identify posterior rib fractures), the pelvis in anteroposterior projection, and each long bone in anteroposterior projection. Additional views (oblique views of the ribs, dedicated views of specific joints) are added when indicated by the initial findings. A follow-up skeletal survey performed approximately 2 weeks after the initial survey identifies fractures that were fresh at the initial survey but that have developed callus and become more radiographically apparent — relevant primarily in living children under evaluation, but the principle informs postmortem reasoning about the sensitivity of the initial survey.

## Blunt Abdominal and Chest Injury in Children

Blunt abdominal and thoracic injuries in children in the setting of suspected abuse follow specific patterns. Abdominal injuries from inflicted blows typically involve solid organs (liver, spleen, pancreas) with characteristic patterns of injury. Pancreatic injury from a focal impact against the vertebral column (as when a child is punched in the abdomen) produces a specific pattern of pancreatic contusion or transection with associated retroperitoneal hemorrhage. Duodenal hematoma from similar mechanism produces a specific pattern of injury with associated bowel obstruction. Hepatic and splenic lacerations produce hemoperitoneum with hypovolemic shock. Thoracic injuries in inflicted child abuse are less common than abdominal but include pulmonary contusion, cardiac injury (uncommon), and rib fractures with pneumothorax or hemothorax.

The reasoning about consistency between injury pattern and reported history is central. Accidental blunt abdominal injury in a young child from typical household mechanisms (a fall from height, a strike against furniture) does not typically produce the deep solid organ injury seen in inflicted mechanism. The reconstruction of the reported mechanism against the injury pattern documents the inconsistency. In cases where the reported history is initially consistent with an accidental mechanism but the injury pattern is not (a small fall producing catastrophic hepatic laceration; a household mechanism producing pancreatic transection), the reasoning identifies the inconsistency and pursues the alternative mechanism.

The delay-to-presentation pattern is a specific reasoning element in abusive abdominal injury. Children with severe inflicted abdominal injury frequently present hours after the injury, with the caregiver history reporting a delayed presentation attributed to the child "not looking right" or "not feeling well" without acute alarm. The delay reflects both the caregiver's reluctance to seek care after inflicting the injury and the progressive nature of the child's decompensation from internal bleeding or peritonitis. Documentation of the timeline against the injury findings supports the reasoning about mechanism.

## Neglect Fatalities

Neglect fatalities in children arise from failure to provide adequate nutrition, hydration, medical care, or safety, with resulting death from the specific deprivation or from complications. The pattern includes deaths from starvation and dehydration, deaths from untreated medical conditions that would have been treatable with adequate care, and deaths from environmental exposure or from injury that adequate supervision would have prevented.

### Starvation and Dehydration Deaths

Death from starvation in children is characterized by severe wasting with reduction of body mass to well below expected for age and length, loss of subcutaneous fat, muscle atrophy, characteristic skin changes (thin, dry, with poor turgor), and specific findings of chronic malnutrition on organ examination (hepatic steatosis with atrophy, intestinal villous atrophy, endocrine changes). Age and length percentiles are calculated and compared with population norms; body weight for length or age below the 3rd percentile or with substantial decline from prior documented weights supports the diagnosis. Dehydration produces additional findings including dry mucous membranes, sunken eyes, hemoconcentration on chemistries, and characteristic changes on serum sodium and other electrolytes.

The reasoning integrates the autopsy findings with the antecedent history including growth records from pediatric visits, feeding history, and any evidence of specific medical conditions that could produce failure to thrive independently. The distinction between neglect-related failure to thrive and medical-cause failure to thrive is important; some cases involve both, with an underlying medical condition worsened by inadequate care. The multidisciplinary evaluation with pediatric abuse specialists and pediatric nutrition specialists supports the reasoning.

### Deaths From Untreated Medical Conditions

Death of a child from an untreated medical condition that would have been treatable with adequate care is a category of neglect fatality that requires specific reasoning. Diabetic ketoacidosis in a child with previously undiagnosed diabetes where medical attention was not sought despite characteristic symptoms; sepsis from an infection that was not treated; complications of an ongoing chronic medical condition where medications were not administered; asthma exacerbation without medical intervention — each represents a category where the underlying medical condition is not the sole cause of death but where the failure to obtain care contributed proximately. The certification typically includes both the medical condition and the neglect contribution, with the manner determination requiring reasoning about the specific circumstances of the failure to seek care.

Figure 13.3: Patterned Contusion from a Recognizable Impacting Object

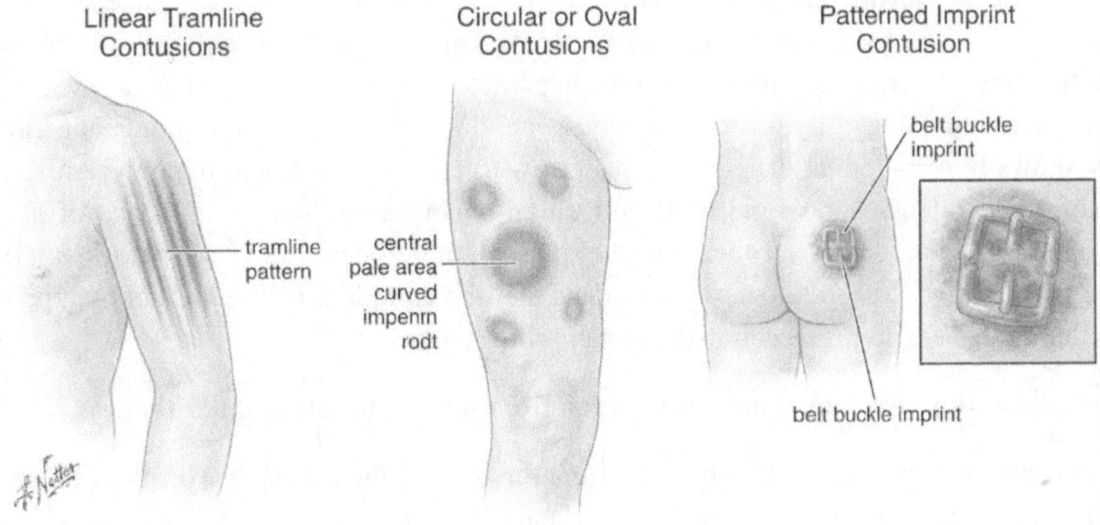


## Environmental Exposure and Supervision Failures

Environmental exposure fatalities in children include drowning in unsecured swimming pools or open water without supervision, hyperthermia from confinement in vehicles or environments without cooling, hypothermia from inadequate shelter or clothing, and injury from unsafe household conditions (accessible firearms, unsecured medications, unsafe sleep environments in older children). Deaths from injury during inadequate supervision include falls from height in inadequately supervised environments, drowning during inadequately supervised bathing, and injury from access to weapons or vehicles. The reasoning about manner determination in these cases depends on the specific circumstances, on the age and developmental stage of the child, and on the reasonable expectations for supervision at that developmental stage. The determinations range from accident (unforeseeable and reasonable-supervision cases) through undetermined (ambiguous circumstances) to homicide (cases where the neglect meets the definition of a criminal act).

## SCENE-TO-CERTIFICATION DECISION SYSTEM — Neglect Fatality Reconstruction Arc

**Presenting Death Scenario:** A 3-year-old child is brought to the emergency department by paramedics after emergency response was called by neighbors reporting concern about the family. The child is found to be markedly emaciated with weight substantially below expected for age. Resuscitation is unsuccessful. The medical examiner's office accepts jurisdiction. The living environment is documented by scene investigators: the residence shows evidence of general disorganization, limited food in the pantry consistent with recent purchases only, and no evidence of ongoing medical care for the child. The mother reports that the child had been vomiting for several days and had been eating less over the preceding weeks.

**Autopsy Signature:** External examination documents severe wasting: body weight approximately 7 kilograms (expected weight for age approximately 14 kilograms), loss of subcutaneous fat, prominent bony prominences, and skin changes of chronic malnutrition. Full-body radiographic skeletal survey shows no fractures. Internal examination shows hepatic steatosis with reduced organ weight, intestinal villous atrophy on histology, thymic atrophy, and generalized findings of chronic malnutrition. Vitreous chemistry shows hyponatremia, dehydration pattern with elevated urea, and hypoglycemia. There is no evidence of acute infection, no significant congenital abnormality, and no evidence of an alternative medical condition that could account for the presentation independent of nutritional deprivation. Toxicology is negative. Records review documents that the child had not been seen by a pediatrician in the preceding two years despite recommended well-child visits.

**Cause Determination:** Starvation and dehydration from severe chronic malnutrition.

**Manner Determination:** Homicide. The determination reflects the extreme severity of the malnutrition, the absence of an alternative medical explanation, and the pattern of failure to seek medical care despite documented symptoms and despite the visibly deteriorating condition of the child. The manner classification is medical; specific criminal charges are the province of law enforcement and the prosecutor.

**Trap Logic:** The distinction between neglect-related failure to thrive and medical-cause failure to thrive requires systematic exclusion of underlying medical conditions. A child with celiac disease, cystic fibrosis, congenital heart disease, or specific endocrine or metabolic disorders may present with severe wasting from the underlying condition. The systematic approach includes: histologic examination for evidence of specific medical cause; metabolic workup for inborn errors; documentation of any physical stigmata of syndromic disease; and integration with prior medical records. When systematic examination excludes alternative causes and documents severe chronic malnutrition without other explanation, the neglect determination is supported.

**Certification Anchor:** Neglect fatalities are certified with reference to the specific mechanism (starvation, dehydration, untreated medical condition, environmental exposure, injury from inadequate supervision) integrated with the exclusion of alternative causes. Manner is homicide when the neglect meets the definition of a criminal act; manner may be classified as accident or undetermined in cases where the neglect reflects genuine incapacity of the caregiver rather than active neglect.

## Reconstruction and the Age-Discrepancy Question

The age-discrepancy question — the mismatch between the reported age of an injury (from the caregiver history) and the age of the injury as identified at autopsy — is a central reasoning question in child abuse investigation. The pathologist estimates injury age from the histologic findings and integrates with the radiographic findings for skeletal injury; when the estimated injury age is inconsistent with the reported history, the inconsistency is documented and reasoned.

### Contusion Aging Revisited

Contusion aging by gross color is unreliable for precise time estimation (as developed in Chapter 5). Histologic contusion aging provides more objective markers with the sequence: acute hemorrhage in the first hours; neutrophilic infiltrate by 24 hours; macrophage infiltrate with hemosiderin appearance by 3 to 7 days; fibroblastic organization by 1 to 2 weeks; complete organization by weeks to months. Multiple contusions of substantially different ages in a child document repeated injury over time and do not fit a single reported event. The pathologist reports contusion aging within broad ranges rather than as specific timepoints, but the ranges are usually adequate to identify substantial mismatches with reported history.

### Skeletal Injury Aging

Skeletal injury aging is estimated from radiographic and histologic findings of callus formation and remodeling. Fresh fractures show a linear defect without callus; early callus formation is visible radiographically at approximately 7 to 10 days; mature callus appears at 3 to 6 weeks; remodeling continues over months to years. Multiple fractures at substantially different stages of healing on a single skeletal survey document repeated injury over weeks to months. The findings are integrated with any reported history; substantial mismatch supports the reasoning about ongoing abuse rather than single event.

## The Case Team Approach

Child abuse investigation requires a multidisciplinary team including forensic pathology, pediatric abuse specialists, law enforcement, child protective services, prosecuting attorneys, and, in many cases, pediatric radiology and other subspecialty consultation. The forensic pathology contribution is central to the reasoning but is not the sole element; integration with the team supports the aggregate determination.

### Coordination With Pediatric Abuse Specialists

The child abuse pediatrician (a subspecialty within pediatrics devoted to evaluation of suspected abuse in living children) provides consultation on the interpretation of findings and on the integration with the developing medical understanding of abuse patterns. The forensic pathologist typically coordinates with the child abuse pediatrician on cases with any complexity, particularly cases involving multiple children in the family and cases where the initial impression may benefit from a second professional perspective.

### Documentation for Legal Proceedings

Child abuse cases proceed to criminal prosecution in many jurisdictions when the pathology findings support inflicted mechanism. The autopsy report is written with substantial rigor because it will be scrutinized by opposing experts and by the court. Photographic documentation is extensive; specimen retention is conservative; second-opinion consultation is often obtained at the time of the autopsy. The report distinguishes objective findings from reasoned opinion, and the reasoning section develops the integration of findings with the case history in transparent form. The pathologist prepares for the reasonable possibility of testimony months or years later and preserves the case documentation accordingly.

### Birth Injury as Differential Consideration

Birth injury is a specific differential consideration in the youngest infants presenting with subdural hemorrhage, retinal hemorrhage, or skeletal injury. Vaginal delivery, particularly instrumented delivery (forceps, vacuum extraction), can produce a range of birth injuries including small subdural hematomas, retinal hemorrhages that resolve over days to weeks, cephalohematoma, clavicular fracture, and less commonly humeral or femoral fractures from the delivery mechanism. The birth-related injuries typically follow a predictable time course — present at birth or in the immediate neonatal period, evolving over days to weeks, and resolved or resolving by the fourth to sixth week of life. The reasoning in an infant presenting after this period with subdural or retinal findings distinguishes between residual birth injury (in a small window of continued interpretability) and new injury. Documented obstetric history, delivery notes, and any postnatal imaging support the distinction. In an infant older than approximately six weeks, birth injury as a differential explanation for extensive subdural or retinal hemorrhage becomes progressively less likely, though prior undiagnosed subdural collections from birth may persist in some cases.

### Coagulopathy and Hematologic Differential

Coagulopathy is a specific differential consideration in cases of infant hemorrhage. Vitamin K deficiency bleeding (previously termed hemorrhagic disease of the newborn) is a documented cause of intracranial hemorrhage in infants who did not receive routine vitamin K prophylaxis at birth; the pattern includes intracranial hemorrhage and may include additional bleeding sites (gastrointestinal, umbilical). Hemophilia and other inherited bleeding disorders can produce recurrent bleeding including intracranial hemorrhage; the family history and coagulation studies (postmortem if the child died) support the diagnosis. Idiopathic thrombocytopenic purpura and disseminated intravascular coagulation from sepsis produce their own bleeding patterns. In a case with unexplained hemorrhage, systematic evaluation for coagulopathy is standard — recovery of blood for coagulation testing where possible, review of the medical history for prior bleeding tendency, and documentation of any other bleeding sites at autopsy that support or exclude a systemic bleeding disorder.

**CLINICAL PEARL:** In an infant presenting with intracranial hemorrhage of unclear mechanism, systematic evaluation for coagulopathy (particularly vitamin K deficiency bleeding in infants who may have missed vitamin K prophylaxis) and for the birth-injury window is essential before concluding abusive head trauma. The differential evaluations do not exclude AHT when present; they identify alternative or contributing mechanisms and support the honest reasoning about the case.

## The Caregiver Stress Context

The context of inflicted infant injury frequently involves specific caregiver stressors that emerge in the investigation. Postpartum depression, chronic sleep deprivation from infant care, unresolved caregiver mental health conditions, substance use, poverty and housing instability, and intimate partner violence in the household are all documented risk factors for infant abuse. Recognition of these contexts does not by itself establish inflicted mechanism in an individual case but supports the reasoning about the family situation. Prevention efforts — particularly the Purple Crying and Period of Purple Crying education programs directed at expected infant fussiness and at caregiver coping — have been developed to address the specific pattern of shaking injury that occurs when a caregiver becomes overwhelmed by inconsolable crying. Forensic pathology contributes to these prevention efforts through the aggregate data generated by the individual case investigations, which support epidemiological understanding of the pattern.

## Pediatric Sexual Abuse Fatalities

Pediatric sexual abuse fatalities are uncommon but require specific investigation protocol. Death may occur from direct injury during the assault (particularly in very young children), from associated blunt or asphyxial injury inflicted during the assault, or from injuries inflicted after the assault to conceal it. The forensic examination includes systematic external and internal genital examination, documentation of any injury (with specific attention to the developmental normal range of pediatric anatomy so that normal variation is not misidentified as injury), collection of specimens for DNA analysis, and integration with pediatric abuse specialist consultation. Sexual assault evidence collection kits appropriate for postmortem use are standard in these cases; the specimens support subsequent perpetrator identification and legal proceedings. The reasoning about sexual abuse in the context of a fatal case is integrated with the overall assault mechanism and manner determination.

## Historical Perspective and the Evolving Literature

The scientific and forensic understanding of child abuse patterns has evolved substantially over the past several decades. The initial description of the battered child syndrome by Kempe and colleagues in 1962 established the medical recognition of inflicted child injury as a specific pattern. The subsequent decades have refined the understanding of skeletal injury specificity, of the constellation of abusive head trauma findings, and of the interpretive limits of individual findings. The current professional understanding, as reflected in position statements from major professional societies, has been developed through peer-reviewed research, retrospective case series, biomechanical modeling, and clinical experience with living children under evaluation. The peer-reviewed literature continues to evolve, and the practicing forensic pathologist maintains familiarity with current evidence to integrate with the case reasoning.

### Fatal Abuse of Older Children

Fatal abuse of older children (school-age through adolescence) presents different patterns than infant abuse. The injury mechanisms are more varied — blunt assault from fists or objects, prolonged confinement with associated environmental deprivation, sexual assault, and injury with weapons. The specific patterns of infant abuse (metaphyseal corner fractures, classic constellation of abusive head trauma) do not typically apply to older children. The forensic examination includes documentation of any external injury with attention to patterned findings that document the mechanism; skeletal survey remains relevant but the specific findings shift toward long bone fractures, skull fractures with mechanism consistent with impact, and injuries at sites reflecting the specific assault. Toxicology may identify substance exposure (including administration of substances to children by caregivers, a specific documented mechanism). The reasoning integrates the injury pattern with the reported history and with the developmental stage of the child; older children may have contributed to case reasoning through statements to medical personnel or investigators before death, and these accounts are integrated into the case file with recognition of their reliability limits.

### Fatal Pediatric Drowning: Bathtub and Pool Contexts

Pediatric drowning deserves specific attention because the manner determination in these cases can be complex. Bathtub drowning of a young child, drowning in a household bucket or wading pool, and drowning in an unsecured swimming pool are documented mechanisms. In supervised bathing, an inattentive supervising adult can produce accidental drowning that meets legal definitions of neglect; in unsupervised bathing (particularly in young children left alone), the negligence pattern is more clearly established. In deliberate drowning of a child — a documented but uncommon homicide mechanism — the autopsy may show additional injury consistent with the assault (contusions from restraint, additional injuries) and the scene may show evidence of struggle. The reasoning integrates the autopsy findings, the scene reconstruction, and the reported history with attention to the developmental capabilities of the child (a young toddler can drown in a few centimeters of water; a school-age child capable of standing typically cannot drown accidentally in a shallow tub without additional mechanism).

### Forensic Photography Standards for Pediatric Cases

Forensic photography in pediatric abuse cases exceeds standard adult protocol. Every skin surface is systematically photographed, with attention to the developmental normal range so that findings are documented accurately without over- or under-interpretation. Overview photographs document the body as a whole and the position of injuries in anatomic context; mid-range photographs document each region with clear anatomic reference; close-up photographs of every injury are taken with a scale in frame and with attention to lighting that reveals the pattern of the finding. Special-lighting photography (side-lighting to reveal subtle contusion patterns, alternate light source examination in some jurisdictions) supplements standard photography when specific findings are subtle. The photographic archive supports later review by pediatric abuse specialists and by opposing experts if the case proceeds to litigation.

## Preserving Evidence for Prosecution

The evidentiary standards for child abuse prosecution have specific requirements that shape the forensic pathology documentation. Photographic documentation is expected to be extensive and organized. Specimen retention is conservative, with tissue blocks and slides retained indefinitely and with additional wet tissue retained per office policy. The chain of custody documentation is meticulous, with each specimen tracked from collection through analysis. The autopsy report is written with attention to the potential audience of jurors and appellate judges as well as of professional colleagues. Second-opinion consultation on the case findings, often obtained at the time of the autopsy from a peer forensic pathologist or from a child abuse pediatric specialist, supports the reasoning and provides evidence of the professional consensus about the findings. The pathologist prepares for the reasonable possibility of testimony months or years after the case and preserves the documentation accordingly.

## SCENE-TO-CERTIFICATION DECISION SYSTEM — Child Abuse Determination Arcs

**Abusive Head Trauma:** The constellation of subdural hemorrhage, retinal hemorrhage, and encephalopathy is highly associated with inflicted head injury but has documented interpretive controversy regarding specific mechanism. The reasoning documents the findings, integrates with reported history, and identifies inflicted versus non-inflicted mechanism without over-specifying the reasoning within the inflicted category.

**Skeletal Injury Patterns:** Metaphyseal corner fractures, posterior rib fractures, spiral fractures of long bones in pre-ambulatory infants, and multiple fractures at various stages of healing are specific patterns supporting inflicted mechanism. Full-body radiographic skeletal survey with pediatric radiologist interpretation is essential.

**Blunt Abdominal and Thoracic Injury:** Inflicted abdominal injury involves solid organs with characteristic patterns (pancreatic transection from focal impact, hepatic and splenic laceration, duodenal hematoma). Reasoning about consistency between injury pattern and reported history is central to identifying inflicted mechanism.

**Neglect Fatalities:** Neglect fatalities include starvation and dehydration deaths, deaths from untreated medical conditions, environmental exposure deaths, and injury from inadequate supervision. Systematic exclusion of alternative medical explanations supports the neglect determination when the pattern is present.

**The Age-Discrepancy Question:** Estimation of injury age from histologic and radiographic findings integrated with reported history identifies substantial mismatches that support ongoing abuse rather than single reported events. Contusion and skeletal injury aging are reported in broad ranges consistent with published limits of specificity.

## Summary and Key Concepts

Abusive head trauma is the leading cause of fatal child abuse in young children and one of the most contested reasoning areas in forensic pathology. The constellation of subdural hemorrhage, retinal hemorrhage, and encephalopathy is highly associated with inflicted head injury; specific mechanism identification within the inflicted category is contested in the literature.

Skeletal injuries characteristic of infant and child abuse include metaphyseal corner fractures (highly specific), posterior rib fractures at the costovertebral junction, spiral fractures in pre-ambulatory infants, and multiple fractures at various stages of healing. Full-body radiographic skeletal survey with pediatric radiologist interpretation identifies the pattern.

Inflicted blunt abdominal and thoracic injuries follow characteristic patterns including pancreatic injury from focal impact against the vertebral column, hepatic and splenic laceration, and duodenal hematoma. Reasoning about consistency between injury pattern and reported history is central.

Neglect fatalities include starvation and dehydration deaths, deaths from untreated medical conditions, environmental exposure deaths, and injury from inadequate supervision. Systematic exclusion of alternative medical explanations supports the neglect determination.

The age-discrepancy question — mismatch between estimated injury age and reported history — supports reasoning about ongoing abuse rather than single reported events. Contusion aging and skeletal injury aging are reported in broad ranges consistent with the documented specificity limits.

Child abuse investigation requires a multidisciplinary team including forensic pathology, pediatric abuse specialists, law enforcement, and prosecuting attorneys. The forensic pathology contribution is central but is one element of the aggregate reasoning.

# CHAPTER 14: ELDER ABUSE, NEGLECT, AND DEATHS IN THE ELDERLY

**Learning Objectives**

1. Articulate the framework for elder death investigation and identify the specific factors that distinguish it from the general adult death investigation.
2. Recognize physical elder abuse patterns and distinguish inflicted injury from the age-related changes and common comorbidities of elderly decedents.
3. Identify the constellation of findings characteristic of elder neglect and failure to care, including malnutrition, dehydration, medication mismanagement, and complications of chronic disease.
4. Interpret falls and fall-related death in the elderly with attention to the mechanism of injury and to any signs suggesting inflicted rather than accidental mechanism.
5. Recognize pressure injury patterns, stage them appropriately, and reason about the caregiving history that supports or contradicts the observed pattern.

## The Elder Death Investigation Framework

Elder death investigation has emerged as a specific focus within forensic pathology over recent decades, driven by demographic shifts (the aging of the American population), by growing recognition of the scale of elder abuse and neglect, and by the increasing number of deaths occurring in institutional long-term care settings where systematic case review has revealed patterns previously undetected. The forensic pathologist encounters elder deaths in a range of contexts: sudden death in the community, death in the residence with delayed discovery, death in a long-term care facility, and death following presentation to a healthcare setting with injuries. Each context has specific reconstruction implications, and the pathologist approaches the elder case with attention to the interpretive challenges specific to the elderly decedent.

The interpretive challenges arise from the intersection of several factors. Elderly decedents typically have multiple comorbid conditions that produce their own findings on autopsy; distinguishing findings of underlying disease from findings of inflicted injury or of neglect requires systematic reasoning. Elderly skin is thin and fragile with reduced subcutaneous fat, producing easy contusion and skin tears from mechanisms that would be unremarkable in younger decedents. Elderly bone is osteopenic or osteoporotic, producing fractures under forces that would not fracture younger bone. Cognitive impairment in many elderly decedents limits the reliability of any history the decedent gave in life and complicates the reasoning about consent, competency, and the appropriate use of restraints in medical care. The pathologist reasons through these factors systematically for each case.

### Epidemiology and the Scale of Elder Abuse

Elder abuse is substantially underreported and undercounted in existing epidemiology, but published studies suggest that approximately one in ten community-dwelling elderly individuals experiences some form of abuse annually, with rates higher in institutional settings. Physical abuse accounts for a fraction of the total; more common categories are financial exploitation, emotional abuse, and neglect. Fatal elder abuse is a smaller category still but is documented, particularly in the specific contexts of caregiver strain, alcohol or substance use in caregivers, and financial exploitation combined with inadequate care. The scale of the underlying problem has led to systematic elder death review teams in many jurisdictions, modeled on the child death review teams that operate in most states.

**KEY POINT:** The elderly decedent presents distinct interpretive challenges: age-related skin fragility, osteoporosis, common comorbidities producing autopsy findings, and cognitive impairment limiting history reliability. Systematic reasoning distinguishes findings of natural disease from findings of inflicted injury or neglect.

## Physical, Sexual, and Financial Elder Abuse

### Physical Abuse Patterns

Physical abuse of an elderly individual can involve a range of mechanisms: assault by hand or by objects, restraint injury from inappropriately applied restraints, injury from inappropriate handling during transfers or bathing, and injury from failure to prevent falls or from active pushing. The autopsy findings vary with the mechanism. The pathologist looks for patterned injuries that document a specific implement (belt marks, tramline contusions from rods, patterned bruising from recognizable objects); for injuries in locations characteristic of restraint (bilateral wrist or ankle abrasions from cuffs or ties, contusions on the anterolateral thighs from restraint chairs); for facial injuries at sites where the decedent could not have injured themselves in a fall (posterior scalp injury with the fall history reported as forward, contusions along the mandible without lower body injury); and for injuries at various stages of healing suggesting an ongoing pattern rather than a single event.

**Figure 14.1: Elderly Skin Fragility and the Distinction from Inflicted Injury**

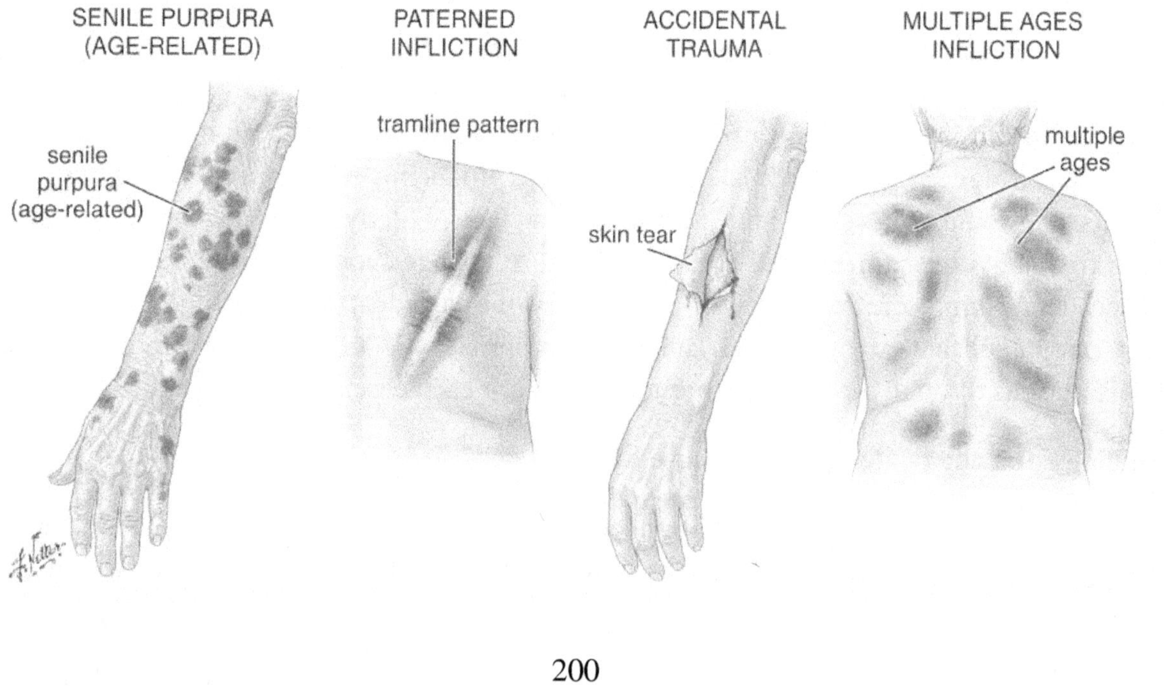

The distinction between inflicted injury and injury reflecting the natural falls that are common in elderly decedents is one of the most demanding reasoning problems in elder death investigation. Elderly individuals fall frequently, and falls produce contusions, abrasions, and, in a substantial fraction, fractures. Not every contusion on an elderly decedent represents abuse. The systematic reasoning documents each injury with reference to location, character, apparent age, and consistency with the reported mechanism; the pattern of injuries (distribution, number, ages) is evaluated for consistency with the reported history. A single contusion on a lower extremity with a documented fall history in a decedent with dementia is different from multiple contusions of variable ages distributed across the body without documented mechanism, and the reasoning distinguishes them.

### Sexual Abuse in Elderly Decedents

Sexual abuse of elderly individuals is documented and requires specific investigation when suspected. The examination includes systematic external and internal genital examination, documentation of any injury, collection of specimens for DNA analysis, and integration with the overall case reasoning. Elderly genital anatomy is atrophic in most postmenopausal decedents and shows characteristic changes that the examiner must distinguish from acute injury. Vaginal atrophy, thinning of the vaginal mucosa, and reduced elasticity of the tissues predispose to injury from any penetration; the presence of injury does not by itself establish assault versus consensual activity, and the reasoning integrates the findings with the case history and with any available witness accounts. In institutional care contexts, sexual abuse of cognitively impaired elderly individuals is a documented pattern that requires specific attention and integration with the aggregate care records.

### Financial Exploitation and Its Consequences

Financial exploitation of elderly individuals is not primarily a forensic pathology concern in the individual death case, but the pathologist should recognize the context because financial exploitation frequently coexists with physical neglect. A decedent whose financial resources have been misappropriated may have been unable to afford adequate care, may have been in an inadequately supported living situation, and may have developed the physical findings of neglect as a direct consequence of the financial exploitation. Documentation of the physical findings supports subsequent civil or criminal proceedings related to the financial exploitation, and coordination with adult protective services and with law enforcement is standard when the aggregate case pattern raises these concerns.

## Elder Neglect and Failure to Care

Elder neglect encompasses failure to provide adequate nutrition, hydration, hygiene, medical care, medication management, or safety by a caregiver responsible for the elderly individual's care. The pattern includes deaths from starvation and dehydration in decedents unable to access food or fluid independently, deaths from complications of untreated medical conditions, deaths from medication mismanagement (both underuse and overuse of prescribed medications), and deaths from environmental exposure or from injury that adequate supervision would have prevented. Neglect fatalities occur both in the home care context and in institutional care settings, and the reasoning depends on the specific context.

### Malnutrition and Dehydration in the Elderly

Malnutrition in an elderly decedent is documented by body weight for height compared to expected values, by loss of subcutaneous fat and muscle mass, by characteristic skin changes (thin, dry, poor turgor), and by histologic and organ findings of chronic nutritional deprivation. The distinction from malnutrition of medical cause — cancer cachexia, chronic heart failure with cardiac cachexia, end-stage renal or hepatic disease — requires systematic evaluation and integration with the medical history. Cancer cachexia produces its own pattern of wasting and is not itself evidence of neglect when the cancer is diagnosed and adequately supported by palliative care; cachexia occurring in an elderly decedent without documented adequate medical support raises the reasoning about neglect contribution. Dehydration is similarly documented by clinical findings (dry mucous membranes, sunken eyes), by vitreous chemistry showing elevated urea and characteristic electrolyte changes, and by evidence of inadequate fluid access or provision.

### Medication Mismanagement

Medication-related deaths in elderly decedents span a spectrum from unintentional overdose in decedents with cognitive impairment (who may take doses in excess of prescribed) through inadequate administration of prescribed medications (missed doses of essential medications with resulting decompensation of chronic disease) to intentional overdose by caregivers (rare but documented). The autopsy identifies elevated drug levels on toxicology in overdose cases and integrates with the medication history; low or absent levels of essential medications support inadequate administration. Common medications involved in elder-specific fatalities include opioid analgesics (both underuse leading to inadequate pain management and overuse leading to respiratory depression), sedative-hypnotics (with elderly individuals particularly vulnerable to falls and to respiratory depression at doses well tolerated in younger patients), antihypertensives (with medication errors producing hypotensive or hypertensive complications), and warfarin (with mismanagement producing bleeding or thromboembolic complications).

### Reasoning About Neglect in the Case Context

The reasoning about whether neglect contributed to the death integrates the physical findings with the caregiving context. The distinction between active neglect (deliberate failure to provide care), passive neglect (failure from caregiver incapacity, lack of knowledge, or resource limitations), and reasonable end-of-life care (comfort-focused care in a decedent with a terminal condition) is not always clearly resolvable at autopsy but affects the eventual manner determination. A decedent with dementia and end-stage disease who died in hospice care with appropriate palliative comfort measures presents a very different case than a decedent with treatable conditions found in unsanitary conditions with evidence of prolonged deprivation. The pathologist documents the physical findings; the reasoning about manner integrates with the broader case investigation including adult protective services, law enforcement, and, where applicable, the healthcare team responsible for the decedent's care.

**SCENE-TO-CERTIFICATION DECISION SYSTEM — Pressure Injury and Neglect Arc**

**Presenting Death Scenario:** An 84-year-old woman with advanced dementia is brought to the emergency department by paramedics from a private residence where she lived with her adult daughter. She is unresponsive and is pronounced dead shortly after arrival. She has multiple pressure ulcers on the sacrum, heels, and posterior scapulae. The daughter reports that her mother had refused to be moved for weeks and that home health nursing had not been retained despite her mother's deteriorating condition. There is no documented history of physician contact in the preceding six months despite her mother's known dementia and cardiovascular disease. Adult protective services becomes involved.

**Autopsy Signature:** External examination documents severe wasting (body weight approximately 38 kilograms for a 1.60 meter body, well below expected), stage IV pressure ulcers on the sacrum (with exposure of underlying bone and osteomyelitis), stage III ulcers on both heels, and stage II ulcers on the posterior scapulae. Multiple ulcers show evidence of chronic infection with purulent exudate. Internal examination shows sepsis with disseminated intravascular coagulation, chronic malnutrition findings, dehydration, and severe atherosclerotic cardiovascular disease consistent with the reported history. Toxicology is negative apart from subtherapeutic levels of prescribed medications documenting inadequate administration.

**Cause Determination:** Sepsis due to chronic pressure ulcers with osteomyelitis, in the setting of chronic malnutrition, dehydration, and inadequate care of an elderly woman with dementia.

**Manner Determination:** Homicide. The pattern of severe pressure injury with underlying osteomyelitis, chronic malnutrition and dehydration, subtherapeutic medication levels, and absence of any documented medical care for a decedent with known dementia and cardiovascular disease supports the determination that inadequate care contributed proximately to the death. The manner determination is medical; specific criminal charges are the province of law enforcement and the prosecutor.

**Trap Logic:** Pressure ulcers can develop in elderly decedents even with adequate care in some end-of-life contexts (particularly in decedents receiving hospice care with appropriate comfort focus), and pressure ulcers by themselves do not automatically establish neglect. The systematic reasoning distinguishes: pressure injury stage (deeper injury with bone involvement suggests prolonged neglect), presence of infection (suggesting inadequate care of established injury), evidence of adequate medical support (documented physician visits, hospice enrollment, home health nursing), and the aggregate care pattern. When the pressure injury is severe (stage III or IV), chronically infected, associated with other neglect findings (malnutrition, dehydration, medication nonadherence), and occurring in the absence of documented adequate care, the neglect determination is supported. When the injury is milder, in the context of documented adequate care, or in a decedent with appropriate hospice enrollment for a terminal condition, the reasoning may support natural manner despite the presence of pressure injury.

**Certification Anchor:** Elder neglect fatalities are certified with reference to the specific mechanism (pressure injury with infection, starvation, dehydration, medication mismanagement, exposure) integrated with the caregiving context. The severity of physical findings and the pattern of caregiving inadequacy together support the manner determination. Coordination with adult protective services and with law enforcement is standard in these cases.

## Falls and Fall-Related Death in the Elderly

Falls are the leading cause of injury-related death in elderly individuals in most epidemiological data. Fall-related deaths span mechanisms including immediate death from severe injury (typically catastrophic head injury or hip fracture with subsequent complications), delayed death from injury sequelae (pulmonary embolism after immobilization, pneumonia after prolonged bed rest), and death from complications of the underlying medical conditions that produced the fall. The forensic pathologist encounters fall-related deaths across all three categories, and the reasoning about the specific mechanism supports the case certification.

### Fall-Related Head Injury

Fall-related head injury in the elderly typically produces subdural hemorrhage from bridging vein tear, cerebral contusion, and, when the fall is from height or with substantial force, skull fracture with more severe intracranial injury. Elderly individuals are particularly vulnerable to subdural hemorrhage from relatively minor mechanisms because cerebral atrophy allows greater stretch of the bridging veins with even small angular acceleration. A ground-level fall with head impact in an elderly decedent can produce a lethal subdural hematoma that would not occur in a younger person with the same mechanism. The autopsy identifies the head injury and integrates with the fall history; substantial mismatch between the mechanism reported and the injury pattern warrants specific reasoning.

Figure 14.2: Acute Subdural Hematoma in the Elderly on Postmortem CT

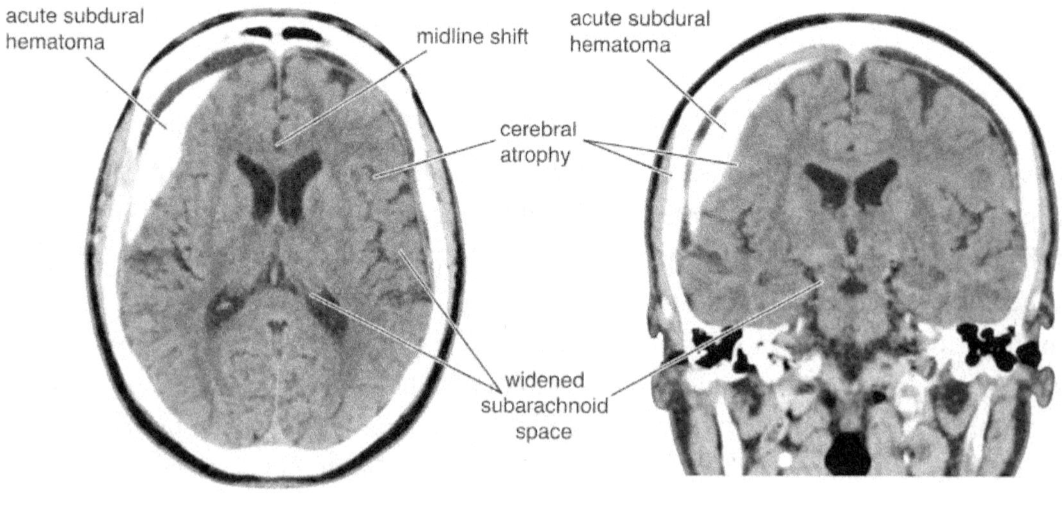

### Hip Fracture and Its Complications

Hip fracture is the classic fall-related injury in the elderly and carries substantial mortality within the year following the injury. Direct death from hip fracture is uncommon; more commonly, death occurs from complications including pulmonary embolism, pneumonia, complications of surgery or of prolonged immobilization, and progression of underlying comorbid disease during the recovery period. The pathologist encountering a decedent who died in the weeks following hip fracture identifies the fracture, its surgical repair status if any, the specific complication that produced death, and the underlying cardiovascular and other comorbidities that contributed. The certification typically includes the fall-related hip fracture with the specific complication (pulmonary embolism following hip fracture and repair; hospital-acquired pneumonia following surgical repair) and the contributing conditions.

### The Mechanism-Injury Consistency Question

The distinction between accidental and inflicted mechanism in an elderly fall is one specific application of the general mechanism-consistency reasoning. Reported falls that produce injury patterns inconsistent with the reported mechanism warrant specific reasoning. A reported ground-level fall producing catastrophic multi-system injury; a reported fall producing injuries only on the posterior body without any contact injuries on the anterior body; a reported fall in a decedent with dementia where the caregiver is the only witness; a reported fall with injuries in patterns suggestive of a push rather than a spontaneous loss of balance — each raises the reasoning about the alternative mechanism. The systematic evaluation documents the injury pattern, the reported history, and the reasoning about consistency; the manner determination reflects the assessment.

### SCENE-TO-CERTIFICATION DECISION SYSTEM — Elder Fall Determination Arc

**Presenting Death Scenario:** A 79-year-old woman is found deceased at the bottom of a residential staircase by her adult son, who reports that he found her when he returned home from work. He states that she must have fallen down the stairs, which she used routinely despite her age and osteoarthritis. Emergency services confirm death at the scene. The medical examiner's office accepts jurisdiction. Prior history documents that the son had recently gained power of attorney and that adult protective services had received a call from a neighbor several weeks earlier expressing concern about the mother's care.

**Autopsy Signature:** External examination documents extensive multi-site injury: a large scalp laceration and depressed skull fracture over the right parietal region; contusions and abrasions distributed on the anterior and lateral body; fractured wrists bilaterally with clinical appearance suggesting defensive positioning during a fall; and, on layered anterior neck dissection performed as standard given the possibility of neck compression, no evidence of cervical soft tissue hemorrhage. Internal examination confirms severe head injury with acute subdural and subarachnoid hemorrhage, extensive cerebral contusion, and no additional injury of suspicious pattern. Postmortem CT confirms the skull fracture and identifies no other skeletal fracture beyond the wrists. Toxicology is negative.

**Cause Determination:** Blunt force head injury with skull fracture and severe intracranial hemorrhage consistent with a fall down a staircase.

**Manner Determination:** Accident. The pattern of injuries is consistent with a fall down the reported staircase: the head injury pattern is characteristic of impact against a firm surface during a tumbling fall; the bilateral wrist fractures are consistent with defensive positioning as the decedent attempted to protect herself; the distribution of contusions on the anterior body is consistent with contact against the stairs during the fall. The absence of any injury pattern suggesting alternative mechanism (no defensive wounds on the hands, no injury to the posterior body inconsistent with the fall, no cervical soft tissue hemorrhage suggesting strangulation) supports the accident determination. The context of caregiver concern reported by adult protective services is documented but does not change the manner determination in the absence of specific evidence of inflicted mechanism.

**Trap Logic:** The context of adult protective services concern raises the possibility of inflicted mechanism, and the case is investigated with attention to that possibility. The systematic evaluation — injury pattern reconstruction, cervical dissection, complete external examination, integration with the reported history — does not identify findings supporting inflicted mechanism. The trap is to certify homicide based on context alone without specific injury evidence, and equally the trap is to accept the reported history without systematic examination. The correct reasoning is the systematic examination with transparent documentation of what was considered and what the findings support.

**Certification Anchor:** Fall-related death in the elderly is certified as accident when the injury pattern is consistent with the reported mechanism, when no findings suggest inflicted alternative, and when the systematic examination has considered and excluded alternative mechanisms. The context of caregiver concern is documented but does not by itself change the manner determination in the absence of specific injury evidence. When findings do support inflicted mechanism (patterned injuries, cervical soft tissue hemorrhage, defensive wounds inconsistent with fall pattern), homicide is the appropriate certification with transparent documentation of the reasoning.

## Pressure Injury and Its Investigation

Pressure injuries — also termed pressure ulcers or decubitus ulcers — are areas of skin and underlying tissue damage produced by prolonged pressure against a bony prominence, typically at sites of skin contact with supporting surfaces during prolonged immobility. Their presence in an elderly decedent has forensic significance because the pattern and severity of pressure injury reflects the adequacy of positional care over the antecedent period.

### Staging and Documentation

Pressure injuries are staged by the National Pressure Injury Advisory Panel classification (updated iterations of which have been developed over decades) into stage I (intact skin with nonblanchable erythema over a bony prominence), stage II (partial-thickness loss with exposed dermis), stage III (full-thickness loss with adipose visible but without exposure of underlying bone, tendon, or muscle), stage IV (full-thickness loss with exposure of underlying bone, tendon, or muscle), unstageable (full-thickness loss where the base is obscured by slough or eschar such that the true depth cannot be assessed), and deep tissue injury (intact or non-intact skin with localized area of persistent nonblanchable deep discoloration, indicating underlying deep tissue damage). The staging supports the reasoning about care adequacy: stage I and mild stage II injuries can develop rapidly over hours in a critically ill decedent even with adequate positional care; stage III and IV injuries typically require prolonged inadequate care to develop.

### Pressure Injury and Care Adequacy

The reasoning about care adequacy from pressure injury requires attention to the decedent's medical condition, to the care setting, and to the timeline of injury development. A decedent with terminal illness receiving hospice care with appropriate comfort focus may develop pressure injuries as an expected finding of the terminal state, particularly if the family has requested a home comfort-focused approach; the injuries are not by themselves evidence of neglect. A decedent in an institutional setting with expected active care who develops stage IV pressure injuries with osteomyelitis raises specific concerns about care adequacy. The reasoning integrates the physical findings, the care documentation, and the specific context; consultation with wound care specialists supports the reasoning in complex cases.

## Deaths in Long-Term Care Facilities

Long-term care facility deaths present specific reconstruction challenges because the decedent has been in institutional care with documented medical records, because staff members are witnesses to the sequence of events, and because the case may involve systemic care quality issues rather than individual perpetrator conduct. The forensic pathology approach in these cases integrates the autopsy findings with the facility records, the staff interviews conducted by law enforcement or by adult protective services, and, where indicated, coordination with state or federal regulators overseeing long-term care.

### Common Case Patterns

Common case patterns in long-term care facility deaths include: unexpected sudden death (which may reflect underlying disease, medication effect, or unrecognized injury); fall-related death with the fall witnessed or unwitnessed and with variable documentation quality; death from complications of chronic disease with reasoning about care adequacy; death associated with restraint use (with attention to the specific restraint and the mechanism); and death associated with medication administration (with attention to medication errors, drug interactions, and medication mismanagement). Each pattern has specific reconstruction implications, and the pathologist integrates the autopsy findings with the facility documentation.

### Restraint-Associated Deaths in Institutional Care

Physical restraints in long-term care facilities — chair restraints, bed rails, restraint chairs — have specific documented risks including asphyxia from entrapment, injury from the restraint itself, and complications from prolonged restricted movement. Deaths associated with restraint use in institutional settings require systematic examination for evidence of the restraint mechanism (patterned marks, specific injury patterns), integration with the facility restraint records, and reasoning about whether the restraint use was appropriate and adequately monitored. The specific pattern of chest wall restraint with resulting positional restriction of respiration is a documented mechanism in institutional restraint deaths and warrants specific attention. The topic overlaps substantially with the deaths-in-custody discussion of Chapter 16.

Figure 14.3

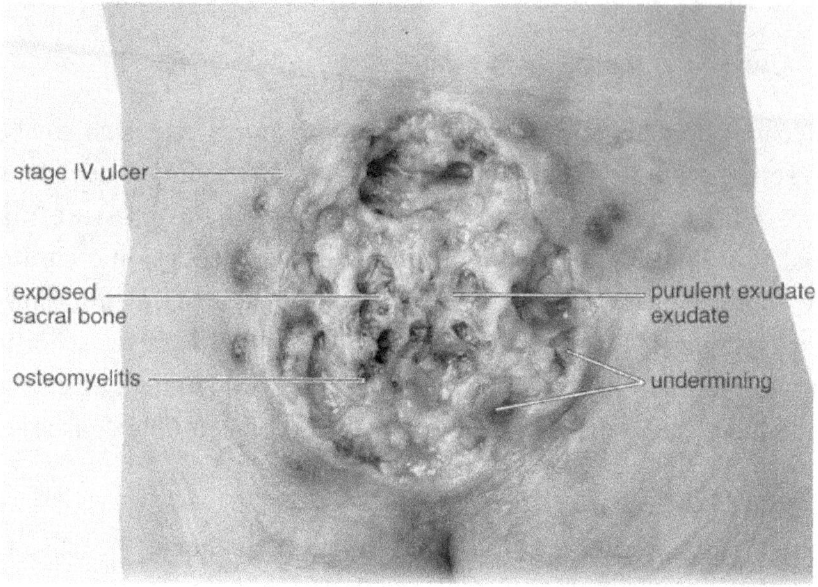


**Serial Deaths in Facility Contexts**

Serial deaths in a single facility or under the care of a single provider have been documented as a specific pattern in institutional care. Medical serial killers, though rare, have caused substantial numbers of deaths in institutional care contexts before detection, typically through administration of lethal medications to vulnerable patients. Recognition depends on aggregate case analysis rather than on individual case investigation — no single case typically identifies the pattern, but review across multiple deaths under the same care may reveal it. Coordination with hospital or facility risk management, with state regulators, and with law enforcement is standard when the pattern emerges. The forensic pathology contribution is the individual case documentation that supports the aggregate analysis.

**CAUTION:** Serial deaths in a long-term care or hospital setting under the care of a single provider warrant specific analysis. No single case may identify the pattern; the analysis is aggregate. Coordination with facility risk management, state regulators, and law enforcement is standard when the pattern is suspected. The forensic pathology contribution is individual case documentation adequate to support the aggregate analysis.

**Self-Neglect and Diogenes Syndrome**

Self-neglect — a pattern in which an elderly individual with capacity fails to provide their own basic needs — is a documented category with substantial forensic implications. Diogenes syndrome, sometimes called senile squalor syndrome, describes an extreme form in which the elderly individual lives in extreme squalor, refuses assistance, hoards materials, and often has associated psychiatric or cognitive impairment. Deaths in self-neglect present differently from caregiver neglect: the scene shows the neglect pattern (unsanitary conditions, spoiled food, inadequate heating or cooling, hoarded materials interfering with movement), but there is no external caregiver whose action or inaction produced the situation. The manner determination in these cases is complex because the decedent retained sufficient capacity to refuse assistance and the intent was not self-destructive in the sense of suicide. Manner is typically classified as natural (when the death is from underlying disease that the decedent refused to treat), accident (in some interpretations), or undetermined depending on office practice. The certification documents the self-neglect context transparently.

The distinction between self-neglect and caregiver neglect is critical. A decedent found in unsanitary conditions might reflect either pattern, and the reasoning integrates the scene evidence, the antecedent history, and the pattern of the decedent's functional capacity. A decedent with dementia who was under a family member's care and who was found in inadequate conditions represents caregiver neglect; a decedent with capacity who refused offered assistance from family or from adult protective services and lived independently in the conditions represents self-neglect. The distinction shapes the manner determination and any subsequent legal proceedings against caregivers.

**Capacity, Consent, and the Elderly Decedent**

The concept of decision-making capacity is central to the reasoning about many elder death cases. Capacity is the ability to understand the nature of a decision, to appreciate its consequences, to reason among alternatives, and to communicate a choice. Capacity may be preserved in some domains and lost in others (a decedent with dementia may retain capacity to make simple daily decisions while having lost capacity for complex financial decisions). Capacity is a legal determination made during life, not a forensic determination made postmortem. However, the pathologist reasoning about a case that involves elder abuse or neglect commonly encounters the capacity question in retrospect — whether the decedent could have consented to the care arrangement, whether the decedent could have refused offered assistance, whether the decedent understood the risks of the decisions being made. Documentation of the decedent's functional and cognitive status from medical records, from family accounts, and from any assessment tools completed during life supports the reasoning. Consultation with geriatric medicine or geriatric psychiatry specialists is available for cases where the capacity question is central.

**Delayed Discovery and Time of Death**

Elderly decedents in community residence, particularly those living alone, are frequently discovered at substantial delay after death. Delayed discovery adds interpretive challenge to the case: postmortem changes are more advanced, injury and disease findings may be obscured or exaggerated by decomposition, time-of-death estimation is less precise, and the specific circumstances leading to death may be less recoverable from scene evidence. Systematic scene documentation before body removal is particularly important in these cases. The pathologist integrates the postmortem findings with the estimated postmortem interval, with any evidence of pre-death illness (medications in the residence, evidence of self-care attempts, evidence of collapse pattern in the scene), and with the antecedent history. Cases of delayed discovery in decedents living alone frequently reflect the aggregate pattern of inadequate community support for elderly individuals living independently — a pattern with policy implications beyond the individual case.

### Polypharmacy and Drug Interactions in the Elderly

Elderly decedents frequently take multiple medications, and drug interactions and adverse effects account for a substantial fraction of medication-related deaths in this population. Polypharmacy — defined variably but commonly as concurrent use of five or more medications — increases the risk of adverse drug reactions and interactions. Specific patterns include: anticholinergic burden from multiple medications with anticholinergic properties producing cognitive decline, falls, and complications; sedative-hypnotic interactions with other central nervous system depressants producing respiratory depression; anticoagulant interactions with other medications producing bleeding complications; and specific interactions such as serotonin syndrome from concurrent serotonergic medications. Toxicology in the elderly decedent frequently identifies multiple medications at therapeutic or slightly elevated levels; the reasoning about whether the medication burden contributed to death integrates the levels, the clinical setting, and any documented interaction pattern. Simplification of medication regimens by geriatric medicine specialists is a documented approach to reducing polypharmacy-related deaths, and the forensic pathology data on these cases supports the epidemiological understanding of the pattern.

### End-of-Life Care and Hospice Patterns

The distinction between neglect-related death and appropriate end-of-life care is a specific reasoning category that requires attention. Hospice-enrolled decedents receive care focused on comfort rather than on curative intervention; the standard of care in hospice does not include treatment aimed at prolonging life against the underlying disease trajectory. Autopsy findings in hospice decedents may include chronic disease at advanced stages, complications of the terminal condition, and, in many cases, pressure injuries and dehydration that reflect the terminal state rather than inadequate care. The reasoning integrates the hospice enrollment status, the specific care plan (which typically includes documented family conferences and specific comfort measures), and the autopsy findings; the presence of hospice care substantially changes the interpretation of findings that might otherwise raise neglect concerns. Family-managed hospice care at home carries additional complexity because the family provides much of the direct care and the boundaries between appropriate comfort care and inadequate care may be less clear-cut than in institutional hospice.

The pathologist encountering a decedent with hospice enrollment reviews the documentation carefully, integrates the specific care approach with the autopsy findings, and reasons about whether the findings are consistent with the appropriate end-of-life trajectory. In most cases, the reasoning supports natural manner with the underlying terminal condition as the primary cause; findings that raise specific concerns (severe injury inconsistent with the reported care, evidence of abuse in addition to the terminal condition) still warrant investigation but the reasoning framework differs from the community-dwelling non-hospice decedent.

## Environmental Disaster Deaths in the Elderly

Environmental disaster deaths — heat waves, cold snaps, hurricanes, wildfires, floods — disproportionately affect elderly populations. The mechanisms include hyperthermia from inadequate cooling in prolonged heat exposure (particularly in decedents in inadequately air-conditioned residences during heat waves), hypothermia from inadequate heating or from exposure during storm-related power loss, and disaster-specific mechanisms (drowning during hurricane flooding, thermal injury during wildfires, injury during storm-related structural damage). The elderly vulnerability reflects reduced physiologic reserve, higher prevalence of chronic conditions that impair adaptation to environmental extremes, greater social isolation reducing rescue during emergencies, and specific limitations (medication requirements for refrigeration, need for medical equipment requiring electricity, immobility limiting evacuation). Deaths during major disasters are typically certified with the specific mechanism and integrated with the aggregate disaster casualty count for public health and policy purposes. Preparedness deficiencies in the response to elderly-specific needs — documented in retrospective analyses of major disasters — have policy implications that the forensic pathology data supports.

## Financial Exploitation and Fatal Consequences

Financial exploitation of elderly decedents — the misappropriation of resources by family members, caregivers, or scam actors — has documented associations with fatal outcomes through several mechanisms. Decedents whose resources have been misappropriated may have been unable to afford medications, adequate food, safe housing, or medical care; the physical findings of the resulting inadequate care are present at autopsy. Decedents subjected to prolonged financial abuse may show psychological decline that contributes to overall deterioration and to inadequate self-care. Scam-related deaths — elderly decedents who died in circumstances related to attempts to comply with fraudulent demands — have been documented. The forensic pathology contribution is documentation of the physical findings that support subsequent civil or criminal proceedings related to the financial exploitation; coordination with adult protective services, law enforcement financial crimes units, and, where applicable, state attorneys general offices supports the aggregate response.

## The Elder Death Review Team

Systematic elder death review teams have been developed in many jurisdictions on the model of child death review teams. The teams typically include forensic pathology, geriatric medicine, adult protective services, law enforcement, prosecutors, long-term care ombudsmen, and, in some jurisdictions, elder advocacy representatives. Review of individual elder death cases and of aggregate patterns supports identification of systemic issues (facility care quality, community support gaps, medication management deficiencies) that individual case investigation would not identify. The forensic pathology contribution is the case documentation and reasoning that supports the aggregate analysis. Participation in the elder death review team supports both the individual case reasoning and the broader public health goal of reducing preventable elder mortality.

**SCENE-TO-CERTIFICATION DECISION SYSTEM — Elder Death Determination Arcs**

**The Elder Investigation Framework:** Elder death investigation requires attention to the interpretive challenges specific to elderly decedents: skin fragility, osteoporosis, common comorbidities producing autopsy findings, and cognitive impairment limiting history reliability. Systematic reasoning distinguishes natural disease findings from findings of inflicted injury or neglect.

**Physical Abuse Recognition:** Physical abuse patterns include patterned injuries documenting specific implements, restraint-associated injuries, injuries at sites inconsistent with reported falls, and multiple injuries of variable ages. The distinction from age-related fragility and from routine handling injury requires systematic examination and integration with the caregiving context.

**Neglect Fatalities:** Elder neglect fatalities include starvation and dehydration deaths, deaths from untreated medical conditions, medication mismanagement deaths, and complications of pressure injuries with inadequate care. Systematic exclusion of alternative medical explanations and integration with the caregiving context supports the manner determination.

**Fall Investigation:** Fall-related death in the elderly is common and typically accidental in mechanism. The distinction from inflicted mechanism (push, assault) depends on systematic examination of the injury pattern for consistency with the reported mechanism, absence of alternative-mechanism findings (defensive injury, cervical soft tissue hemorrhage), and integration with the caregiving context.

**Long-Term Care Facility Deaths:** Long-term care facility deaths integrate autopsy findings with facility records, staff interviews, and coordination with regulators. Common patterns include unexpected sudden death, fall-related death, restraint-associated death, and medication-related death. Serial deaths under single-provider care warrant specific aggregate analysis with facility and law enforcement coordination.

## Summary and Key Concepts

Elder death investigation presents specific interpretive challenges arising from age-related skin fragility, osteoporosis, common comorbidities producing autopsy findings, and cognitive impairment limiting history reliability. Systematic reasoning distinguishes natural disease from inflicted injury and from neglect.

Physical elder abuse patterns include patterned injuries documenting specific implements, restraint-associated injuries, and injuries at sites inconsistent with reported falls. The distinction from age-related fragility requires systematic examination and integration with the caregiving context.

Elder neglect fatalities include starvation and dehydration deaths, deaths from untreated medical conditions, medication mismanagement deaths, and complications of pressure injuries with inadequate care. The reasoning integrates physical findings with the caregiving context.

Fall-related deaths in the elderly are common and typically accidental in mechanism. Elderly individuals are particularly vulnerable to subdural hemorrhage from ground-level falls because of cerebral atrophy. The distinction from inflicted mechanism depends on systematic examination and injury pattern consistency reasoning.

Pressure injuries are staged from I through IV and unstageable, with severity reflecting the adequacy of positional care over the antecedent period. Stage III and IV injuries with associated infection support the reasoning about inadequate care when the caregiving context supports it.

Long-term care facility deaths integrate autopsy findings with facility documentation, staff interviews, and coordination with regulators. Serial deaths under single-provider care warrant specific aggregate analysis with facility risk management and law enforcement involvement.

# CHAPTER 15: SEXUAL ASSAULT AND THE POSTMORTEM SEXUAL ASSAULT EXAMINATION

**Learning Objectives**

1. Articulate the framework for postmortem sexual assault examination and its integration with the broader forensic autopsy.
2. Perform the standard postmortem sexual assault evidence collection protocol with attention to specimen preservation and chain of custody.
3. Recognize anogenital injury patterns and reason about consistency with reported or reconstructed assault mechanism, with attention to the normal anatomic variation that must not be misidentified as injury.
4. Interpret toxicological findings in the context of drug-facilitated sexual assault cases and articulate the specimen collection and analytical considerations.
5. Reason systematically about the assault-homicide case, integrating the sexual assault findings with the overall injury pattern and manner determination.

## The Postmortem Sexual Assault Examination Framework

Postmortem sexual assault examination is a specialized element of the forensic autopsy that arises whenever the case history, scene evidence, or autopsy findings suggest that sexual assault may have preceded death or accompanied the fatal mechanism. The examination follows a standardized protocol modeled on the sexual assault examination performed in living survivors, adapted for the postmortem context. The purpose is to identify and preserve evidence supporting perpetrator identification, to document injury patterns consistent with assault mechanism, and to integrate the findings with the overall case reasoning. The examination is performed with the same professional dignity accorded to every other autopsy element.

The framework recognizes that sexual assault preceding or accompanying death occurs across a broad range of case types: assault-homicide where the fatal mechanism is directly connected to the assault; homicide with concurrent sexual assault where the sexual assault is one element of the overall violence; sexual assault of a decedent (necrophilic assault, a documented but uncommon pattern); and cases where sexual assault occurred at some point in the antecedent period and may or may not connect to the immediate mechanism of death. The pathologist reasons about each case with attention to the specific pattern and to what the physical evidence supports.

The pathologist encountering a case with any indication of possible sexual assault performs the postmortem sexual assault examination in every such case, regardless of the initially estimated probability. Missed opportunities for evidence collection cannot be recovered later, and cases that initially appear to have no sexual assault component may reveal on complete workup that assault occurred. The systematic protocol is applied with the same discipline as every other element of the autopsy.

### When the Sexual Assault Examination Is Indicated

Specific indications for the postmortem sexual assault examination include: scene evidence suggesting sexual assault (disarrayed clothing, evidence of struggle in a sexual context, victim discovered in a state consistent with assault); homicide with any evidence of sexual motivation or context; deaths of individuals in specific vulnerable populations where assault is a documented pattern (elderly individuals in some institutional care contexts, individuals with substantial cognitive impairment, children with any concerning findings); deaths in circumstances where drug-facilitated sexual assault is a differential (unexplained deaths of individuals in social contexts with alcohol or drug availability); and any death where investigators have identified specific evidence supporting sexual assault as a case element. The pathologist follows the office protocol for the specific indications and applies conservative judgment in favor of performing the examination when uncertainty exists.

## Evidence Collection Protocol

The postmortem sexual assault evidence collection kit is a standardized set of specimens collected in a defined sequence and preserved in specific containers with chain of custody documentation. The kit content varies by jurisdiction but the core elements are consistent across current practice.

### External Specimens

External specimens include: swabs of the mouth, external skin surfaces potentially exposed to biological material from a perpetrator (breasts, buttocks, thighs), and any specific areas identified as suspicious (bite marks, contusions from grip, areas with identifiable biological deposits). Combings of scalp hair, pubic hair (when present), and axillary hair collect trace material from a perpetrator. Fingernail scrapings or fingernail cuttings preserve material scraped from a perpetrator during defensive struggle; the specimens are collected before any handling of the hands that could dislodge material. Clothing worn by the decedent is preserved intact when possible, or specific portions containing biological deposits or damage are preserved. Alternate light source examination — illumination of the body surface with ultraviolet or other alternative light sources — identifies biological deposits (semen, saliva) that are not visible under standard lighting; identified deposits are collected with dedicated swabs.

### Internal Specimens

Internal specimens include: oral swabs (buccal and posterior pharyngeal, with attention to sites where oral penetration would have deposited material); vaginal swabs (external, distal, and posterior fornix, collected in sequence to identify material at different sites); anal and rectal swabs (external, distal, and proximal, similarly collected in sequence); and, when indicated, urethral specimens. Speculum examination supports adequate specimen collection from the vaginal fornix in decedents where speculum insertion does not damage evidence; in some cases, digital examination is used to guide swab placement. Each specimen is collected on a specific swab, air-dried according to standard protocol (typically at least 30 minutes of drying), packaged in a specifically labeled envelope, and integrated into the sealed evidence collection kit.

### Blood, Vitreous, and Toxicology Specimens

Blood specimens for toxicology in sexual assault cases include the standard toxicology specimens (peripheral and central blood, vitreous, gastric contents, urine when available) with attention to preservation for drug-facilitated sexual assault analysis. Specific specimens collected for drug-facilitated sexual assault analysis include urine (with attention to the time from suspected exposure to death, because many facilitating agents have short half-lives) and hair (for retrospective identification of chronic exposure or of exposure preceding the recent event beyond the window of blood or urine detection). The specimens are preserved with standard chain of custody and are analyzed with focused drug panels reflecting the facilitating agents commonly identified in these cases.

Figure 15.1: Anogenital Injury Patterns in Sexual Assault: Documented Sites

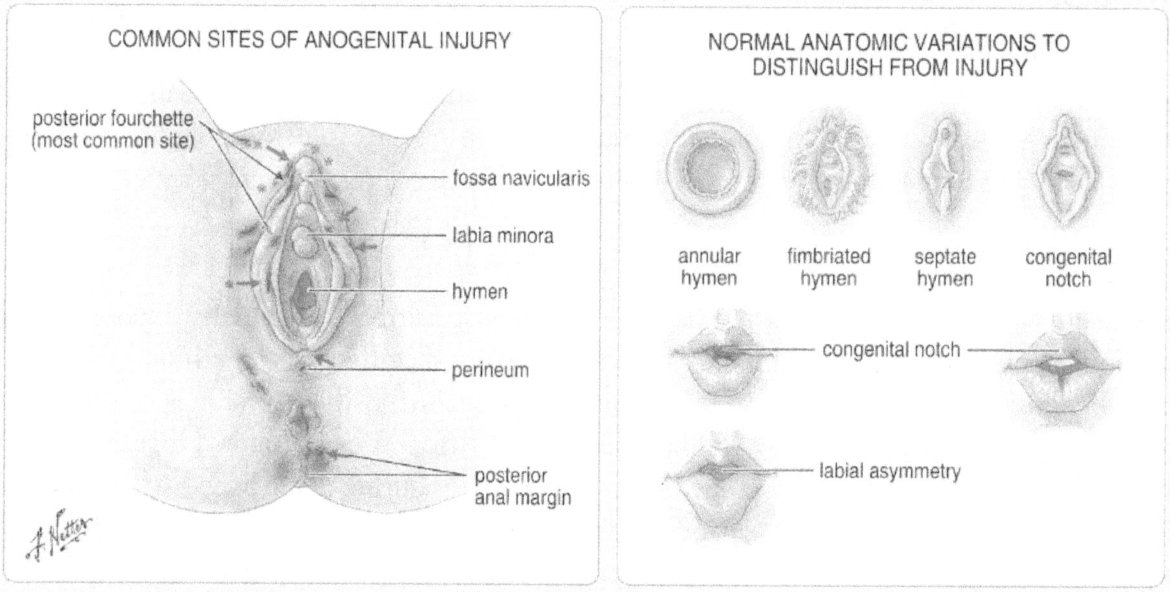


### Chain of Custody Documentation

Chain of custody documentation for sexual assault evidence begins at the moment of specimen collection and continues through every transfer, storage, and analysis event. Each specimen is labeled at the time of collection with the case identifier, specimen description, collection date and time, and collector identity. The specimens are packaged in the sealed kit with tamper-evident seals. Transfer to the crime laboratory or to other analytical facilities is documented with signed transfer forms. Storage at each site is documented with temperature logs and access records. The pathologist's role is to establish the beginning of the chain with rigorous specimen collection and packaging; the subsequent chain is maintained by law enforcement and by laboratory personnel.

## Anogenital Injury Patterns

Anogenital injury interpretation in sexual assault cases is one of the more contested areas of forensic examination. The findings range from clearly documented injury (lacerations, contusions, avulsions with obvious mechanism) through subtle findings requiring careful documentation to normal anatomic variation that must not be misidentified as injury. The examination requires familiarity with normal anatomy and its variation as well as with the injury patterns documented in assault cases.

### Sites of Injury and Their Interpretation

In female genital assault, the most commonly documented site of injury is the posterior fourchette, followed by the fossa navicularis, the labia minora, and the hymen (in pre-pubertal and some adult cases). Posterior fourchette lacerations are documented in a substantial fraction of vaginal assault cases and are among the more reliable indicators of assault mechanism when found. Fossa navicularis abrasions are similarly documented. Injuries to the labia minora may be contusions, abrasions, or lacerations. Hymenal findings require particular care because hymenal anatomy varies substantially in normal individuals and because the interpretation of hymenal findings in prepubertal and adolescent cases has evolved substantially in the peer-reviewed literature; consultation with pediatric child abuse specialists is standard in cases where hymenal findings are central to the case reasoning.

Anal injuries in sexual assault cases include contusions and abrasions of the perianal skin, lacerations of the posterior anal margin (typically at the 6 o'clock and 12 o'clock positions with the decedent in supine position, reflecting the mechanical stress points of anal penetration), and, in cases of severe injury, more extensive laceration or avulsion. Anal injury is distinguished from the findings of chronic anal disease (hemorrhoids, fissures from constipation or other causes) and from postmortem changes; consultation and second-opinion review support the interpretation in complex cases.

### Normal Variations That Must Not Be Misidentified

Normal anatomic variations that must not be misidentified as injury include: normal variation in hymenal morphology (crescentic, annular, fimbriated, septate, and other variants documented in normal individuals); normal variation in labial size and shape; skin tags, papillae, and other normal skin projections that must not be confused with lesions; normal pigmentation variation; and postmortem changes that can produce apparent findings not present in life. The examiner is trained in normal variation to a level adequate for reliable distinction; consultation with pediatric abuse specialists or with sexual assault nurse examiners is available for cases where the distinction is difficult. Documentation of findings that are ambiguous is preserved as ambiguous, with the interpretation reasoning transparent in the report.

**CLINICAL PEARL:** The interpretation of hymenal findings and of subtle anogenital abnormalities in sexual assault cases has evolved substantially in the peer-reviewed literature. Findings previously described as pathognomonic have been shown to be normal variants; findings previously overlooked have been identified as significant. Consultation with pediatric abuse specialists, with sexual assault nurse examiners, and with peer forensic pathologists supports the interpretation in complex cases.

Figure 15.2: Sexual Assault Evidence Collection Sequence: Standardized Protocol

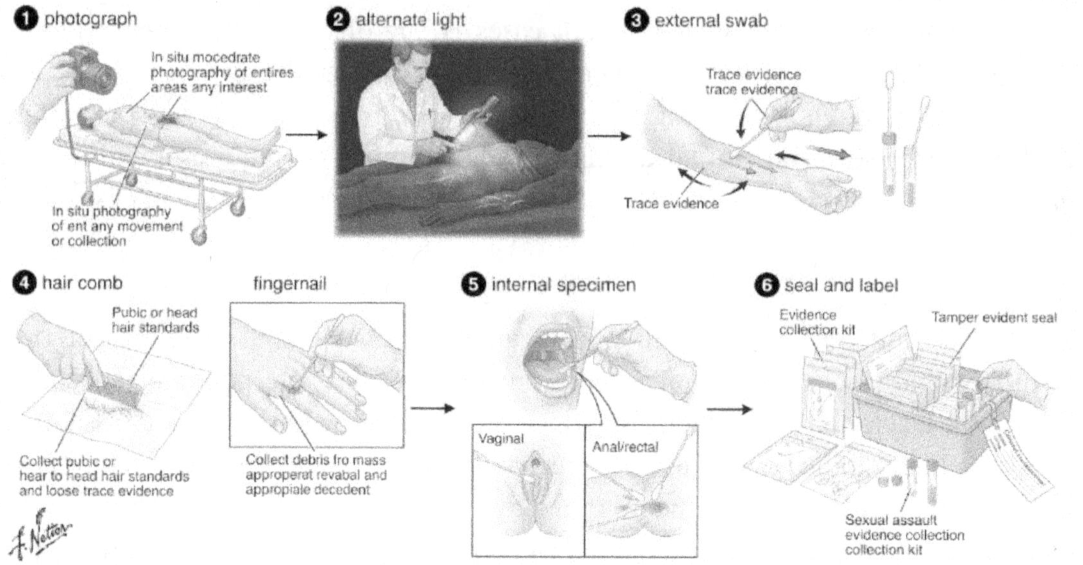


### The Absence of Injury Does Not Exclude Assault

A specific reasoning point deserves emphasis: the absence of anogenital injury does not exclude sexual assault. Consensual sexual activity produces variable findings, some assault mechanisms produce minimal or no anatomic injury (particularly when the decedent was unconscious or incapacitated at the time of the assault), and postmortem changes can obscure injuries that were present in life. The absence of injury is documented; the absence is not read as evidence excluding assault. Conversely, the presence of injury does not by itself establish that the injury was assault-related; the interpretation integrates injury with the case context. The reasoning discipline is the same as elsewhere in forensic pathology — findings are documented, alternatives are considered, and reasoning is transparent.

## Toxicology in Sexual Assault Cases

Toxicological analysis in sexual assault cases addresses two related questions: whether the decedent was under the influence of alcohol or drugs at the time of the assault (voluntary or involuntary), and whether specific drug-facilitated sexual assault agents can be identified. The distinction matters because the analytical approach differs — comprehensive drug screening for the first question, focused analysis for specific facilitating agents for the second question.

### Drug-Facilitated Sexual Assault

Drug-facilitated sexual assault refers to assault in which the perpetrator administered a substance to the victim to produce incapacitation or amnesia facilitating the assault. Common facilitating agents include ethanol (frequently combined with other agents), benzodiazepines (particularly flunitrazepam, though it is not licensed in the United States and is uncommonly identified in American cases; other benzodiazepines are more common), gamma-hydroxybutyrate (GHB, with short half-life and rapid metabolism producing a narrow window of detection), ketamine, opioids (both prescription and illicit), and various other sedative-hypnotic agents. The window of detection for each agent varies substantially, and the reasoning about drug-facilitated sexual assault depends on collection of appropriate specimens as early as possible in the case investigation.

### Specimen Collection for Drug-Facilitated Analysis

Specimen collection for drug-facilitated sexual assault analysis includes urine (the primary specimen for many facilitating agents due to their concentration and prolonged detection window in urine), blood (for agents with adequate blood detection windows), and hair (for retrospective analysis of exposure preceding the death by weeks or months, useful when the specific exposure event predates the detection window in blood or urine). Sample size for urine analysis is important because some analytical techniques for facilitating agents require larger volumes than standard toxicology screens. The pathologist coordinates with the analytical laboratory to ensure adequate specimen for the specific tests being requested.

### SCENE-TO-CERTIFICATION DECISION SYSTEM — Postmortem Sexual Assault Evidence Arc

**Presenting Death Scenario:** A 22-year-old woman is found deceased in her residence by her roommate the morning after attending a party. The decedent was last seen at the party approximately 12 hours before discovery. Scene documentation shows her fully clothed on her bed, without evidence of struggle at the scene. The roommate reports that the decedent had been drinking at the party and had left with a person the roommate did not recognize. The medical examiner's office accepts jurisdiction on the unexpected death of a young person, and the postmortem sexual assault examination is initiated as a standard element given the circumstances.

**Autopsy Signature:** External examination is unremarkable apart from small perianal contusions and a small labial contusion; there is no other significant external injury. Postmortem sexual assault evidence collection kit is completed with standard protocol including external, oral, vaginal, and anal specimens; alternate light source examination identifies biological deposits on the anterior thigh and perineum which are collected on dedicated swabs. Internal examination shows nonspecific findings without acute pathology. Toxicology shows blood ethanol of 0.22 grams per deciliter and detection of gamma-hydroxybutyrate in urine at a level consistent with recent exogenous administration. Additional drug screen is otherwise negative. Vaginal swabs subsequently confirm the presence of male DNA consistent with an unknown individual who is not the decedent.

**Cause Determination:** Acute combined ethanol and gamma-hydroxybutyrate toxicity, with contributing hypoxic injury from respiratory depression.

**Manner Determination:** Homicide. The determination reflects: the constellation of findings including anogenital injuries consistent with sexual assault, biological evidence of a male perpetrator, evidence of drug-facilitated assault with GHB administration, and death from the combined toxicity produced by the exogenously administered substance. The specific criminal characterization is the province of law enforcement and the prosecutor; the manner classification reflects the medical determination that the death resulted from another person's actions.

**Trap Logic:** The trap in cases of young women found dead after social contexts involving alcohol is to attribute the death to voluntary alcohol intoxication without pursuing the drug-facilitated sexual assault differential. Voluntary ethanol intoxication to a level of 0.22 is generally not lethal in an otherwise healthy young person and warrants investigation for contributing factors. The systematic protocol includes: postmortem sexual assault evidence collection whenever the circumstances support the differential; focused toxicological analysis for facilitating agents; and integration of the findings. The GHB detection in this case establishes the drug-facilitated component; without the specific analysis, the case might have been certified as acute ethanol toxicity of undetermined manner. A related trap is failure to preserve the evidence collection kit properly, which forecloses the DNA analysis that identified the male biological material.

**Certification Anchor:** Postmortem sexual assault examination is performed whenever the circumstances support the differential, regardless of the initially estimated probability. Toxicology in sexual assault cases includes focused analysis for facilitating agents. Chain of custody preservation supports the subsequent DNA analysis that identifies perpetrators. The systematic protocol prevents case closure on incomplete workup.

## The Assault-Homicide Case

The assault-homicide case — in which sexual assault is one component of an assault ending in death — is the specific case type where the sexual assault findings integrate with the overall assault pattern to support the aggregate reconstruction. The examination proceeds through the standard autopsy elements together with the sexual assault protocol, and the reasoning integrates all findings.

### The Combined Injury Pattern

Assault-homicide cases commonly show combined injury patterns including: fatal mechanism injuries (typically neck compression, blunt head injury, or gunshot wound); defensive injuries on the hands and forearms from the decedent's attempt to defend against the assault; contusions and abrasions from the mechanical struggle; and anogenital injuries from the sexual component. The specific combination varies with the case; some assault-homicides show extensive combined injury while others show a fatal mechanism with only limited additional injury. The pathologist documents each element and integrates them for the aggregate reasoning.

### Reconstruction Reasoning

Reconstruction reasoning in assault-homicide cases addresses several questions: what was the sequence of events, what was the fatal mechanism, when did the sexual assault occur relative to the fatal mechanism, and what physical evidence supports the reconstruction. The sequence question is often central because it affects the criminal characterization: assault occurring before death has different legal implications than assault occurring after death. Physical evidence supporting sequence includes: vital reaction at injury sites (tissue response indicating the injuries occurred antemortem), the pattern of hemorrhage in the assault injuries (arterial spurting or extensive tissue hemorrhage supporting antemortem injury; minimal hemorrhage supporting near-death or postmortem injury), and specific tissue findings on histology of injury margins. The reasoning integrates these elements to construct the most defensible reconstruction.

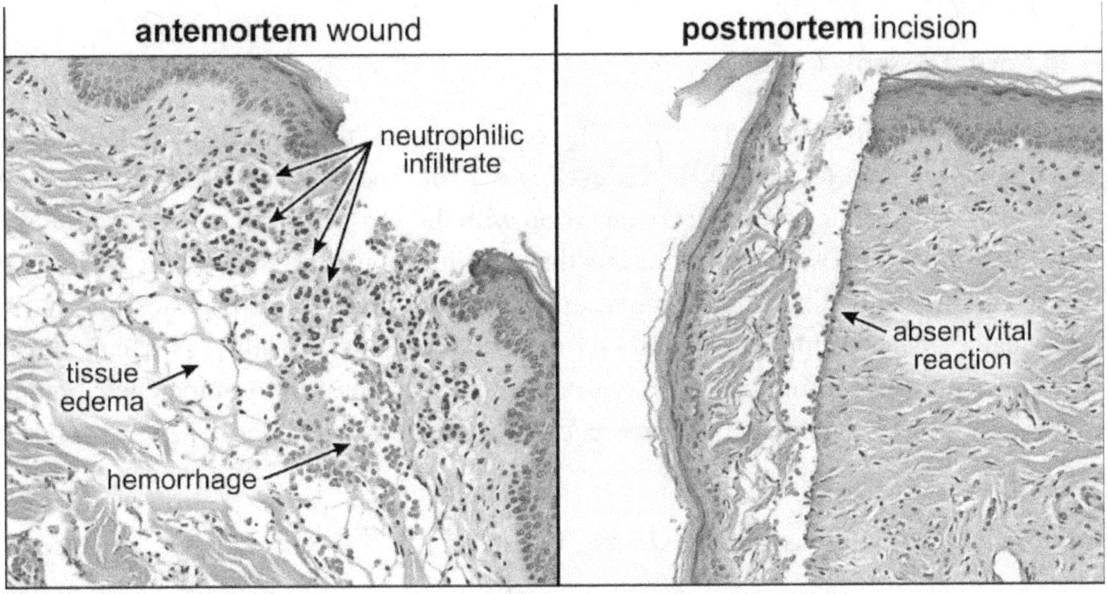


**Figure 15.3.** Histopathology of antemortem and postmortem injury margins (100x)

### Necrophilic Assault

Necrophilic sexual assault — sexual assault of a decedent after death — is uncommon but documented. The pattern arises in specific contexts including morgue or funeral home settings (a documented but rare pattern), and in scenes where a perpetrator returned to a victim after killing them. The distinction between antemortem and postmortem sexual assault depends on the vital reaction reasoning applied to any assault injuries: antemortem assault injuries show vital reaction (hemorrhage, tissue response); postmortem assault injuries do not. Biological evidence of assault may be recovered regardless of the timing, so evidence collection is performed with the same protocol whether antemortem or postmortem assault is the differential.

## Documentation, Chain of Custody, and Testimony

The documentation of sexual assault cases is prepared with particular attention to the potential legal use of the findings. The report clearly distinguishes objective observations (documented injuries, collected specimens, laboratory results) from reasoned opinions (interpretation of injury patterns, conclusions about assault mechanism). The photographic documentation is extensive and organized. The chain of custody documentation for evidence supports the admissibility of the physical evidence at trial.

### The Autopsy Report in Sexual Assault Cases

The autopsy report in sexual assault cases follows the standard structure with additional detail in specific sections. The findings section documents every relevant injury with anatomic location, dimension, character, and photographic reference. The evidence collection section documents the specimens collected, the collection sequence, and the packaging and chain of custody. The interpretation section develops the reasoning about injury mechanism, consistency with reported or reconstructed assault, and integration with the other autopsy findings. The pathologist writes with clarity for the professional and lay audiences that may read the report.

### Testimony in Sexual Assault Cases

Sexual assault cases frequently proceed to criminal prosecution, and the forensic pathologist is often called to testify. Preparation for testimony includes review of the autopsy report, the photographic documentation, and the laboratory results; consultation with the prosecutor to understand the specific case theory; and review of any opposing expert reports that may have been produced. The pathologist testifies about objective findings and about the reasoned opinions developed at autopsy; testimony is limited to what the physical evidence supports. Cross-examination in sexual assault cases can be challenging because the defense may attack findings, opinions, and general professional competence; preparation with the prosecutor and, where available, with more experienced pathology colleagues supports effective testimony.

### The Multidisciplinary Sexual Assault Response Team

Sexual assault investigation typically involves a multidisciplinary team including forensic pathology, sexual assault nurse examiners (for living survivor cases), law enforcement sex crimes investigators, forensic biologists analyzing biological evidence, prosecutors, victim advocates, and, in appropriate cases, mental health professionals supporting the victim's family. The forensic pathology contribution in fatal cases is the autopsy documentation and reasoning; integration with the broader team supports the aggregate case reasoning and the effective prosecution when the case proceeds to trial. Participation in sexual assault response team meetings and in the aggregate case review supports both the individual case reasoning and the broader systemic response.

### SCENE-TO-CERTIFICATION DECISION SYSTEM — Assault-Homicide Reconstruction Arc

**Presenting Death Scenario:** A 34-year-old woman is reported missing by her family after she failed to arrive at work. Two days later her body is discovered in a wooded area approximately 3 kilometers from a bar she was known to frequent. The scene documentation identifies extensive scene evidence: disarrayed clothing partially removed from the body, evidence of struggle in the surrounding vegetation, and a discarded item of the decedent's clothing at a location approximately 15 meters from the body. Postmortem interval is estimated at approximately 40 to 48 hours based on ambient temperature and postmortem changes. Law enforcement identifies the case immediately as a homicide with likely sexual assault component. The medical examiner's office accepts jurisdiction and initiates full sexual assault examination as part of the autopsy.

**Autopsy Signature:** External examination documents extensive injuries: contusions and abrasions on the face, defensive-pattern injuries on the hands and forearms (small crescent-shaped abrasions on the volar surfaces of the fingers consistent with grip on an assailant's hand, contusions on the dorsum of the hands consistent with defensive strikes), a horizontal ligature furrow on the neck approximately 1 centimeter wide, contusions on the anterior neck consistent with digital pressure, and multiple contusions and abrasions on the anterior trunk. Anogenital examination identifies posterior fourchette laceration approximately 1 centimeter in length with adjacent contusion, contusions on both labia, and perianal contusions. Full sexual assault evidence collection kit is completed including alternate light source examination which identifies multiple biological deposits on the body surface. Internal examination confirms cervical soft tissue hemorrhage with a fracture of the right greater cornu of the hyoid. Histology of the anogenital injuries and of the ligature furrow shows vital reaction supporting antemortem injury. Toxicology shows blood ethanol of 0.15 grams per deciliter with no other drugs detected.

**Cause Determination:** Asphyxia due to ligature strangulation, in the context of sexual assault.

**Manner Determination:** Homicide. The determination reflects the constellation of findings: fatal ligature strangulation mechanism with confirmatory internal findings; extensive assault injuries including defensive-pattern findings supporting resistance; anogenital injuries with vital reaction supporting antemortem sexual assault; and the scene evidence of struggle and body disposition.

**Trap Logic:** The trap in assault-homicide cases is either to focus on the fatal mechanism (strangulation in this case) without systematic sexual assault examination and evidence collection, or to focus on the sexual assault without adequate reconstruction of the fatal mechanism. The systematic approach performs the complete autopsy and the complete sexual assault examination, with each element documented for the aggregate reasoning. The sequence reasoning — whether the sexual assault occurred before, during, or after the fatal mechanism — is supported by the histologic finding of vital reaction at the anogenital injury margins, which confirms antemortem timing. A related trap is failure to preserve evidence adequately in cases where the scene evidence is extensive; the integration of scene, autopsy, and biological evidence supports both the reconstruction and the eventual prosecution.

**Certification Anchor:** Assault-homicide cases are certified with reference to the fatal mechanism (strangulation, blunt injury, gunshot wound, etc.) with documentation of the sexual assault component in the report narrative. The manner is homicide. Vital reaction reasoning at injury margins supports the sequence reconstruction. Systematic evidence collection preserves the biological evidence supporting perpetrator identification.

### Pediatric Sexual Assault Fatalities

Pediatric sexual assault fatalities represent a specific and demanding subcategory. The examination is performed with the standard postmortem sexual assault protocol adapted for pediatric anatomy. Consultation with pediatric child abuse specialists is standard for the interpretation of pediatric anogenital findings, which have a substantial and evolving peer-reviewed literature separate from adult findings. Specific injury patterns in pediatric cases include hymenal injury (with attention to normal developmental variation), perianal injury, and injuries to the labia minora and posterior fourchette. The pathologist reasons about pediatric findings with awareness of the specific interpretive framework developed for this population and consultation supports the interpretation.

### Male Sexual Assault Cases

Male sexual assault cases follow similar protocol adapted for anatomy. External and internal specimen collection includes oral, anal, and genital specimens. Injury patterns in anal assault include contusions and abrasions of the perianal skin, lacerations at the 6 and 12 o'clock positions, and, in cases of severe assault, more extensive injury. Injury to the genitalia including the scrotum and penis may occur in assault cases and is documented systematically. The reasoning about male sexual assault cases parallels the reasoning for female cases, with attention to the specific anatomic patterns and to the epidemiological understanding of assault in male victims.

### Institutional Sexual Assault Contexts

Sexual assault in institutional care contexts — long-term care facilities, hospitals, correctional facilities, and other congregate settings — has been documented as a specific pattern requiring recognition. Elderly individuals with cognitive impairment, individuals with significant disability, and individuals in confinement environments have documented vulnerabilities to sexual assault by care providers, staff members, or other residents. Recognition of these patterns requires specific attention: the pathologist encountering an elderly decedent with cognitive impairment or an individual in institutional care performs the postmortem sexual assault examination when any circumstance supports the differential, without dismissing the possibility based on the setting alone. Coordination with facility administration, with adult protective services or child protective services as applicable, and with law enforcement is standard when the pattern emerges.

### The Evolving Peer-Reviewed Literature

The forensic pathology understanding of sexual assault has evolved substantially over the past several decades. Specific findings previously considered pathognomonic have been reinterpreted based on studies of normal variation and consensual sexual activity. Studies of injury patterns in reported sexual assault cases have refined understanding of frequency and character of specific findings. The interpretation of pediatric anogenital findings has evolved substantially. The practicing forensic pathologist maintains familiarity with current peer-reviewed literature to integrate with the case reasoning and updates practice as the evidence base develops. Attendance at specialty meetings, participation in continuing medical education, and consultation with colleagues supports ongoing professional currency.

### Bite Mark Identification and Preservation

Bite marks are documented findings in some sexual assault cases and require specific preservation protocol. When identified, bite marks are photographed with a scale in frame, at multiple angles, and under both standard and alternate light source examination. Swabs of the bite mark surface collect saliva that may contain the perpetrator's DNA. In some cases, forensic odontologist consultation supports the interpretation of the bite mark for comparison with a suspect's dentition, though the reliability of bite mark comparison has been substantially challenged in the peer-reviewed literature and the National Academy of Sciences reports; comparison-based conclusions are treated with appropriate caution. The DNA analysis of the bite mark swab is a more objective forensic contribution than the geometric bite mark comparison and is the primary use of bite mark preservation in current practice. Photographic documentation of the bite mark is preserved regardless of the intended analytical use, because the finding itself supports the reasoning about assault mechanism.

### Manual Assault Injury Patterns

Manual assault findings frequently accompany sexual assault cases and warrant specific documentation. Contusion patterns on the medial thighs are documented in a substantial fraction of sexual assault cases and reflect the mechanical force required to separate the decedent's legs during the assault. Contusions on the arms reflect the assailant's grip during the assault. Contusions and abrasions on the shoulders, upper back, and buttocks reflect the mechanical contact during the assault. Petechial hemorrhages of the face and conjunctivae in a sexual assault case without documented strangulation may reflect chest compression during the assault with impaired venous return; the finding warrants specific reasoning about the assault mechanism. Documentation of manual assault findings integrates with the sexual assault findings for the aggregate case reasoning.

### The Sexual Assault Evidence Backlog Issue

The delayed analysis of sexual assault evidence collection kits has been a substantial systemic issue in American forensic practice. Documented backlogs at crime laboratories have resulted in kits collected in the postmortem examination remaining unanalyzed for months to years in some jurisdictions. The delay has substantial implications: perpetrators identified from other cases may not be connected to the current case within the window when prosecution is timely; the biological evidence may degrade during storage, though modern preservation standards have reduced this problem; and family closure on the case is delayed. The forensic pathologist's role is to collect the evidence with rigorous protocol and to advocate through office administrative channels and through professional societies for timely analysis; the pathologist does not control the analytical laboratory queue but supports the case by ensuring the evidence is collected properly and communicated as an appropriate priority.

### Historical Perspective on Sexual Assault Investigation

The systematic postmortem sexual assault examination is a relatively recent development in forensic practice. Earlier practice frequently omitted sexual assault examination unless the case history explicitly identified the assault as an element; the recognition that sexual assault frequently accompanies homicide of women and vulnerable individuals, and that systematic examination identifies cases where the assault would otherwise be missed, has driven the current standard of routine examination when circumstances support it. Similarly, the recognition that drug-facilitated sexual assault is a documented pattern requiring specific analytical approach has driven the development of focused toxicological analysis. The forensic pathology practice continues to evolve as the peer-reviewed literature develops and as the aggregate case experience refines the understanding of what the examination reliably identifies and what its interpretive limits are.

### The Autopsy Report in Sexual Assault Cases: Extended Format

Beyond the standard autopsy report structure, sexual assault cases benefit from specific documentation elements. A discrete section describing the evidence collection with specimen inventory supports the chain of custody documentation for the analytical laboratory and for later legal proceedings. A discrete section describing anogenital findings with reference to normal variation supports the interpretation for reviewing pathologists and for legal proceedings. Photographic documentation is organized systematically with an index supporting later retrieval of specific views. Consultation reports (from pediatric abuse specialists, sexual assault nurse examiners, or peer forensic pathologists) are integrated with the primary report. The extended format supports the multiple audiences of the report — the investigating law enforcement agency, the prosecutor, the defense (through discovery), and, in some cases, appellate review — with the documentation each audience requires.

### SCENE-TO-CERTIFICATION DECISION SYSTEM — Sexual Assault Determination Arcs

**The Examination Framework:** Postmortem sexual assault examination is a standardized element of the forensic autopsy performed whenever case circumstances support the differential. The examination follows the sexual assault evidence collection kit protocol adapted for the postmortem context, with rigorous chain of custody documentation supporting subsequent analysis and legal proceedings.

**Evidence Collection:** The evidence collection kit includes external and internal specimens (swabs from oral, vaginal, anal, and skin sites), hair combings, fingernail specimens, clothing preservation, and specimens for toxicology including drug-facilitated sexual assault analysis. The collection sequence and packaging follow standardized protocol; the chain of custody begins at collection and continues through analysis.

**Anogenital Injury Interpretation:** Anogenital injury interpretation integrates the injury findings with the case context. The absence of injury does not exclude assault, and the presence of injury does not by itself establish assault mechanism. Normal anatomic variation must not be misidentified as injury; consultation supports interpretation in complex cases.

**Toxicology and Drug-Facilitated Cases:** Toxicology in sexual assault cases addresses voluntary intoxication and drug-facilitated assault. Focused analysis for specific facilitating agents (GHB, benzodiazepines, ketamine, others) requires appropriate specimens and analytical techniques. Detection windows vary by agent, and prompt specimen collection supports subsequent analysis.

**The Assault-Homicide Reconstruction:** The assault-homicide case integrates sexual assault findings with the overall injury pattern for aggregate reasoning. Sequence reasoning (assault before, during, or after fatal mechanism) is supported by vital reaction findings at injury margins. Documentation and testimony are prepared with attention to the legal use of the findings.

## Summary and Key Concepts

Postmortem sexual assault examination is a standardized element of the forensic autopsy performed whenever case circumstances support the sexual assault differential. The examination follows a rigorous protocol with standardized evidence collection, chain of custody documentation, and integration with the overall case reasoning.

The sexual assault evidence collection kit includes external and internal specimens, hair combings, fingernail specimens, clothing preservation, and specific toxicology specimens for drug-facilitated sexual assault analysis. Collection sequence, packaging, and chain of custody follow standardized protocol.

Anogenital injury interpretation integrates the injury findings with case context. Common sites of injury in vaginal assault include the posterior fourchette, fossa navicularis, and labia minora. Anal injuries typically occur at the 6 and 12 o'clock positions. Normal anatomic variation must be distinguished from injury; consultation supports interpretation in complex cases.

The absence of anogenital injury does not exclude sexual assault; a substantial fraction of assault cases show minimal or no anatomic injury, particularly when the victim was incapacitated. The presence of injury does not by itself establish assault mechanism.

Toxicological analysis in sexual assault cases addresses voluntary intoxication and drug-facilitated assault. Common facilitating agents include ethanol, benzodiazepines, gamma-hydroxybutyrate, ketamine, and opioids. Focused analysis with appropriate specimen collection is required for detection of specific facilitating agents.

The assault-homicide case integrates sexual assault findings with the overall injury pattern. Vital reaction at injury margins supports the sequence reasoning (antemortem versus postmortem timing of assault relative to fatal mechanism). Documentation and testimony are prepared with attention to the legal use of findings.

# CHAPTER 16: DEATHS IN CUSTODY, RESTRAINT, AND SUDDEN DEATH DURING STRUGGLE

**Learning Objectives**

1. Articulate the framework for custodial death investigation and its integration with law enforcement, community, and civil rights considerations.
2. Recognize positional asphyxia and restraint-associated mechanical asphyxia mechanisms in the context of law enforcement or institutional restraint.
3. Reason systematically about sudden death during struggle, integrating cardiovascular substrate, drug intoxication, and physiologic stress as contributing factors.
4. Articulate the controversy surrounding excited delirium as a diagnostic entity and reason about how to certify these cases with appropriate professional caution.
5. Recognize the injury patterns associated with conducted electrical weapon deployment and reason about the role of the weapon in cause of death.

## The Custodial Death Framework

Deaths in custody — during law enforcement contact, during arrest, in police detention facilities, in jails, and in prisons — constitute a specific and demanding category of forensic pathology practice. The medical, legal, social, and political stakes are all substantial. Families of decedents seek understanding of what happened to their loved ones. Law enforcement agencies seek accountability for their personnel and defense against unwarranted allegations. Civil rights communities scrutinize the individual case and the aggregate pattern for evidence of systemic problems. Courts and prosecutors depend on the medical determination to inform charging decisions. The pathologist reasons with attention to all these audiences and produces a determination that reflects the physical evidence and the professional reasoning transparently.

The framework for custodial death investigation begins with recognition that the case is not a routine death — the involvement of law enforcement at the death or preceding the death creates specific requirements for evidence documentation, for scene reconstruction, for the autopsy protocol, and for the ultimate certification. Many jurisdictions have specific protocols for in-custody deaths that exceed the standard autopsy protocol and that require specific documentation. The pathologist encountering a custodial death applies the protocol systematically and reasons through the specific issues that these cases raise.

The forensic pathologist working on custodial death cases is subject to substantial external scrutiny. The determinations produced will be reviewed by attorneys representing the decedent's family in civil litigation, by defense attorneys representing law enforcement officers in criminal proceedings, by civil rights investigators, by expert witnesses retained by any of these parties, and, in some cases, by academic researchers analyzing aggregate patterns. The pathologist prepares for this scrutiny by systematic documentation, transparent reasoning, and consultation with colleagues on the more difficult cases. The professional standards for these cases exceed those for routine autopsies.

### Terminology and Definitional Care

The terminology in this area matters and has evolved. The general category of "death in custody" encompasses deaths during initial law enforcement contact, deaths during arrest, deaths in transport, deaths in detention or booking facilities, and deaths in jails and prisons. The specific subcategory of "restraint-associated death" refers to deaths temporally connected to restraint by law enforcement or institutional personnel. "Sudden death during struggle" (sometimes abbreviated SDDS) refers to unexplained sudden cardiovascular collapse during physical altercation, often in the context of restraint or arrest. Each term has specific implications, and the pathologist uses terminology with attention to its definitional precision.

## Positional Asphyxia and Restraint Mechanics

Positional asphyxia refers to death from a body position that mechanically restricts respiration to a degree that produces fatal hypoxia. The concept has substantial historical and contested status in the specialty. The proposed mechanism is that prone positioning, particularly with restraint of the extremities behind the body, mechanically impairs chest wall excursion sufficient to produce hypoxia over minutes when the position is maintained. Additional weight applied to the back (a knee, a body, or restraint pressure) exacerbates the mechanical restriction.

### The Physiologic Question

The physiologic question is whether prone positional restraint in the absence of other physiologic stressors is sufficient to produce fatal hypoxia. Multiple laboratory studies have measured pulmonary function and gas exchange in volunteers subjected to prone restraint positions and have found variable results: some studies show substantial reduction in ventilatory capacity while others find only modest effects. The interpretive controversy in the specialty reflects both this variable experimental data and the fundamental difficulty of translating experimental findings in cooperative volunteers to the real-world context of restrained struggling individuals. The peer-reviewed literature contains both position statements supporting positional asphyxia as a documented lethal mechanism and analyses questioning whether the mechanism alone accounts for restraint-associated deaths.

The current professional consensus, to the extent that consensus exists, is that prone restraint is one of multiple physiologic stressors that can contribute to death during restraint, and that most restraint-associated deaths involve multiple contributing factors rather than positional asphyxia as the sole mechanism. The pathologist reasons about individual cases with attention to the specific circumstances, the physical findings, and the integration of all elements rather than to a categorical framework.

### Physical Findings in Restraint-Associated Death

The physical findings in restraint-associated death are typically limited. Petechial hemorrhages of the face, conjunctivae, and mucous membranes may be present and reflect the increased venous pressure of struggle and restraint; the finding is nonspecific and occurs in many cardiovascular deaths. Contusions from the restraint mechanism (marks on the wrists and ankles from handcuffs and shackles; contusions on the back or chest from the restraining forces; contusions on the head or face from the struggle) are documented and integrated with the reported mechanism. In some cases with specific mechanisms (neck compression, chokehold restraint), findings characteristic of neck compression — layered cervical soft tissue hemorrhage, hyoid or thyroid cartilage fracture, ligature-pattern marks — are present and specifically documented.

Figure 16.1: Restraint-Associated Injury Patterns

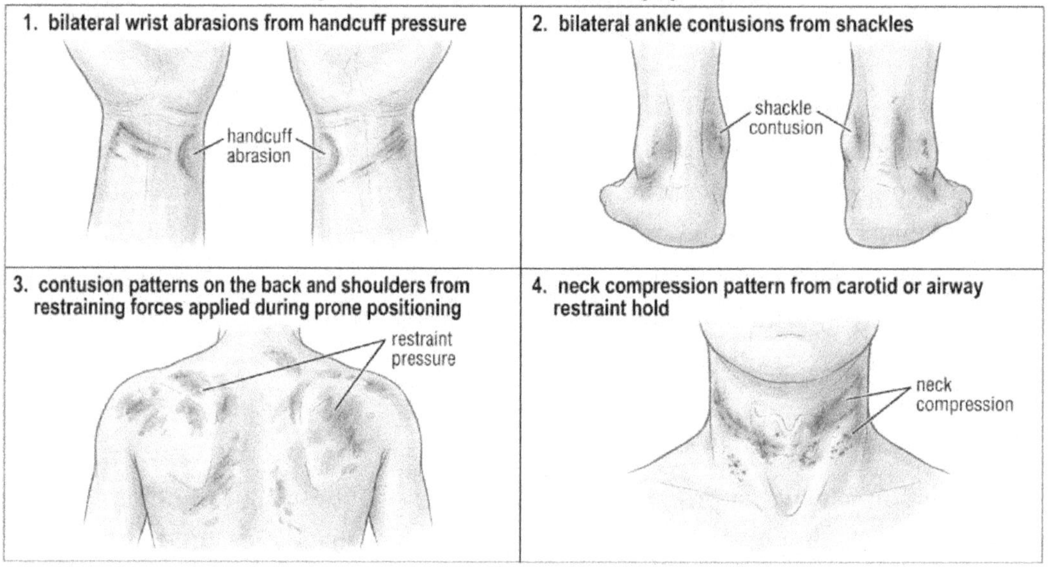


## Sudden Death During Struggle

Sudden death during struggle is a specific pattern in which an individual collapses and dies during physical altercation, typically during law enforcement contact or restraint but also documented in other contexts (bar fights, physical altercations in institutional settings, agitated states during medical intervention). The mechanism reflects the intersection of multiple physiologic stressors on a vulnerable substrate, with cardiovascular collapse as the terminal event.

### The Substrate and the Triggers

The substrate for sudden death during struggle typically includes: underlying cardiovascular disease (coronary atherosclerosis, cardiomyopathy, hypertensive heart disease with left ventricular hypertrophy, congenital abnormalities); acute drug intoxication (particularly with sympathomimetic drugs — cocaine, methamphetamine, MDMA, synthetic cathinones — that produce catecholamine excess); acute psychiatric decompensation with severe agitation; chronic drug or alcohol use with associated cardiovascular effects; and, in some cases, coexisting acute medical conditions. The triggers include the physical struggle itself with substantial catecholamine surge, the physical exertion, the physiologic stress of restraint, and, in some cases, the specific effects of applied restraint mechanisms.

The mechanism synthesizes these elements: acute catecholamine surge in an individual with an arrhythmic substrate, exacerbated by drug-induced catecholamine excess and by physiologic stress, produces sudden arrhythmic death. The specific arrhythmia is not directly observed in the field death (there is no continuous monitoring at the time of collapse), but the pattern is inferred from the aggregate case findings and from the peer-reviewed literature on the syndrome. The autopsy findings support the substrate identification (severity and type of cardiovascular disease, presence of hypertrophy, presence of drug intoxication on toxicology); the reasoning integrates the substrate with the triggers to produce the mechanistic explanation.

FIGURE 16.2: LEFT VENTRICULAR HYPERTROPHY AS SUBSTRATE FOR ARRHYTHMIC SUDDEN DEATH

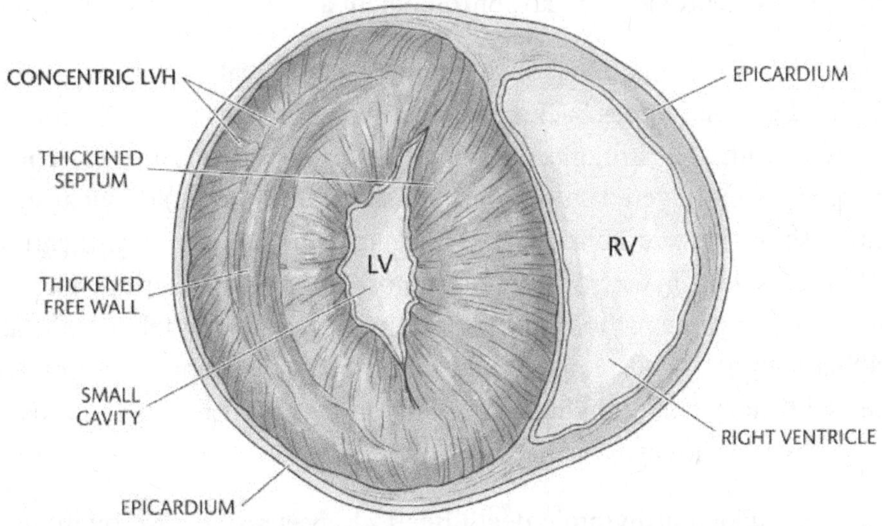


## The Certification Challenge

The certification of sudden death during struggle presents specific challenges because the case typically shows: underlying cardiovascular disease of variable severity (often significant but not by itself acutely fatal); drug intoxication of variable severity (often significant contribution but rarely at levels that would independently be fatal); and physical restraint or struggle immediately preceding the death. The certification approach varies among offices and among individual practitioners; some certify these cases as natural (with attribution to the underlying cardiovascular disease as the primary cause and the struggle and restraint as contributing factors), some certify as accident (attributing to the drug intoxication or to the specific mechanism), some certify as homicide (attributing to the actions of the restraining personnel), and some certify as undetermined. The determinations have substantial consequences for legal proceedings and for the decedent's family, and the reasoning is documented transparently in the report regardless of the specific classification.

**EVIDENCE:** The certification of sudden-death-during-struggle cases shows documented variation among forensic pathologists and among jurisdictions. Published analyses have shown that the same fact pattern may be classified differently by different pathologists. Transparent reasoning in the report, consultation with colleagues, and willingness to acknowledge the interpretive controversy support both the individual case and the professional integrity of the determinations.

**SCENE-TO-CERTIFICATION DECISION SYSTEM — Sudden Death During Struggle Arc**

---

**Presenting Death Scenario:** A 38-year-old man is encountered by law enforcement responding to a report of an agitated individual in a public setting. The individual is behaving erratically, sweating profusely, and speaking incoherently. Law enforcement attempts to detain him and physical struggle ensues. He is restrained in prone position by multiple officers and handcuffed. Within several minutes of restraint, he becomes unresponsive. Resuscitation is initiated at the scene and continued during emergency transport; he is pronounced dead at the emergency department. The medical examiner's office accepts jurisdiction. Body-worn camera footage is provided by law enforcement and reviewed as part of the case investigation.

**Autopsy Signature:** External examination documents bilateral wrist abrasions from handcuffs, contusions on the shoulders and upper back consistent with restraint pressure, contusions and abrasions on the face consistent with the struggle, and no findings suggesting neck compression or airway obstruction as the mechanism. Layered anterior neck dissection shows no cervical soft tissue hemorrhage. Internal examination shows severe concentric left ventricular hypertrophy (heart weight 520 grams), moderate coronary atherosclerosis with 50 percent stenosis in the left anterior descending artery, no acute coronary event, and no other acute pathology. Toxicology shows methamphetamine at 480 nanograms per milliliter in peripheral blood and amphetamine at 160 nanograms per milliliter (metabolite of methamphetamine) with no other drugs detected. Histology confirms myocyte hypertrophy consistent with chronic hypertensive cardiovascular disease.

**Cause Determination:** Sudden arrhythmic death due to hypertensive cardiovascular disease with acute methamphetamine intoxication, during physical restraint. The cause statement identifies the substrate (hypertensive cardiovascular disease with left ventricular hypertrophy), the trigger (acute methamphetamine intoxication with associated catecholamine excess), and the context (physical restraint with associated physiologic stress and struggle).

**Manner Determination:** The manner determination in this case is one of the most contested in the specialty. Options include: natural (attributing to the underlying hypertensive cardiovascular disease), accident (attributing to the methamphetamine intoxication), homicide (attributing to the actions of the restraining personnel), and undetermined. This case would be certified differently by different practitioners, and the certification decision must be transparently reasoned in the report regardless of the specific classification chosen. Some offices have developed guidelines specifying the preferred certification approach for these cases; the individual practitioner works within the office guidelines while preserving the option to certify differently in cases where the specific facts warrant.

**Trap Logic:** The trap in these cases operates in multiple directions. Certification as natural without acknowledging the contribution of restraint and struggle understates the role of the physical actions of the restraining personnel. Certification as homicide without adequate substrate reasoning risks attributing to restraint what is fundamentally arrhythmic death from cardiovascular substrate. Certification as accident without acknowledging the physical restraint context understates the contribution of the specific mechanism. The systematic approach is transparent reasoning about each element (substrate, trigger, context) and honest acknowledgment of the interpretive controversy where it exists. Second-opinion consultation is standard in these cases at most offices. Body-worn camera review is standard when footage is available and provides context that scene evidence alone does not.

**Certification Anchor:** Sudden death during struggle in the context of law enforcement restraint requires transparent documentation of substrate, trigger, and context; systematic examination for evidence of specific mechanism (neck compression, positional restriction, weapon injury); integration with body-worn camera and scene evidence; and honest reasoning about the manner classification. The determination is documented so the reasoning is reconstructible from the record, and consultation supports the decision.

## Excited Delirium and Its Controversy

Excited delirium is a term used in the older forensic pathology and law enforcement literature to describe a syndrome of severe agitation, delirium, incoherent speech, elevated body temperature, and sudden collapse, often occurring in the context of stimulant drug intoxication or acute psychiatric decompensation. The term has been used as a diagnostic category for cases of sudden death during struggle particularly in cases involving stimulant drug intoxication. The current status of the term is contested in the peer-reviewed literature and in major professional organizations.

### The Controversy

The controversy over excited delirium has multiple dimensions. Medical and psychiatric professional organizations — including the American Psychiatric Association, the American Medical Association, and the American College of Emergency Physicians — have issued position statements questioning or repudiating the term as a diagnostic category. The concerns include: the lack of consistent diagnostic criteria across cases labeled as excited delirium; the racial disparities in application of the term, with disproportionate use in cases involving Black decedents; the association of the term with sudden death during law enforcement restraint, potentially serving to shift causal attribution from the restraint to the decedent's presumed medical condition; and the lack of a coherent underlying pathophysiological mechanism that would define excited delirium as distinct from other agitated states with cardiovascular collapse.

The National Association of Medical Examiners has more recently indicated that the term excited delirium should not be used as an official cause of death, and many offices have moved away from the term in current practice. The current recommended approach is to certify the case with specific mechanisms (acute stimulant intoxication, hypertensive cardiovascular disease, sudden arrhythmic death during struggle) rather than with the umbrella term. The change reflects the broader recognition that the label historically served to obscure specific mechanistic reasoning that a case-by-case approach would produce.

**CAUTION:** The term "excited delirium" has been repudiated by major professional organizations and is being phased out of forensic pathology practice. Current recommended approach is to certify with specific mechanisms rather than the umbrella term. The pathologist adopts the current professional standard and reasons through cases previously labeled as excited delirium with the current mechanistic framework.

## Conducted Electrical Weapon Deaths

Conducted electrical weapons (CEWs), including the widely deployed TASER, deliver a brief high-voltage electrical impulse that produces involuntary muscle contraction and incapacitation, allowing law enforcement personnel to restrain a subject without physical hand-to-hand combat. The weapons have been generally considered safe as less-lethal alternatives to firearms or physical strikes, and the substantial majority of deployments do not result in death. However, deaths temporally associated with CEW deployment have been documented and require specific reasoning.

### The Physical Findings

The physical findings of CEW deployment include the barb sites on the skin where the probes contacted the body — typically small punctate marks with surrounding erythema; the retained probes may be present at autopsy if not removed at the scene. Multiple deployments are documented by multiple barb sites. Contact deployment (with the weapon applied directly to the skin rather than fired) produces a paired burn pattern reflecting the two electrical contacts on the weapon housing. Documentation of the barb sites, of any retained probes, of the deployment history from law enforcement records, and of the timeline of collapse relative to deployment supports the case reasoning.

**Figure 16.3:** Conducted Electrical Weapon Deployment: Barb Sites and Contact Marks

**Probe Barb Sites** | **Contact Deployment Marks**

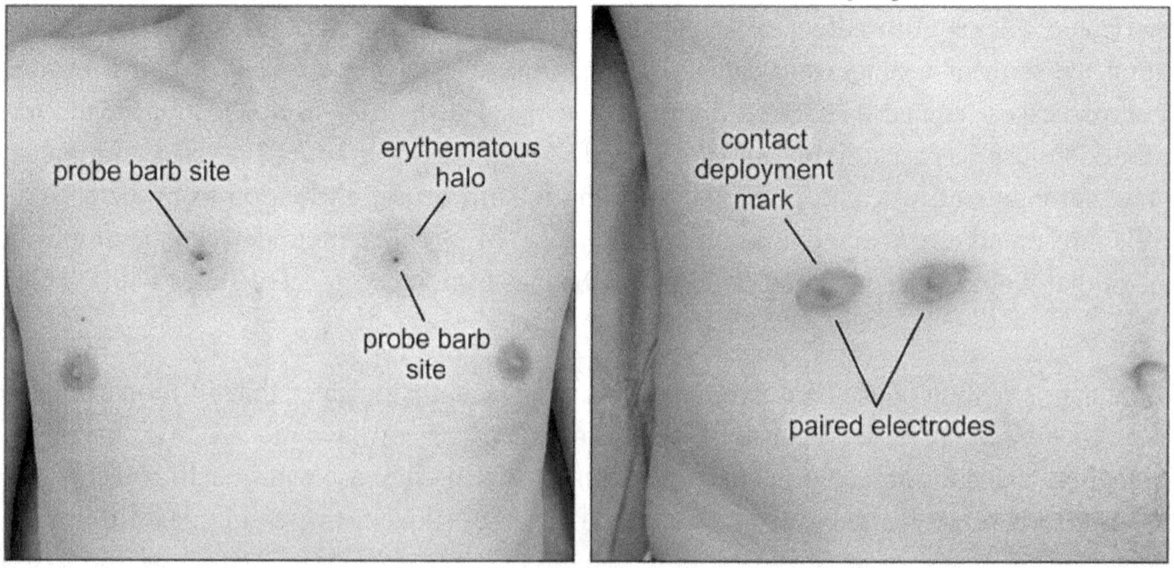

### The Causal Reasoning

The causal reasoning about whether the CEW deployment contributed to death is contested in the peer-reviewed literature. Manufacturer studies and some peer-reviewed research have suggested that the electrical pulse is unlikely to produce lethal cardiac arrhythmia in typical deployments; other analyses have identified specific circumstances (chest deployment near the cardiac silhouette, deployment during specific phases of the cardiac cycle, deployment on individuals with specific cardiovascular substrate) where arrhythmia is more plausibly associated. The pathologist reasoning about a specific case integrates the timeline of collapse relative to deployment, the underlying cardiovascular substrate, and any concurrent drug intoxication with the deployment details. Certification varies from natural (with cardiovascular substrate as the primary cause and the CEW deployment as one contributor) through undetermined to homicide depending on the specific findings and the office practice.

## Autopsy and Investigation Protocol for In-Custody Deaths

The autopsy protocol for in-custody deaths follows the standard forensic autopsy protocol with specific additions and rigor. Photographic documentation is extensive and organized. The external examination documents all injuries with reference to the reported restraint mechanism, the reported deployments of any weapons, and any prior injuries. The internal examination proceeds with attention to cardiovascular substrate identification, to any injuries not apparent on external examination, and to the specific findings that might support alternative mechanisms.

### Specific Protocol Elements

Specific protocol elements for in-custody deaths include: layered anterior neck dissection performed as standard given the frequent inclusion of neck restraint in the case questions; systematic cardiovascular examination including heart weight, wall thickness measurements, coronary artery examination, and histology; comprehensive toxicology including drug screening at the levels adequate for forensic determination; retention of specimens for later analysis; and, where indicated, retention of the eyes for postmortem ophthalmologic examination when the case reasoning involves head trauma or asphyxial mechanism. Consultation with peer forensic pathologists is standard for the more complex cases; second-opinion review at the time of autopsy supports the primary determination.

### Integration With Body-Worn Camera and Other Recordings

Body-worn camera footage, dashboard camera footage, and civilian bystander recordings are increasingly available in law enforcement contact deaths. The pathologist reviewing footage as part of the case investigation observes the specific interactions, the sequence of events, the applied restraint mechanisms, the timeline of collapse relative to specific interventions, and the emergency response. The footage is integrated with the autopsy findings and with witness accounts for the aggregate case reconstruction. The pathologist notes the footage review in the report and integrates the observations into the reasoning; the footage does not replace the medical determination but informs it.

### External Review and Second Opinions

In-custody deaths frequently receive external review — from independent forensic pathologists retained by the decedent's family, from experts retained by law enforcement agencies or their legal representatives, from civil rights investigators, or from academic reviewers. The primary pathologist prepares for this external review by systematic documentation, transparent reasoning, and, in many cases, by proactive engagement with external reviewers to explain the reasoning and answer questions. The willingness to acknowledge the interpretive controversy in these cases, to explain the reasoning, and to modify determinations when subsequent evidence supports modification is a professional strength rather than a weakness.

### SCENE-TO-CERTIFICATION DECISION SYSTEM — Restraint-Associated Death Reasoning Arc

---

**Presenting Death Scenario:** A 46-year-old man is arrested during a traffic stop that escalated into physical confrontation. Body-worn camera footage shows the officer applying an arm-based hold that includes pressure against the anterior neck for approximately 2 minutes during struggle. The decedent becomes unresponsive during the restraint. Resuscitation is initiated at the scene and continued during emergency transport; he is pronounced dead at the emergency department approximately 45 minutes after the initial restraint. The medical examiner's office accepts jurisdiction. Body-worn camera footage from multiple angles is reviewed as part of the case investigation. The decedent has a documented history of hypertension and asthma.

**Autopsy Signature:** External examination documents bilateral wrist abrasions from handcuffs, contusions on the neck and face consistent with the restraint hold and struggle, contusions on the shoulders and upper back, and no additional significant external injury. Layered anterior neck dissection identifies extensive hemorrhage in the sternocleidomastoid muscles bilaterally, hemorrhage in the strap muscles, hemorrhage in the periesophageal soft tissue, and a small fracture of the right superior horn of the thyroid cartilage. The airway is patent without foreign body. Internal examination shows moderate concentric left ventricular hypertrophy (heart weight 440 grams), mild coronary atherosclerosis without acute event, and no other significant pathology. Toxicology is negative apart from levels of prescribed antihypertensive medication.

**Cause Determination:** Asphyxia due to compression of the neck during restraint, on the substrate of hypertensive cardiovascular disease. The cause statement identifies both the acute mechanism (neck compression producing airway or vascular obstruction sufficient to interrupt consciousness and adequate ventilation) and the substrate (hypertensive cardiovascular disease that reduced cardiovascular reserve). Layered neck dissection confirms the mechanism through the documented soft tissue hemorrhage and cartilage fracture.

**Manner Determination:** Homicide. The determination reflects that death resulted from the actions of another person (the restraining officer) applying pressure to the neck sufficient to produce fatal asphyxia. The manner classification is medical; specific criminal or civil determinations are the province of law enforcement, prosecutors, and courts. Manner classification as homicide in a law enforcement context does not imply criminal wrongdoing; the classification reflects the medical determination that death resulted from another person's actions.

**Trap Logic:** The reasoning about restraint-associated neck compression deaths depends on the specific findings integrated with the reported and recorded mechanism. Layered anterior neck dissection is the standard technique for identifying internal soft tissue hemorrhage; the technique may show hemorrhage even when external findings are limited. The trap is either to certify as natural death based on the underlying cardiovascular disease without acknowledging the neck compression mechanism, or to certify as homicide without adequate physical evidence of the specific mechanism claimed. In this case, the dissection findings support neck compression as the mechanism, and the reasoning is transparent about the integration of substrate with the specific mechanism.

**Certification Anchor:** Restraint-associated deaths with a neck compression component are certified with reference to the specific mechanism identified by systematic examination (layered neck dissection), with substrate reasoning transparent in the report. The manner classification reflects the medical determination of whether death resulted from another person's actions; the classification is medical rather than legal, and criminal or civil consequences are the province of law enforcement and courts.

### Chokehold and Vascular Neck Restraint

Neck restraint holds employed by law enforcement have evolved over recent decades with substantial policy attention. The airway chokehold applies pressure across the anterior neck to occlude the trachea and produce respiratory arrest; the vascular neck restraint (sometimes called a lateral vascular neck restraint or carotid hold) applies pressure to the lateral neck to compress the carotid arteries and produce cerebral hypoperfusion with loss of consciousness. The two mechanisms produce different physiologic effects and different case reasoning. Airway chokeholds are frequently associated with cervical soft tissue hemorrhage in the anterior neck and with cartilage fracture; vascular neck restraints may show more limited findings but can still produce cerebral hypoxic injury and death. Many law enforcement agencies have restricted or prohibited both categories of neck restraint in recent policy revisions, and the specific hold used in a case (identified from body-worn camera footage and from officer accounts) is central to the reasoning.

### Jail and Prison Deaths

Deaths in jails and prisons — as distinct from deaths during arrest or law enforcement contact — present their own reconstruction challenges. Deaths in jails frequently involve individuals with acute substance intoxication or withdrawal, individuals with untreated medical conditions, individuals with acute psychiatric decompensation, and individuals subject to suicide in confinement. The pattern of deaths in prisons is dominated by natural deaths of the aging incarcerated population, with cardiovascular disease, cancer, and other chronic conditions as the common causes. Specific patterns include suicide by hanging from cell fixtures, deaths from drug overdose using contraband substances, deaths from delayed medical care in confinement contexts, deaths during use of force by correctional staff, and deaths from violence by other incarcerated individuals. The autopsy protocol adapts to the specific circumstances but preserves the systematic approach: complete external and internal examination, layered neck dissection when indicated, comprehensive toxicology, integration with facility records and staff accounts.

### Suicide in Custody

Suicide in custody — typically by hanging from cell fixtures, sheets, or clothing — is a documented pattern with substantial epidemiological data. Jail suicides occur most frequently in the initial days of confinement, particularly in individuals awaiting adjudication with no prior confinement history. Prison suicides distribute across the population with specific patterns in solitary confinement and in individuals with mental health conditions. The autopsy identifies the mechanism (typically ligature hanging with associated furrow and internal findings), integrates with the facility documentation of the discovery, and reasons about the manner determination. Suicide is the typical manner determination; the reasoning is systematic even in cases where suicide is the presumed manner because staged homicidal hanging — in which a homicide is staged as a suicide — is a documented pattern in institutional settings that requires exclusion by systematic examination.

### Documentation for Civil Rights and Federal Investigation

In-custody deaths in the United States are subject to federal review through mechanisms including the Death in Custody Reporting Act, civil rights investigation by the Department of Justice, and, in aggregate, federal statistical reporting on in-custody deaths. The forensic pathology report supports these mechanisms with systematic documentation of the mechanism, the injuries, and the case reasoning. The pathologist preserves the documentation with attention to the potential federal review that these cases may receive; the professional standard is transparent, well-supported determinations that withstand external scrutiny from multiple review sources.

### The National Association of Medical Examiners Position

The National Association of Medical Examiners has issued position statements on multiple aspects of in-custody death investigation, including the recommendation against the use of excited delirium as a cause of death, guidance on the layered anterior neck dissection technique, guidance on the certification of restraint-associated deaths, and general principles for the conduct of in-custody death autopsies. The individual practitioner refers to these position statements as authoritative guidance and integrates them with local office practice. Departures from the NAME guidance should be reasoned and documented; adherence to the guidance supports both the individual case and the broader professional standards.

### Hog-Tie and Hobble Restraints

The hog-tie or hobble restraint — a specific restraint method in which the wrists and ankles are bound behind the body and connected — has substantial documented association with restraint-associated deaths. The mechanism combines prone positioning with mechanical restriction of the extremities behind the body, which can further restrict respiratory excursion and prevents the decedent from repositioning to relieve mechanical restriction. Many law enforcement agencies have prohibited or substantially restricted the hobble restraint in recent policy changes, reflecting the accumulated experience with restraint-associated deaths where hog-tying was documented as a factor. The pathologist reasoning about a case with hobble restraint documented in the mechanism integrates the specific restraint with the general reasoning about restraint-associated death; the specific mechanism supports greater weight on the physical restraint as a contributor when a hobble is documented.

### Chemical Agents in Custodial Encounters

Chemical agents used in custodial encounters include oleoresin capsicum (OC or pepper spray), tear gases (CS, CN), and, less commonly, other agents. The typical physiological effects are irritation of the eyes, upper airway, and skin, with rapid clearance and limited long-term effects. Deaths temporally associated with OC deployment have been documented in individuals with severe asthma (where the airway irritation may precipitate severe bronchospasm), individuals with cardiovascular disease (where the catecholamine response to the exposure may contribute to arrhythmic events), and individuals with other specific vulnerabilities. The pathologist reasoning about a case involving OC or other chemical agent deployment integrates the deployment with the general case reasoning; the agent alone is rarely the sole cause of death but may contribute in specific vulnerable individuals. Documentation of the deployment timing, quantity, and site of application supports the reasoning.

### Medical Emergency Response During Arrest

The timeliness and adequacy of medical emergency response during and after arrest is a specific reasoning element in in-custody death cases. Delayed recognition of medical emergency (the decedent appearing to be resisting when actually experiencing agonal breathing or cardiovascular collapse), delayed initiation of resuscitation, and delayed transport to emergency medical facilities all contribute to the aggregate outcome. Body-worn camera footage frequently documents the timeline of collapse, recognition of collapse, initiation of resuscitation, and arrival of emergency medical services. The pathologist reviewing the case integrates the medical response timeline with the autopsy findings; delayed recognition or intervention that likely contributed to the outcome is documented, though the specific causal attribution to the delay is often difficult to quantify. Recent training initiatives for law enforcement personnel emphasize recognition of medical emergency during restraint and rapid transition from restraint to resuscitation when the individual becomes unresponsive; the aggregate case data supports the value of these training initiatives.

### Body-Worn Camera Integration in Case Analysis

The systematic integration of body-worn camera footage into forensic pathology case analysis has developed rapidly with the widespread deployment of the technology. The pathologist reviewing footage as part of the case reconstruction observes the specific interactions, sequences of events, applied mechanisms, and timing of collapse. The methodology of review benefits from a systematic approach: initial review of the complete footage to understand the case overall; targeted review of specific segments where restraint or force was applied; targeted review of the collapse and subsequent medical response;

and, where multiple camera angles are available, comparative review of the different perspectives. Documentation of the observations in the report supports the transparency of the reasoning; the footage is a source of evidence that the pathologist integrates with the physical findings rather than a source that replaces them. Some offices have developed formal protocols for BWC review with checklists for the elements to be documented and integrated; the approach reflects the recognition that the footage is now a standard element of many custodial death cases and that systematic integration supports the professional standards for these determinations.

### The Impact of Public and Legal Scrutiny on the Specialty

The public and legal scrutiny of custodial death determinations, particularly following widely reported cases in the past decade, has substantially affected forensic pathology practice in this area. Individual practitioners have been publicly criticized, professionally challenged, and subjected to disciplinary review based on their determinations in these cases. The specialty has responded with more explicit position statements from professional societies, with development of consensus standards for the certification of specific case types, and with recognition of the interpretive controversy as a topic warranting explicit treatment rather than avoidance. The individual practitioner navigates this environment by rigorous documentation, transparent reasoning, adherence to professional standards, and willingness to acknowledge the limits of certainty in interpretation. The specialty's credibility depends on the professional integrity of the individual determinations and on the collective willingness to engage the difficult questions rather than to retreat from them.

### Preservation of Evidence Chain in Custody Cases

The evidence chain in custody cases is subject to heightened scrutiny because of the litigation potential. The pathologist preserves the autopsy documentation with attention to the potential future legal use: photographic archive is comprehensive and organized; specimen retention is conservative with tissue blocks, slides, and retained frozen tissue preserved indefinitely; the autopsy report is written with clarity for professional and lay audiences; and consultation notes from second-opinion review are preserved. The chain of custody for physical evidence collected at the autopsy — clothing, weapons or restraint devices if provided, retained specimens for later analysis — is maintained with rigorous documentation. Some offices retain the autopsy specimens under evidentiary custody separate from routine specimen retention to preserve the chain adequately for potential legal use.

### SCENE-TO-CERTIFICATION DECISION SYSTEM — Custodial Death Determination Arcs

**The Custodial Death Framework:** Deaths in custody require systematic protocol exceeding routine autopsy standards, transparent reasoning, and integration with body-worn camera and other recording evidence. External scrutiny of the determinations is standard, and preparation for this scrutiny supports the professional integrity of the case.

**Positional Asphyxia and Restraint:** Positional asphyxia is one of multiple contributing mechanisms in restraint-associated deaths, with contested experimental support for its role as sole mechanism. Physical findings in restraint deaths are typically limited to restraint marks and nonspecific findings; the reasoning integrates findings with the reported mechanism.

**Sudden Death During Struggle:** Sudden death during struggle reflects the intersection of cardiovascular substrate, drug-induced catecholamine excess, and physiologic stress. The certification is contested among practitioners, and transparent reasoning about substrate, trigger, and context supports honest determinations regardless of the specific manner classification chosen.

**Excited Delirium: Repudiated Terminology:** The term excited delirium has been repudiated by major professional organizations and is being phased out of forensic pathology practice. Current recommended approach is certification with specific mechanisms (acute stimulant intoxication, hypertensive cardiovascular disease) rather than the umbrella term.

**Conducted Electrical Weapons:** CEW deployment findings include probe barb sites and, in contact deployment, paired burn marks. The causal reasoning about whether deployment contributed to death integrates deployment specifics, cardiovascular substrate, drug intoxication, and timeline; determination approaches vary among practitioners and offices.

## Summary and Key Concepts

Deaths in custody require specific protocol exceeding routine autopsy standards. The professional standards for these cases reflect the substantial external scrutiny to which the determinations will be subjected, from families, from law enforcement, from civil rights investigators, and from courts.

Positional asphyxia is a contested mechanism in the specialty. Current understanding is that prone restraint is one of multiple contributing mechanisms in restraint-associated deaths rather than the sole cause. Physical findings are typically limited, and the reasoning integrates findings with the reported mechanism.

Sudden death during struggle reflects the intersection of cardiovascular substrate (particularly hypertensive left ventricular hypertrophy, cardiomyopathy, and coronary disease), drug-induced catecholamine excess (particularly sympathomimetic drugs), and physiologic stress. The certification varies among practitioners and is documented with transparent reasoning about substrate, trigger, and context.

The term “excited delirium” has been repudiated by major professional organizations. Current recommended approach is certification with specific mechanisms rather than the umbrella term; the change reflects concerns about the term's diagnostic incoherence and about racial disparities in its application.

Conducted electrical weapons produce identifiable findings including probe barb sites and, in contact deployment, paired burn marks. The causal reasoning about whether deployment contributed to death is contested and integrates deployment specifics with cardiovascular substrate and drug intoxication.

The autopsy protocol for in-custody deaths includes layered neck dissection as standard, systematic cardiovascular examination, comprehensive toxicology, specimen retention, and consultation with colleagues on complex cases. Integration with body-worn camera footage and preparation for external review are standard elements.

# CHAPTER 17: POSTMORTEM TOXICOLOGY: SPECIMEN COLLECTION, INTERPRETATION, AND REDISTRIBUTION

**Learning Objectives**

1. Articulate the fundamental principles of postmortem toxicology and how they differ from clinical toxicology in living patients.
2. Perform the standard postmortem toxicology specimen collection protocol with attention to the specimen types most useful for different analytical questions.
3. Interpret postmortem blood drug concentrations with recognition of the specific challenges that distinguish postmortem from antemortem interpretation.
4. Recognize postmortem redistribution and its effects on blood concentrations of specific drugs, and reason about the reliability of central versus peripheral blood measurements.
5. Integrate toxicological findings with autopsy findings and clinical history to reach cause and manner determinations grounded in the full case reasoning rather than in isolated toxicology results.

## Principles of Postmortem Toxicology

Postmortem toxicology is the analytical identification and quantification of drugs, poisons, and other exogenous substances in specimens collected at autopsy, integrated with the case reasoning to support cause and manner determinations. The discipline shares fundamental analytical techniques with clinical toxicology but differs substantially in the interpretive framework. In clinical toxicology, blood drug concentrations reflect the antemortem physiological state of a living patient, are interpreted against published therapeutic and toxic ranges established in living subjects, and inform ongoing clinical management. In postmortem toxicology, blood drug concentrations reflect a complex combination of the antemortem physiological state plus postmortem changes including redistribution from tissue reservoirs, degradation of specific compounds, and postmortem production of substances (ethanol from bacterial fermentation, gases from decomposition). The pathologist reasoning about a postmortem toxicology result works within this framework.

The interpretive framework for postmortem toxicology has developed substantially over recent decades through peer-reviewed research examining specific drugs, specific specimen types, and specific reconstructions. The pathologist maintains familiarity with the current literature and integrates the specific findings with the recognized interpretive frameworks. The determination in a toxicology-related death is not a matter of comparing a blood concentration to a published lethal range — the framework is substantially more complex — but rather of integrating the specific finding with the case context to reach the most defensible reconstruction.

The forensic pathologist directs the toxicology workup by ordering specific analyses appropriate to the case reasoning, by ensuring appropriate specimen collection, and by interpreting the returned results in the case context. The analytical work itself is performed by forensic toxicologists in dedicated laboratories; the pathologist collaborates with the toxicologist on complex cases and on specimen and analytical decisions. This chapter addresses the pathologist's role — specimen collection, interpretation of results, and integration with autopsy findings — rather than the analytical chemistry of the laboratory.

### The Toxicology Question and the Case Context

The toxicology workup in a forensic case is directed by the specific questions the case reasoning requires. Was the decedent under the influence of drugs or alcohol at the time of death? Did drug intoxication contribute to the mechanism of death? Was a specific drug (a common therapeutic, a substance of abuse, a poison) present at levels adequate to cause death? Was drug administration by another person a factor? Each question drives specific analytical approaches. A comprehensive drug screen for a decedent found dead of unclear cause differs from focused analysis for a specific drug in a case with a known clinical context. Ordering the specific analysis appropriate to the case supports both efficient use of laboratory resources and the specific reasoning the case requires.

**KEY POINT:** Postmortem toxicology results are interpreted within the case context, not against published lethal ranges in isolation. The pathologist reasoning about a specific drug concentration integrates the level with the specimen source, with the recognized postmortem redistribution behavior of the drug, with any relevant tolerance or chronic use history, and with the autopsy findings supporting or contradicting the toxicological cause.

## Specimen Collection Protocol

The standard postmortem toxicology specimen collection protocol includes multiple specimen types collected in defined manner at defined sites. Each specimen has specific analytical utility, and the pathologist collects each systematically because subsequent case questions may not be predictable at the time of autopsy.

### Blood: Peripheral and Central

Blood is the primary specimen for drug identification and quantification. Two blood collection sites are used: peripheral blood (from the femoral vein, collected by needle aspiration from the vein under direct visualization or from the exposed vessel) and central blood (from the heart chambers, aorta, or vena cava). The distinction matters because postmortem redistribution affects central blood more than peripheral blood for many drugs — central blood concentrations are commonly elevated over peripheral concentrations as drugs redistribute from tissue reservoirs into the great vessels and heart during the postmortem interval. Peripheral blood is generally more reliable for quantitative interpretation of blood concentrations that will be compared to antemortem therapeutic or toxic ranges. Both specimens are collected in every case; the pathologist may use central blood when peripheral is unavailable (from decomposition, from prior blood loss) but recognizes the interpretive limits.

### Vitreous Humor

Vitreous humor from the eye is a specimen with specific analytical utility. Vitreous is relatively protected from postmortem redistribution because of its anatomic isolation from the vascular system, and it is analytically useful for specific substances including glucose (elevated in diabetic ketoacidosis), ketones (elevated in DKA and starvation ketosis), and electrolytes (with specific patterns supporting antemortem chemistry). Vitreous ethanol is more specific for antemortem ethanol exposure than blood ethanol because vitreous is less subject to postmortem bacterial ethanol production; vitreous ethanol substantially exceeding blood ethanol is unusual antemortem and typically reflects analytical or collection issues, while blood ethanol substantially exceeding vitreous ethanol raises the concern of postmortem production. The specimen is collected by needle aspiration from each eye separately (with the specimens combined for analysis if adequate volume from a single eye is not available).

### Urine

Urine when available is a valuable specimen for drug screening because most drugs are concentrated in urine relative to blood and because urine reflects an integration of exposure over the preceding hours to days. Urine drug screening identifies many substances that may be below the detection limit in blood, and urine is the primary specimen for detection of specific drug-facilitated sexual assault agents including gamma-hydroxybutyrate. Urine is collected by catheterization of the bladder before evisceration when available; some decedents have no urine present at autopsy (decedents with prolonged dying process with reduced urine output, decedents with obstructive uropathy), in which case the urine analytical opportunity is unavailable.

### Gastric Contents

Gastric contents provide evidence of recent oral drug ingestion including drug tablets or capsules that may be identifiable by inspection or by analytical identification. In a decedent with recent oral drug overdose, the gastric contents may contain substantial quantities of the ingested drug in identifiable form; identification supports both the drug identification and the mechanism reconstruction. The specimen is collected by measuring the total gastric volume and preserving both a fluid aliquot and any solid material identified. Gastric contents are typically not used for quantitative interpretation of drug concentrations because the concentration in the stomach reflects local physical distribution rather than the systemic level.

### Bile

Bile is a specimen with specific utility for opioid identification, particularly for identifying prior exposure to opioids that may be below detection limits in blood. Morphine and other opioids are excreted in bile and can be identified in this specimen with sensitivity exceeding that of blood in some cases. Bile is collected by aspiration from the gallbladder as a standard specimen in the routine autopsy.

## Hair and Nails

Hair and nails provide retrospective evidence of drug exposure over weeks to months preceding death. Drugs incorporated into growing hair remain detectable for the growth period of the specific hair segment; head hair growth of approximately 1 centimeter per month allows retrospective analysis of exposure timing when hair segments are analyzed sequentially. Hair analysis identifies chronic drug use (particularly relevant in some death investigations), documents exposure that may predate the acute event beyond the window of blood or urine detection, and supports the reasoning about chronic tolerance in specific cases. Hair is collected from the vertex of the scalp (with the growth root end identifiable) in adequate volume for the intended analysis; the specimen is preserved dry in labeled containers.

## Tissue Specimens

Tissue specimens from liver, brain, kidney, and other organs support drug analysis in specific circumstances. Liver tissue is particularly useful for identification of drugs concentrated in the liver (many therapeutic drugs, some drugs of abuse) and for cases where blood specimens are inadequate. Brain tissue is useful for evaluation of central nervous system-active drugs, particularly in cases where the specific concentration at the site of action is relevant. Tissue specimens are typically retained frozen for later analysis rather than analyzed routinely; the retention supports subsequent workup as the case questions develop.

**Figure 17.1: Postmortem Toxicology Specimen Collection Sites**

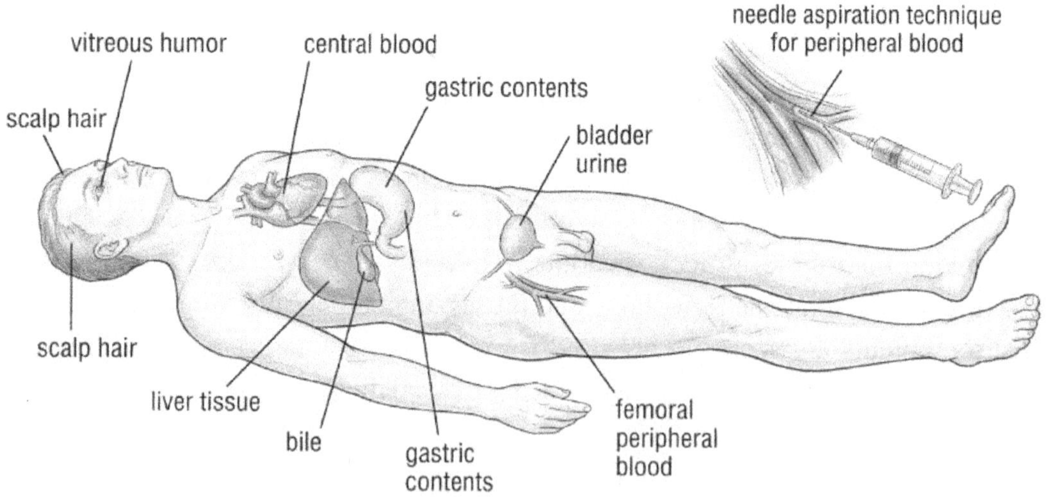


Figure 17.1: Postmortem Toxicology Specimen Collection Sites

## Interpretation of Postmortem Blood Levels

The interpretation of postmortem blood drug concentrations is one of the more sophisticated reasoning tasks in forensic pathology. The interpretation integrates several factors: the specific drug and its known postmortem redistribution behavior, the specimen source (peripheral versus central), any relevant tolerance history, the presence of other drugs producing additive or interactive effects, the autopsy findings supporting or contradicting the mechanism, and the case context. No single blood concentration determines the interpretation; the reasoning is integrative.

### Reference Ranges and Their Limits

Published reference ranges for drug concentrations exist for many substances and are widely used in postmortem interpretation. Typical published ranges include therapeutic (concentrations expected in patients receiving the drug at prescribed doses), toxic (concentrations associated with clinical toxicity in living patients), lethal (concentrations reported in cases where the drug was the primary cause of death), and, for specific drugs, ranges reported in individuals with chronic exposure and tolerance. These ranges are useful starting points but have substantial limits when applied to specific cases: they are typically based on antemortem samples in living patients, they do not fully account for postmortem redistribution, they do not fully account for tolerance in chronic users, and they overlap substantially between categories (particularly between toxic and lethal). The pathologist uses reference ranges as one line of evidence within the aggregate reasoning.

### Tolerance and the Chronic User

Tolerance to specific drug categories — particularly opioids, benzodiazepines, and other central nervous system depressants — substantially affects the interpretation of postmortem blood concentrations. A drug concentration that would be lethal in an opioid-naive individual may be within a range compatible with chronic tolerance in an individual with prolonged high-dose use; conversely, sudden increased exposure in a chronic user who has lost tolerance (after a period of abstinence, after incarceration, after hospitalization) can produce lethal outcome at concentrations that would have been tolerated during ongoing use. The pathologist reasons about tolerance from the history (documented prescribed opioid therapy, documented chronic substance use, documented recent period of abstinence), from the physical evidence (track marks, prescription bottles, drug paraphernalia at scene), and from any prior toxicology results if available. Chronic tolerance shifts the interpretive framework substantially and is a specific consideration in every opioid-related death.

### The Multiple-Drug Case

Many drug-related deaths in current American practice involve multiple substances rather than a single drug. Combinations of opioids and benzodiazepines, opioids with alcohol, stimulants with opioids, and various other multi-drug patterns are common. The interpretation of multi-drug cases is not simply the summation of individual drug interpretations; the specific interactions produce combined effects that exceed the sum of individual contributions. Opioid-benzodiazepine combinations produce more severe respiratory depression than either alone. Opioid-alcohol combinations similarly produce more severe central nervous system depression. Fentanyl analogs mixed with heroin have produced substantial numbers of overdose deaths where the fentanyl analog contribution was not apparent from the initial history. The pathologist reasoning about a multi-drug case integrates each drug with the specific interaction pattern and with the aggregate contribution to the death.

## Postmortem Redistribution

Postmortem redistribution refers to the movement of drugs from tissue reservoirs into blood after death, producing elevated blood concentrations compared to antemortem values. The phenomenon reflects the diffusion of drugs from tissues where they were concentrated during life (particularly the myocardium, lung, and liver) into blood in adjacent great vessels and heart chambers during the postmortem period. The effect is more pronounced in central blood than in peripheral blood and is more pronounced for drugs with specific characteristics.

### Drugs Affected by Redistribution

Drugs particularly affected by postmortem redistribution include many with basic physicochemical properties, high volume of distribution, and substantial tissue binding. Tricyclic antidepressants (amitriptyline, nortriptyline, and others) are classic examples with substantial documented postmortem redistribution where central blood concentrations may exceed antemortem levels by fold-differences. Cocaine is affected by redistribution with additional complication of postmortem enzymatic degradation. Many other cardioactive and psychoactive drugs show variable redistribution behavior. Published lists of drugs with documented postmortem redistribution behavior are available and are consulted in cases where the specific drug is central to the reasoning.

### Peripheral Versus Central Blood

The reasoning about peripheral versus central blood specimens reflects the redistribution phenomenon. Peripheral blood (from the femoral vein) is more distant from the tissue reservoirs from which drugs redistribute and better preserves the antemortem concentration. Central blood (from heart chambers, great vessels) reflects redistribution more substantially. For quantitative interpretation of drug concentrations that will be compared to antemortem therapeutic or toxic ranges, peripheral blood is generally more reliable. The pathologist collects both specimens in every case and uses peripheral blood for the primary quantitative interpretation when both are available.

### Interpretive Limits of Central Blood

Central blood remains valuable in specific circumstances: when peripheral blood is unavailable (from body decomposition, from prior blood loss, from technical difficulty), when comparison of central to peripheral blood specifically addresses the redistribution question, and when analysis of a drug not substantially affected by redistribution is being performed. The interpretation of central blood concentrations recognizes the redistribution effect: an elevated central blood concentration of a redistribution-affected drug does not necessarily indicate an antemortem toxic level, and the reasoning integrates the finding with the drug's specific redistribution behavior and with other case elements.

**SCENE-TO-CERTIFICATION DECISION SYSTEM — Postmortem Redistribution Reasoning Arc**

**Presenting Death Scenario:** A 34-year-old woman is found deceased in her home by her partner. She has a documented history of major depression and has been on stable oral amitriptyline therapy for two years without dose changes. The scene shows no evidence of injury, no signs of struggle, and no evidence of intentional overdose (medications in expected quantities in the prescribed containers). The medical examiner's office accepts jurisdiction. Postmortem interval is estimated at approximately 24 hours based on postmortem changes.

**Autopsy Signature:** External examination is unremarkable. Internal examination shows structurally normal heart of appropriate size, no acute pathology, and no other significant findings on gross or histologic examination. Peripheral (femoral) blood amitriptyline is 120 nanograms per milliliter (within the published therapeutic range of 50 to 300 ng/mL). Central (heart) blood amitriptyline is 480 nanograms per milliliter (elevated above the therapeutic range but consistent with documented postmortem redistribution behavior of amitriptyline). Peripheral blood nortriptyline (the active metabolite) is 90 nanograms per milliliter (within therapeutic range). Other toxicology is negative.

**Cause Determination:** The autopsy and toxicology findings do not identify a cause of death to reasonable medical certainty. Peripheral blood tricyclic antidepressant levels are within the therapeutic range and are not adequate to explain sudden death. Central blood levels are elevated but reflect documented postmortem redistribution rather than antemortem toxic exposure. No alternative structural cause of death is identified. Cause of death is undetermined; the reasoning documents the systematic evaluation and the interpretive limits of the tricyclic redistribution behavior.

**Manner Determination:** Undetermined. The manner cannot be determined without cause of death being determined; systematic examination has not identified either a natural cause or evidence of external cause. Some offices might certify as presumed natural pending molecular workup or other extended workup; the specific certification approach reflects office practice.

**Trap Logic:** The trap in this case is to interpret the elevated central blood amitriptyline as evidence of overdose without recognition of the postmortem redistribution behavior. Certification as tricyclic overdose based on central blood level alone would misattribute the death. The correct interpretation uses peripheral blood as the more reliable indicator of antemortem concentration and recognizes that central blood elevation is expected with amitriptyline. The absence of other evidence supporting overdose (scene evidence of ingestion, gastric contents with tablets, appropriate structural findings) further supports the interpretation that the central blood elevation reflects redistribution rather than intoxication. Cases like this are common and the systematic reasoning is essential.

**Certification Anchor:** Postmortem blood drug interpretation uses peripheral blood as the primary quantitative source when available; central blood is interpreted with reference to the specific drug's redistribution behavior. Elevated central blood concentrations of redistribution-affected drugs do not by themselves establish antemortem toxic exposure. The reasoning integrates blood concentrations with case context, with the drug's specific redistribution behavior, and with the absence or presence of supporting evidence for overdose.

## Analytical Methods

The analytical methods used in postmortem toxicology have evolved substantially over recent decades. Modern practice combines screening methods (immunoassay, targeted screening by mass spectrometry) with confirmatory quantitative methods (gas chromatography-mass spectrometry, liquid chromatography-tandem mass spectrometry). The specific methods used at a given laboratory reflect available equipment, workflow, and the specific analytes of interest.

### Screening Approaches

Screening approaches identify the presence or absence of drugs in a specimen without necessarily quantifying them. Common screens include comprehensive drug panels covering common drugs of abuse (opioids, cocaine, amphetamines, benzodiazepines, others), targeted screens for specific drug classes based on case context, and screens for specific drug-facilitated sexual assault agents. Screening is generally more efficient than comprehensive analysis for negative cases (where no drug is present) and identifies drugs requiring confirmatory analysis in positive cases. Immunoassay-based screens have documented false-positive and false-negative rates for specific drugs; confirmatory analysis is required before reporting positive findings.

**Figure 17.2: Peripheral Versus Central Blood Concentrations: The Redistribution Effect**

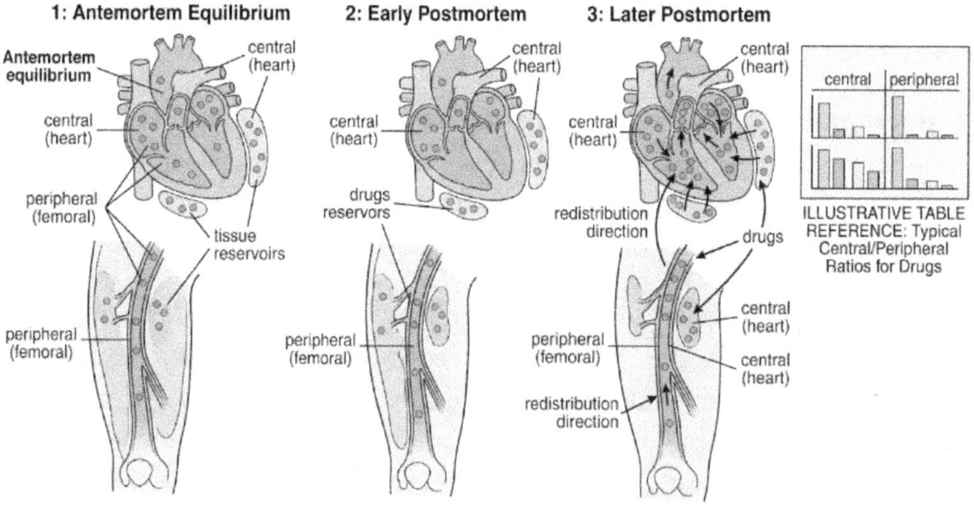


### Confirmatory and Quantitative Analysis

Confirmatory analysis identifies specific drugs with high specificity (using mass spectrometry with characteristic fragmentation patterns) and quantifies them (against calibrated standards). Modern practice uses liquid chromatography-tandem mass spectrometry (LC-MS/MS) as the workhorse technique for most drug analyses; gas chromatography-mass spectrometry (GC-MS) remains standard for some analyses including ethanol quantification. Specialized techniques including inductively coupled plasma-mass spectrometry (ICP-MS) support analysis for heavy metals in specific cases (arsenic, thallium, others). The specific method chosen reflects the analyte, the specimen, and the specific concentration range of interest.

## Toxicology in the Context of the Autopsy Determination

The final integration of toxicology into the autopsy determination is the pathologist's responsibility and integrates the toxicological findings with the autopsy findings, the scene evidence, the antecedent history, and the case reasoning. The toxicology laboratory produces analytical results; the pathologist produces the determination. The distinction matters because a positive toxicology result does not automatically establish drug-related death and a negative result does not automatically exclude it.

### The Integration

The integration considers each element: the toxicological findings (which drugs, at what concentrations, in what specimens, with what interpretive limits); the autopsy findings (structural pathology supporting or contradicting drug-related mechanism, absence of alternative structural causes); the scene evidence (drug paraphernalia, medication containers, evidence of ingestion, evidence of injection); the antecedent history (documented prescription therapy, documented substance use disorder, recent healthcare encounters, mental health status); and the case context (findings suggesting suicide, accident, homicide, or natural). The determination reflects the integration and is reasoned transparently in the report.

### The Suicide, Accident, and Homicide Determinations in Drug Cases

Drug-related deaths distribute across suicide, accident, and, less commonly, homicide manner categories. Suicide by drug overdose typically involves intentional ingestion of a substantial dose of a specific medication with associated scene evidence (a suicide note, prior communication of intent, purposeful assembly of the ingested materials, discrete scene). Accident is the manner classification for most drug overdose deaths in the current American opioid epidemic — unintentional overdose in an individual with drug use disorder using drugs for their intended personal effect rather than with intent to die. Homicide is the manner when a drug was administered to the decedent by another person with intent to harm (documented but uncommon). The pathologist's reasoning integrates the toxicology, autopsy, and scene evidence to support the specific manner determination.

### The Presumptive Certification

In many drug-related death cases, the pathologist certifies at initial autopsy with the specific finding pending toxicology completion. The presumptive certification acknowledges the pending workup and updates when the toxicology results are available. The practice supports timely case closure while preserving accuracy. The pathologist ensures the presumptive certification is documented as presumptive rather than as final and updates the certificate as findings mature.

### Postmortem Ethanol Production

Postmortem production of ethanol by bacterial fermentation is a specific interpretive challenge for blood ethanol measurements. Bacteria present in the body after death (from the intestinal tract, from environmental exposure of the body) can produce ethanol through fermentation of glucose and other substrates during the postmortem period, particularly in conditions of warm ambient temperature and delayed refrigeration of the body. The produced ethanol appears in blood at concentrations that can reach clinically significant levels; distinguishing antemortem ethanol exposure from postmortem production requires specific reasoning. Vitreous ethanol is less subject to postmortem production because of its anatomic isolation and is used as a check on blood ethanol interpretation — when vitreous ethanol is markedly lower than blood ethanol (or absent when blood is significantly elevated), postmortem ethanol production should be suspected. Additional analytical support for the distinction includes measurement of other markers of postmortem microbial activity and comparison with the ratio of urinary ethanol to blood ethanol. The pathologist recognizes the challenge and applies systematic reasoning; the certification of ethanol-related deaths considers both the analytical results and the plausibility of antemortem exposure.

### The Body Packer and Body Stuffer

The body packer is an individual who has ingested sealed drug packets for smuggling purposes, typically with careful preparation to withstand gastric transit and to deliver the drugs intact to a receiving party. Body stuffing is a related but distinct pattern in which drugs are ingested in less secure form during an emergency (typically to hide evidence during police encounter). Both patterns can produce fatal outcome when packet rupture releases the contained drug in mass quantity. The autopsy identifies the ingested packets by direct examination of the gastrointestinal tract or by postmortem imaging performed before evisceration; the finding is documented photographically and the packets are collected for identification and evidence. Body packer deaths characteristically show massive toxicological findings for the packed substance at concentrations well above typical overdose levels, reflecting the rupture of a packet designed to contain the drug during transit. Body stuffing shows more variable presentation because the ingested materials are less protected. Recognition of the pattern requires attention to the specific findings and to the case context.

### The Current American Opioid Epidemic Context

The current American opioid epidemic has substantially affected forensic pathology practice. Opioid overdose deaths have been the leading category of drug-related deaths for over a decade, with fentanyl and fentanyl analogs increasingly dominating the specific agents identified. The pattern reflects the transition of the illicit opioid supply from prescription opioids (early 2000s) through heroin (2010s) to fentanyl-adulterated substances (current). Deaths from fentanyl-adulterated substances often involve individuals who did not intentionally consume fentanyl — the fentanyl was mixed into other substances (heroin, cocaine, methamphetamine, counterfeit prescription tablets) by suppliers upstream. The pathologist encountering the case pattern (young decedent, drug paraphernalia at scene, characteristic pulmonary edema on autopsy, positive fentanyl on toxicology) certifies with reference to the specific pattern and contributes to the aggregate epidemic surveillance data through the state and federal reporting systems. The public health significance of the individual case reporting is substantial — the aggregate patterns support the policy response to the epidemic.

### Analysis of Novel and Unknown Substances

The forensic toxicology response to novel psychoactive substances has evolved with the substances themselves. Synthetic cannabinoids, synthetic cathinones, novel benzodiazepines, novel opioids (including nitazenes and other emerging substances), and other novel psychoactive substances present analytical challenges: standard drug screens do not include them, structural variations are introduced by suppliers to avoid legal control, and reference material for identification may be limited. Modern forensic toxicology laboratories have adapted to the challenge with high-resolution mass spectrometry approaches that can identify novel substances based on their exact mass and fragmentation patterns even without pre-existing reference material. Communication between forensic pathology and forensic toxicology is essential for identifying novel substance cases; the pathologist encountering an unexpected clinical presentation without conventional explanation communicates with the toxicology laboratory to guide the analytical approach. Documentation of the case reasoning and of the analytical findings supports both the individual case and the broader epidemiological surveillance.

### Poisoning Cases and Their Specific Reasoning

Poisoning cases — deaths from exposure to substances not part of the routine drug of abuse or therapeutic pattern — present specific reasoning challenges. The differential includes intentional homicidal poisoning (documented but uncommon in current American practice), intentional suicidal poisoning, accidental exposure (from environmental sources, from occupational exposure, from mistaken ingestion), and, in specific contexts, iatrogenic exposure. Common poisoning agents include heavy metals (arsenic, lead, thallium in specific historical patterns), household chemicals (with characteristic ingestion patterns), agricultural chemicals (organophosphate and carbamate pesticides, rodenticides), industrial chemicals (in occupational exposures), and specific natural toxins (plant alkaloids, mushroom toxins, marine biotoxins). Each agent has specific analytical approaches and characteristic autopsy findings that support the diagnosis when the exposure is identified as a differential consideration. The reasoning depends on the pathologist including poisoning in the differential when the clinical presentation is unusual, and communicating with the toxicology laboratory to guide the specific analytical approach.

### Cocaine and Its Postmortem Analytical Complexity

Cocaine presents specific analytical complexity in postmortem interpretation. Cocaine is subject to postmortem enzymatic degradation to benzoylecgonine and other metabolites; the rate of this degradation depends on temperature, time, and specific factors. Blood cocaine measured at autopsy typically underestimates antemortem cocaine exposure because of the degradation. Benzoylecgonine, the primary metabolite, is more stable postmortem and is often present at higher concentrations than cocaine itself. The interpretation of a positive cocaine result integrates the parent-metabolite ratio (a high metabolite-to-parent ratio suggests the exposure was hours before death; a low ratio suggests recent exposure), the specific concentration in an appropriate specimen, and the case context. Sodium fluoride preservative in the collection tube reduces postmortem cocaine degradation and is standard for cocaine analysis; unpreserved specimens can show substantial degradation between collection and analysis. Cocaine deaths are typically classified by the specific clinical mechanism (arrhythmic death from acute cardiotoxicity, complications of chronic use, or hyperthermic crisis with sudden collapse) integrated with the toxicological finding.

### Vitreous Ethanol Interpretation

Vitreous humor ethanol is a specific analytical tool with substantial utility. The specimen is protected from postmortem microbial ethanol production more than blood, and the ratio of vitreous ethanol to blood ethanol provides interpretive support. When the ratio approximates 1.0 to 1.2 (with vitreous slightly higher than blood, reflecting the redistribution of ethanol from blood to vitreous during death), antemortem ethanol exposure is supported. When blood substantially exceeds vitreous (or vitreous is negative while blood is elevated), postmortem microbial ethanol production is more likely. When vitreous substantially exceeds blood by more than physiological ratios, other issues — including analytical or collection issues, or specific pharmacokinetic circumstances — warrant consideration. The systematic use of vitreous ethanol as a check on blood ethanol interpretation supports certification of ethanol-related deaths and reduces the risk of overinterpreting elevated blood ethanol as antemortem when postmortem production accounts for it.

### Novel Synthetic Substances and the Evolving Landscape

The landscape of substances encountered in forensic toxicology has evolved substantially over recent years, with novel synthetic substances continuously introduced into the illicit market. Categories include: synthetic cannabinoids (spice, K2, and successive generations of chemical variants); synthetic cathinones ("bath salts" and related compounds); designer benzodiazepines (etizolam, flualprazolam, and others); novel opioids beyond fentanyl (nitazenes including isotonitazene and etonitazene, protonitazene, and evolving analog structures); and specific psychoactive substances developed for a variety of purposes. The illicit market response to each new legal control is to introduce new chemical variants that fall outside the specific control while producing similar effects; the analytical response is to develop reference material and identification methods for the new substances. The pathologist reasoning about a case with an unusual clinical presentation and unclear toxicological findings considers novel synthetic substance exposure as a differential and communicates with the toxicology laboratory to guide the analytical approach. Documentation of such cases in the aggregate epidemiological surveillance supports the public health response to emerging substances.

### Postmortem Imaging and Toxicology Integration

Postmortem imaging (particularly postmortem CT) has developed as a complement to autopsy in many offices, and its integration with toxicological reasoning has specific value. In cases of suspected body packing, postmortem CT identifies ingested packets before evisceration disturbs them, supports counting of packets, and identifies rupture. In cases of overdose, postmortem CT can identify pulmonary edema (a characteristic finding of opioid overdose), can identify gastrointestinal contents suggesting recent oral ingestion, and can identify other findings supporting the clinical mechanism. Postmortem CT does not replace toxicological analysis but complements it. Some offices have integrated postmortem imaging as a routine element of overdose case workup; others reserve it for specific case questions. The integration reflects office practice and available resources.

### Communication With the Forensic Toxicology Laboratory

The communication between the forensic pathologist and the forensic toxicology laboratory is central to the effective use of the analytical workup. The pathologist provides case context (clinical history, autopsy findings, specific reasoning questions) that guides the analytical approach. The toxicologist provides analytical expertise on the specific tests available, on the interpretive limits of the results, and on specific reasoning questions arising from the analysis. Complex cases benefit from direct discussion between pathologist and toxicologist; standard cases proceed through routine analytical protocols with communication limited to the analytical result reporting. Building the professional relationship between pathology and toxicology at an office supports both effective individual case workup and the broader quality of the analytical practice.

Figure 17.3: Ingested Drug Packets in Body Packer at Autopsy

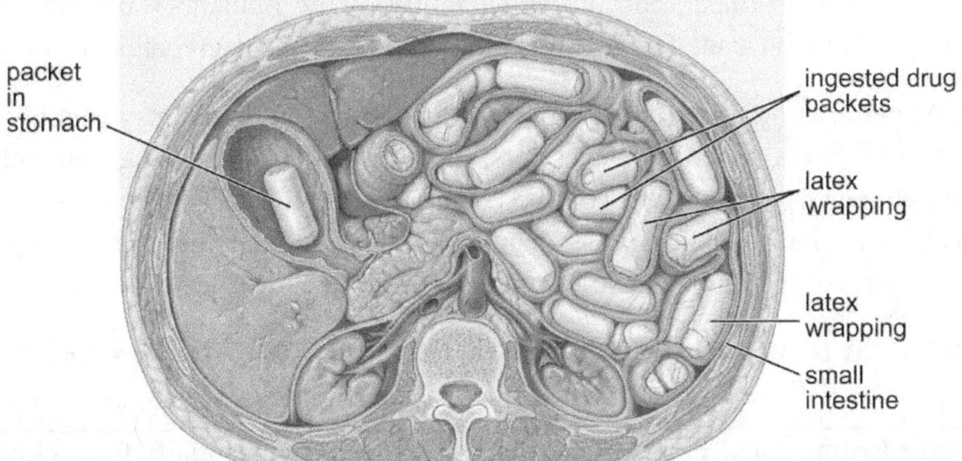


## SCENE-TO-CERTIFICATION DECISION SYSTEM — Toxicology-Cause Integration Arc

**Presenting Death Scenario:** A 28-year-old man with a documented history of opioid use disorder is found deceased in his residence by his roommate. Scene evidence includes drug paraphernalia (syringe, tourniquet, small aluminum foil piece with charred residue) on a table near the decedent. He had been in a residential treatment program with documented abstinence for three months preceding the death, having completed the program approximately 1 week before. The medical examiner's office accepts jurisdiction.

**Autopsy Signature:** External examination documents fresh injection track at the antecubital fossa; multiple healed track marks on both arms consistent with prior chronic injection use. Internal examination shows pulmonary edema of characteristic pattern for opioid overdose, no other acute pathology. Toxicology on peripheral blood: fentanyl 12 nanograms per milliliter, norfentanyl (metabolite) 4 nanograms per milliliter, no other significant drugs detected. Autopsy fluid from the aluminum foil residue at scene confirmed as fentanyl. Central blood fentanyl approximately 20 nanograms per milliliter, consistent with modest redistribution behavior.

**Cause Determination:** Acute fentanyl intoxication.

**Manner Determination:** Accident. The determination reflects: recent completion of residential treatment with associated loss of opioid tolerance; return to opioid use with a dose that would have been tolerated during ongoing use but was fatal after the abstinence period; absence of any evidence suggesting intent to die; and pattern consistent with the well-documented accidental opioid overdose during the post-treatment vulnerable window.

**Trap Logic:** The trap in interpreting opioid deaths of individuals recently discharged from treatment is either to certify as suicide (based on the fatal outcome without consideration of the tolerance context) or to certify as natural (without recognizing the acute drug cause). The correct interpretation integrates the toxicology finding of fentanyl at a concentration consistent with acute intoxication, the autopsy findings supporting opioid overdose mechanism, the scene evidence of active drug use, the antecedent history of use disorder and recent treatment, and the vulnerability of the immediate post-treatment period. The certification as accident with acute fentanyl intoxication reflects the aggregate reasoning.

**Certification Anchor:** Drug-related deaths integrate toxicology with autopsy findings, scene evidence, and antecedent history. The specific manner determination (suicide, accident, homicide, undetermined) reflects the case context. Accident is the common determination for opioid overdose deaths in the current epidemic; the classification is medical rather than legal, and criminal or civil proceedings arising from the death are matters for law enforcement and the prosecutor.

## SCENE-TO-CERTIFICATION DECISION SYSTEM — Postmortem Toxicology Determination Arcs

**The Interpretive Framework:** Postmortem toxicology differs substantially from clinical toxicology in the interpretive framework. Blood drug concentrations reflect antemortem physiology plus postmortem changes including redistribution. The pathologist integrates toxicology with autopsy findings, scene evidence, and history for the specific determination.

**Standard Specimen Collection:** The standard collection protocol includes peripheral and central blood, vitreous humor, urine when available, gastric contents, bile, hair, and retained tissue for later analysis. Each specimen has specific analytical utility, and comprehensive collection supports the subsequent workup as case questions develop.

**Peripheral Blood as Primary Source:** Peripheral blood (femoral) is the primary specimen for quantitative interpretation because it is less affected by postmortem redistribution. Central blood is preserved for comparison and for use when peripheral is unavailable. The specific drug's redistribution behavior informs the interpretation of central-to-peripheral ratios.

**Multiple-Drug Cases:** Multiple-drug deaths are common in current American practice and require specific reasoning about interactive effects. Opioid-benzodiazepine and opioid-alcohol combinations produce combined respiratory and central nervous system depression exceeding either alone. Fentanyl analog contamination of other drug supplies is a common current pattern.

**The Manner Determination:** Drug-related deaths distribute across suicide, accident, and homicide manners with specific reasoning for each. Accident is the common current determination for opioid overdose deaths in the epidemic. Suicide requires evidence of intent; homicide requires evidence of administration by another with intent to harm. Undetermined is appropriate when the workup cannot establish either cause or manner to reasonable medical certainty.

## Summary and Key Concepts

Postmortem toxicology is the identification and quantification of drugs and other substances in specimens collected at autopsy, integrated with the case reasoning for cause and manner determination. The interpretive framework differs substantially from clinical toxicology and requires attention to postmortem changes including redistribution and postmortem production.

The standard specimen collection protocol includes peripheral and central blood, vitreous humor, urine when available, gastric contents, bile, hair, and retained tissue. Comprehensive collection supports the subsequent workup as case questions develop.

Peripheral blood from the femoral vein is the primary specimen for quantitative interpretation because it is less affected by postmortem redistribution. Central blood is preserved for comparison and for use when peripheral is unavailable; interpretation reflects the specific drug's redistribution behavior.

Multiple-drug deaths are common and require specific reasoning about interactive effects. Opioid-benzodiazepine and opioid-alcohol combinations produce combined effects exceeding either alone; fentanyl analog contamination of other drug supplies is a current concern.

Analytical methods combine screening (immunoassay, targeted screens) with confirmatory quantitative analysis (LC-MS/MS, GC-MS). Screening identifies substances requiring confirmatory analysis; confirmatory analysis provides specific identification and quantification for the case interpretation.

The pathologist integrates toxicology with autopsy findings, scene evidence, and history for the specific determination. Positive toxicology does not automatically establish drug-related death, and negative results do not automatically exclude it. The reasoning is documented transparently in the report.

# CHAPTER 18: DRUG AND ALCOHOL DEATHS

**Learning Objectives**

1. Articulate the epidemiology of drug-related deaths in current American practice and the framework for their forensic investigation.
2. Recognize the constellation of findings characteristic of opioid overdose deaths and reason about specific opioid agents including fentanyl analogs.
3. Identify stimulant overdose death patterns including cocaine, methamphetamine, and MDMA, with attention to their specific mechanisms.
4. Distinguish acute alcohol intoxication deaths, chronic alcohol-related deaths, and alcohol withdrawal deaths, and reason about certification for each.
5. Interpret prescription medication deaths with attention to therapeutic versus toxic reasoning and to the multi-drug interaction pattern common in current practice.

## The Epidemiology and Framework of Drug-Related Deaths

Drug-related deaths in the United States have reached levels unprecedented in the modern era of forensic pathology practice. Annual drug overdose deaths have exceeded 100,000 for multiple recent years, with opioids accounting for the substantial majority and stimulants accounting for a growing fraction. The pattern reflects the sequential phases of the American drug crisis: the prescription opioid phase of the early 2000s, the heroin phase of the 2010s, and the fentanyl and fentanyl-analog phase of the current period. Superimposed on this pattern are the deaths from stimulants (particularly methamphetamine), from alcohol (which remains the substance with the largest aggregate mortality burden in most classifications), from prescription medications, and from the polydrug combinations that account for most current overdose deaths.

The forensic pathologist encountering drug-related deaths in the current caseload sees the aggregate pattern reflected in the individual cases: the substantial numbers of accidental overdose deaths in individuals with substance use disorder; the deaths of individuals in the immediate post-treatment or post-incarceration windows when tolerance has decreased; the deaths from unexpected substances (fentanyl contamination of other drug supplies, novel synthetic opioids); and the deaths of older decedents from combinations of prescribed medications and alcohol. Each case has its individual reasoning, and the aggregate case data supports the public health response to the ongoing crisis.

The framework for drug-related death investigation combines the general forensic autopsy protocol with the specific toxicology framework developed in Chapter 17 and with the specific reasoning about mechanism, manner, and case context. The pathologist ordering the toxicology workup, integrating the results with autopsy findings, and reasoning about the specific determination follows the general framework with attention to the specific drug or drug combination involved.

### The Aggregate Case Reporting Function

The forensic pathology contribution to the drug crisis response is not only individual case certification but also the aggregate case reporting that supports public health surveillance. State and federal reporting systems capture the drug overdose deaths with specific detail: the substances involved, the demographic pattern, the specific circumstances, and the case context. The aggregate data supports policy response (naloxone distribution, treatment access, harm reduction programming, drug supply intervention). The pathologist certifying an individual case with specificity about the substances involved contributes to the aggregate data; certifications that lack this specificity limit the public health value of the case.

**KEY POINT:** Individual drug-related death certifications contribute to aggregate public health surveillance that supports the response to the ongoing drug crisis. Specific documentation of substances involved and case context supports both the individual case and the broader response. Vague certifications (e.g., "mixed drug toxicity" without specification) limit the value of the aggregate data.

## Opioid Overdose Deaths

Opioid overdose is the leading category of drug-related death in current American practice. The mechanism is respiratory depression from opioid receptor-mediated central inhibition of respiratory drive; the terminal event is respiratory arrest with subsequent cardiac arrest. The physiologic pattern produces a specific constellation of autopsy findings that supports the diagnosis when identified.

**Figure 18.1:** Opioid Overdose: Pulmonary Foam Cone and Injection Track Marks

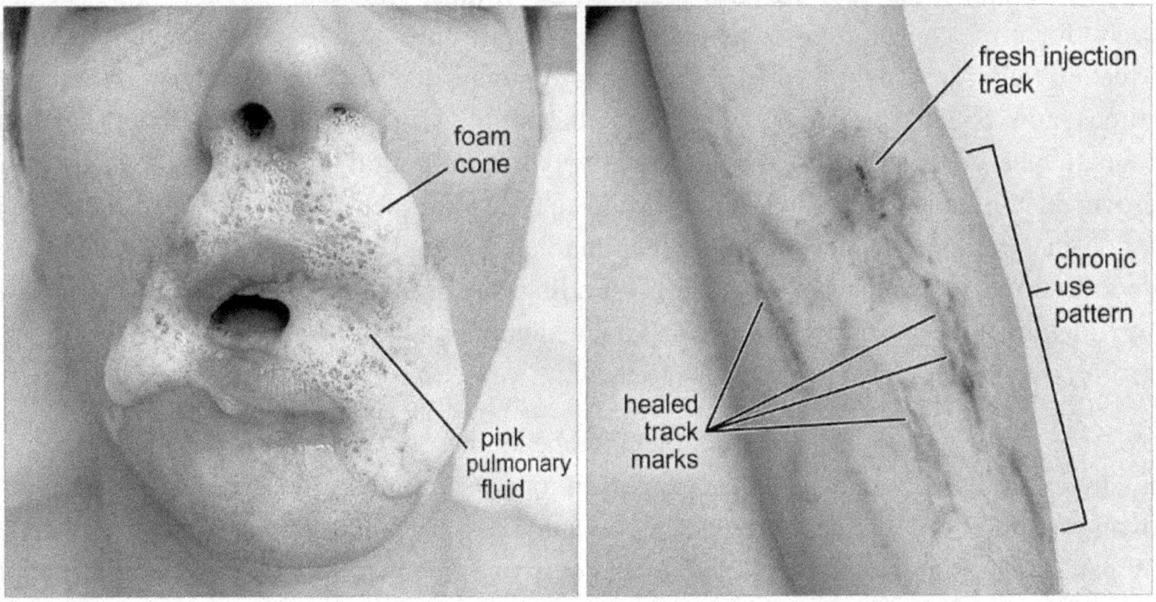

## The Classic Autopsy Findings

The autopsy findings in opioid overdose include: pulmonary edema, often with characteristic frothy fluid emerging from the airway (the foam cone) similar to but generally less voluminous than drowning; pulmonary congestion with heavy, boggy lungs; cerebral edema; and, in cases with prolonged terminal course, evidence of hypoxic organ injury. External findings depend on the specific route of exposure: fresh and healed injection tracks in intravenous users, punctate marks and burns on the fingers or lips from smoking apparatus in decedents who smoke opioids, or no external route findings in decedents who took opioids orally. Scene evidence — syringes, drug packaging, aluminum foil pieces, medication containers — supports the reconstruction and often identifies the specific substance.

The finding of the foam cone at the airway in opioid overdose deserves specific attention. The foam represents pulmonary edema fluid mixed with air from the terminal respiratory effort. The finding is not specific for opioid overdose (occurs in other causes of severe pulmonary edema including cardiac failure, other overdose types, and drowning) but is highly consistent with the pattern when the case context supports it. Documentation of the foam cone at the initial scene examination and at autopsy is standard; the finding may be less prominent by autopsy if hours have elapsed since collapse. Photographic documentation of the foam cone at scene, when available, supports the case reconstruction.

## Fentanyl and Fentanyl Analogs

Fentanyl and its analogs (carfentanil, acetylfentanyl, furanylfentanyl, and successive novel structural variants) now dominate the opioid overdose landscape in most American jurisdictions. The substances have several features relevant to forensic reasoning: they are substantially more potent than morphine or heroin (fentanyl approximately 80 to 100 times more potent than morphine; carfentanil approximately 10,000 times more potent), producing lethal doses that are physically small and difficult for illicit market participants to measure accurately; they have relatively short duration of action, so the acute intoxication may be over in the hours preceding autopsy; and they are frequently mixed into other drug supplies (heroin, cocaine, counterfeit prescription tablets marketed as oxycodone or benzodiazepines) with the mixing not disclosed to purchasers. The autopsy findings are similar to those of other opioid overdoses; toxicology identifies the specific substance and its metabolites.

The pattern of unexpected fentanyl exposure has substantial implications. A decedent who consumed a substance they believed to be cocaine, methamphetamine, or a prescription tablet but that was contaminated with fentanyl may have had no reason to expect opioid effect and may not have arranged for naloxone availability or witness presence that would have supported rescue. The unexpected fentanyl exposure pattern is a significant component of the current epidemic, and identification of the pattern in the individual case contributes to the aggregate surveillance.

**Injection Findings and Track Marks**

Injection track marks reflect the chronic use pattern of intravenous drug users. Fresh injection tracks (linear or punctate scab, adjacent contusion or skin discoloration) document recent injection. Healed injection tracks (linear hyperpigmented scars, sometimes with adjacent skin atrophy) document prior chronic injection. Multiple sites across the antecubital fossa, forearms, hands, feet, and, in advanced chronic use, the neck, thighs, and other sites reflect the progression of vein sclerosis with prolonged use; users move to progressively less accessible sites as veins become unusable. Documentation of the injection findings supports the reasoning about chronic use, which is relevant to the tolerance context and to the case reconstruction.

**SCENE-TO-CERTIFICATION DECISION SYSTEM — Opioid Overdose Reconstruction Arc**

---

**Presenting Death Scenario:** A 42-year-old man is found deceased in the bathroom of a convenience store by an employee. Scene documentation identifies a syringe on the floor beside the decedent and a small aluminum foil piece with charred residue. The decedent is in a slumped position on the floor consistent with collapse during use. Emergency response confirms death at scene. Records review documents a history of opioid use disorder with multiple prior nonfatal overdose episodes.

**Autopsy Signature:** External examination documents multiple healed injection track marks on both antecubital fossae and forearms, a fresh injection track at the left antecubital fossa, and a persistent foam cone at the mouth. Internal examination shows extensive pulmonary edema with the lungs heavy and boggy (right lung 800 grams, left lung 750 grams; expected range 300-400 each), pulmonary congestion, and cerebral edema. Peripheral blood toxicology: fentanyl 18 nanograms per milliliter; norfentanyl (metabolite) 6 nanograms per milliliter; morphine 40 nanograms per milliliter (free); 6-monoacetylmorphine detected (specific metabolite of heroin, confirming recent heroin use); other drugs negative. The aluminum foil residue is subsequently confirmed as containing fentanyl.

**Cause Determination:** Acute combined fentanyl and heroin toxicity.

**Manner Determination:** Accident. The determination reflects: the pattern consistent with accidental overdose in an individual with documented opioid use disorder; the scene evidence of active drug use immediately preceding collapse; the toxicological findings supporting acute intoxication with both intentionally consumed heroin and fentanyl contamination; the absence of evidence suggesting intent to die; and the aggregate pattern consistent with the current opioid epidemic.

**Trap Logic:** The trap in interpreting fentanyl-associated overdose deaths is either to attribute to a single agent when combinations are present, or to certify without documenting the fentanyl contamination pattern that characterizes many current cases. The systematic reasoning: comprehensive toxicological analysis identifying all substances present, confirmation of specific metabolites supporting the intended use (6-monoacetylmorphine confirms heroin as the intended substance; fentanyl was present as contamination or additive); integration with scene evidence supporting the specific pattern; and documentation of the aggregate finding in the report supporting subsequent epidemiological surveillance.

Certification as combined fentanyl and heroin toxicity accurately reflects the finding; certification only as fentanyl or only as heroin would omit relevant information.

**Certification Anchor:** Opioid overdose deaths are certified with specific reference to the substances involved. Combined substance intoxication (fentanyl plus heroin, opioid plus benzodiazepine, opioid plus alcohol) is documented as such rather than reduced to a single substance for reporting simplicity. The aggregate data supports the public health response, and specific documentation contributes to the surveillance.

## Stimulant Overdose Deaths

Stimulant overdose deaths include cocaine, methamphetamine, MDMA, and synthetic cathinones ("bath salts"). The mechanisms differ from opioid overdose — stimulants produce catecholamine excess with sympathomimetic effects rather than respiratory depression, and the mechanism of death is cardiovascular (arrhythmia, hypertensive emergency, hyperthermic crisis) rather than respiratory.

### Cocaine

Cocaine produces sympathomimetic effects through inhibition of catecholamine reuptake. Acute effects include tachycardia, hypertension, hyperthermia, and, in overdose, potentially fatal cardiovascular events including arrhythmia, myocardial ischemia and infarction (in decedents with coronary vulnerability), aortic dissection, and hyperthermic crisis. Chronic effects include cardiovascular pathology (cardiomyopathy, coronary atherosclerosis accelerated by chronic cocaine use, hypertensive vascular changes), pulmonary pathology in specific route-of-use patterns (crack lung in individuals who smoke cocaine), and various systemic effects. Autopsy findings in cocaine death may include the cardiovascular pathology, evidence of chronic use, and specific findings supporting the acute mechanism. Toxicology identifies cocaine and its metabolites; the parent-metabolite ratio (cocaine to benzoylecgonine) informs the timing of recent exposure.

### Methamphetamine and Amphetamines

Methamphetamine produces sympathomimetic effects similar to cocaine but with substantially longer duration of action (hours rather than minutes for the acute effects). The mechanism of death in methamphetamine overdose parallels cocaine: cardiovascular events on a background of catecholamine excess, hyperthermic crisis, and, in some cases, direct cardiotoxicity from chronic use. Methamphetamine has emerged in the past decade as a substantial component of the drug crisis in some regions, with mortality rates that have grown substantially. Combined methamphetamine and opioid deaths ("speedball" combinations of stimulant and depressant) are increasingly common in current caseloads. The autopsy findings include those of the cardiovascular event, evidence of chronic use (dental disease, skin lesions from chronic scratching, weight loss and appearance changes), and specific findings supporting the acute mechanism.

### MDMA and Novel Stimulants

MDMA (3,4-methylenedioxymethamphetamine, "ecstasy") produces stimulant effects with additional serotonergic activity that can produce specific complications including hyperthermic crisis, hyponatremia (from combined effects of the drug and, in some cases, excessive water intake by users trying to avoid dehydration), and serotonin syndrome. Deaths from MDMA typically occur in the context of use at social events (music festivals, concerts, clubs) and reflect the combination of drug effect with environmental factors (high ambient temperature, physical exertion from dancing, inadequate hydration or excessive water intake). Novel stimulants including synthetic cathinones present specific analytical challenges and are documented as emerging causes of stimulant-related death; the analytical response to novel stimulants parallels the response to novel opioids developed in Chapter 17.

## Alcohol-Related Deaths

Alcohol-related deaths span multiple categories: acute alcohol intoxication with fatal outcome from the intoxication itself; deaths from the medical complications of chronic alcohol use (liver disease, cardiovascular disease, others); deaths from alcohol withdrawal (delirium tremens with associated cardiovascular collapse or seizure); and deaths from injury and accident related to alcohol impairment (motor vehicle collisions, falls, drownings). The forensic pathology encounters each category and applies the specific reasoning for the mechanism identified.

### Acute Alcohol Intoxication Deaths

Acute alcohol intoxication can produce fatal outcome through respiratory depression (at blood ethanol concentrations typically above 0.30 to 0.40 grams per deciliter in non-tolerant individuals), through aspiration of gastric contents during vomiting in a decedent with impaired airway protection, through complications in individuals with cardiovascular disease (arrhythmia in the acute intoxication setting), and through the specific pattern of aspiration and asphyxial mechanism in decedents who lost consciousness in circumstances allowing airway compromise. The tolerance context matters substantially: an individual with chronic heavy alcohol use may tolerate blood ethanol concentrations well above 0.40 without acute lethality, while a non-tolerant individual can have fatal outcome at concentrations that would produce only clinically apparent intoxication in a tolerant individual. Blood ethanol interpretation integrates the specific concentration with the tolerance context.

### Chronic Alcohol-Related Disease

Chronic alcohol use produces a substantial spectrum of pathology that contributes to death in many individuals with alcohol use disorder. Cirrhosis with associated complications (variceal hemorrhage, hepatic failure, hepatocellular carcinoma, hepatorenal syndrome) accounts for many chronic alcohol-related deaths. Alcoholic cardiomyopathy contributes to sudden cardiac death and to heart failure deaths. Chronic pancreatitis with associated malabsorption and diabetes contributes to overall morbidity. Wernicke encephalopathy and Korsakoff syndrome from chronic thiamine deficiency contribute to neurologic morbidity. Chronic alcohol use also accelerates cardiovascular disease and specifically increases cancer risk for several sites. The pathologist encountering an alcohol-related death identifies the specific pathology and integrates with the case history.

### Alcohol Withdrawal Deaths

Alcohol withdrawal in individuals with substantial chronic dependence can produce delirium tremens — severe withdrawal with autonomic instability, cardiovascular collapse, seizure, and, in untreated or inadequately treated cases, death. The pattern occurs classically in individuals who suddenly stop drinking after prolonged heavy use, often in the context of hospitalization for another reason, incarceration, or attempts at cessation without medical support. The autopsy findings are typically nonspecific; the reasoning depends on the antecedent history of chronic alcohol use, the temporal association of the withdrawal syndrome with cessation of drinking, and the exclusion of alternative causes.

Figure 18.2: Hepatic Steatosis and Alcoholic Cirrhosis on Histology

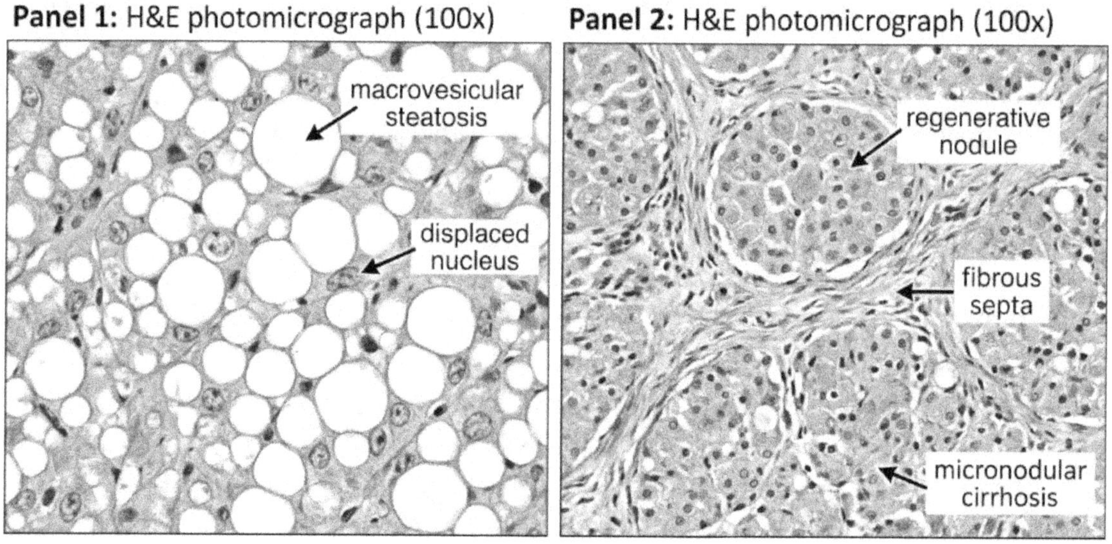


### SCENE-TO-CERTIFICATION DECISION SYSTEM — Alcohol-Related Death Determination Arc

**Presenting Death Scenario:** A 56-year-old man is admitted to the emergency department for altered mental status. He is a documented heavy chronic alcohol user who was hospitalized four days earlier for an unrelated infection and has not consumed alcohol during the admission. During the current admission he develops tremor, agitation, hypertension, tachycardia, and, over the following 12 hours, progresses to seizure and cardiovascular collapse despite aggressive medical management including benzodiazepines and other supportive care. He is pronounced dead approximately 24 hours after transfer for the altered mental status. The medical examiner's office accepts jurisdiction on the in-hospital death of a documented alcohol-dependent individual.

**Autopsy Signature:** External examination is unremarkable apart from resuscitation-related injuries. Internal examination shows moderate hepatic steatosis with early cirrhotic changes, moderate cardiovascular disease with left ventricular hypertrophy consistent with chronic alcohol-related cardiomyopathy, and no acute pathology adequate to explain the terminal syndrome independently. Toxicology is negative for alcohol at the time of death (consistent with several days of abstinence during the hospitalization), negative for other drugs of abuse, and shows the therapeutic levels of the medications administered during hospitalization.

**Cause Determination:** Delirium tremens due to alcohol withdrawal, with contributing chronic alcohol-related cardiovascular disease. The determination reflects the classic clinical pattern of severe withdrawal syndrome in an individual with documented chronic dependence, occurring in the setting of forced abstinence during hospitalization, with the autopsy findings supporting the substrate of chronic alcohol-related disease.

**Manner Determination:** Natural. The cause of death is a natural process (alcohol withdrawal syndrome) occurring in the context of medical care; the manner is natural despite the association with the hospitalization. Some offices might classify as accident given the withdrawal context; the specific determination reflects office practice. Documentation of the reasoning in the report supports the transparent understanding of the classification.

**Trap Logic:** The trap in interpreting alcohol withdrawal deaths in medical care settings is either to attribute to the underlying medical condition (missing the specific withdrawal pattern) or to attribute to medical care (missing the natural progression of the withdrawal syndrome). The systematic reasoning identifies: the documented history of chronic alcohol dependence; the temporal association of the withdrawal syndrome with cessation of drinking during the admission; the clinical progression consistent with delirium tremens; and the autopsy findings supporting the chronic substrate. Certification as delirium tremens with contributing chronic disease reflects the aggregate reasoning.

**Certification Anchor:** Alcohol-related deaths span acute intoxication, chronic disease complications, withdrawal syndromes, and injury-related deaths. Each category has specific reasoning integrating the toxicological findings (or their absence in withdrawal cases with prior abstinence), autopsy findings, and case history. The determination reflects the specific pattern rather than a generic "alcohol-related" classification.

## Prescription Medication Deaths

Deaths involving prescription medications span multiple patterns: intentional suicidal overdose using prescribed medications; accidental overdose (through drug interactions, dosing errors, or unrecognized combinations); adverse drug reactions to appropriately prescribed medications; and, less commonly, medication-related deaths involving another person's prescriptions (diverted medications). The reasoning about each requires attention to the specific medication, to the dose, to the tolerance and health status of the decedent, and to the case context.

### Prescription Opioids

Deaths from prescription opioids follow patterns similar to those of illicit opioids but with specific reasoning about the therapeutic context. A decedent under active prescription opioid therapy for chronic pain who dies from opioid overdose may have died from unintentional overdose during appropriate therapeutic use, from intentional overdose using prescribed medication, from adverse reaction to a stable dose, or from combined effects of the prescribed medication with other substances. The reasoning integrates: the specific medication prescribed and its stability over recent history; the blood concentration at autopsy against the therapeutic and toxic ranges for the tolerant patient; any other substances identified; the antecedent history of pain management; and any evidence supporting suicidal intent. Chronic pain patients are a specific vulnerable population where the reasoning about specific manner is nuanced.

**Figure 18.3:** Prescription Medication Overdose Scene Evidence Documentation

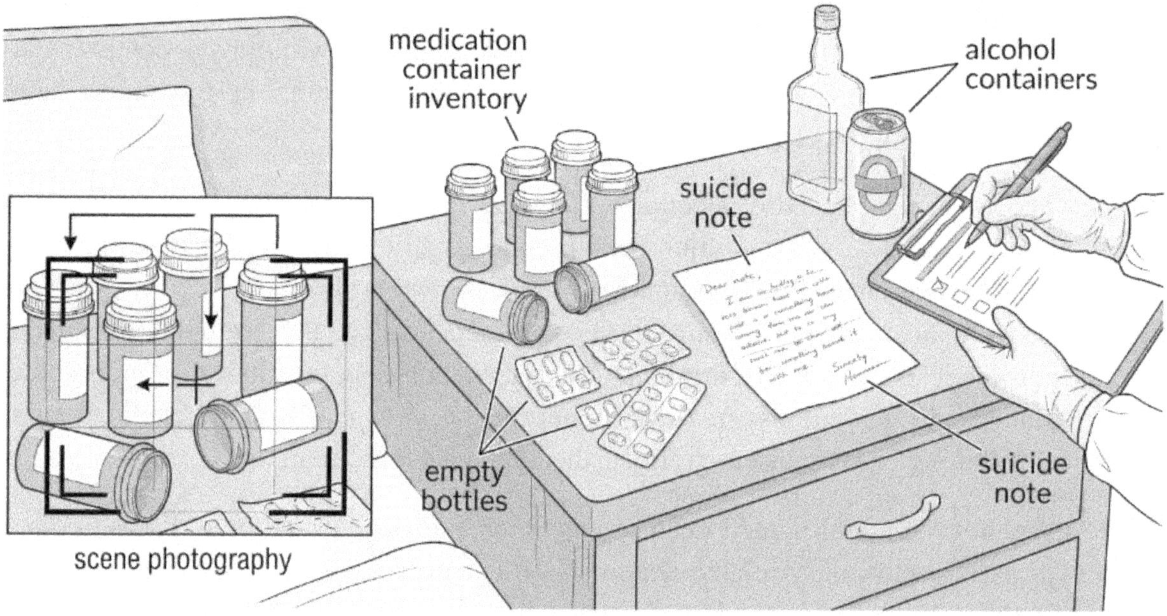


### Benzodiazepines

Benzodiazepines alone are rarely fatal in overdose because of the wide therapeutic window and relatively selective anxiolytic-sedative effect. Benzodiazepine deaths typically involve combination with other central nervous system depressants (opioids, alcohol) with combined respiratory depression producing the fatal mechanism. Prescription benzodiazepine deaths in this pattern often reflect polypharmacy in elderly patients (prescription benzodiazepine with prescription opioid and alcohol use), unrecognized combinations, or intentional combination in suicide attempts. The reasoning about a benzodiazepine finding in a fatal case identifies the combined substances and the interactive effects.

### Antidepressants and Antipsychotics

Antidepressants and antipsychotics present a range of specific patterns. Tricyclic antidepressants (amitriptyline, nortriptyline) have narrow therapeutic windows and can be fatal in overdose through cardiovascular arrhythmia; substantial postmortem redistribution complicates the interpretation as developed in Chapter 17. Selective serotonin reuptake inhibitors are relatively safe in overdose alone but can produce serotonin syndrome in combination with other serotonergic agents. Antipsychotics can produce QT prolongation with arrhythmic risk and can produce neuroleptic malignant syndrome. The reasoning about each specific medication incorporates the specific mechanism and interactive potential.

## The Manner Determination in Drug-Related Deaths

The manner determination in drug-related deaths is one of the more contested areas of forensic pathology and requires transparent reasoning about the specific case.

### Suicide

Suicide by drug overdose is certified when the case reasoning supports intent to die. Supporting evidence includes: a suicide note or documented prior communication of intent; a discrete pattern of drug accumulation (multiple prescriptions filled shortly before, unused portions of medications consolidated at the scene); a pattern of solitary consumption in a location and circumstances arranged for the outcome; toxicological findings supporting substantial ingestion of a substance selected for lethality rather than for personal drug use; and, in cases where alternatives are available, choice of the drug method over less lethal alternatives. Suicide by prescription medication in individuals with documented mental health disease is a specific pattern with substantial epidemiological data. The manner determination as suicide requires the integration of evidence rather than reliance on any single element.

### Accident

Accident is the manner classification for most drug overdose deaths in the current American opioid epidemic. The specific pattern is unintentional overdose in an individual with substance use disorder using drugs for their intended personal effect rather than with intent to die. Evidence supporting accident includes: use in a social or shared context inconsistent with suicidal intent; drug quantity and pattern consistent with use rather than with lethal intent; scene evidence supporting active use rather than accumulated ingestion; absence of documented suicidal intent; and the aggregate epidemiological pattern of accidental overdose in individuals with use disorder. Accident is documented despite the presence of substance use disorder because the decedent's intent was to use the substance rather than to die.

### Homicide

Homicide by drug overdose is documented but uncommon. The pattern requires evidence of administration by another person with intent to harm. In American practice, the most common scenario is administration of drugs to a decedent by an assailant to facilitate assault (developed in Chapter 15 in the sexual assault context) or to produce incapacitation for other purposes. Deaths from illicit drug supply (in which the supplier is aware of contamination or lethal potency and delivers the drug knowing the risk) have been increasingly prosecuted in some jurisdictions as drug-induced homicide; the medical examiner's manner determination in these cases is typically accident based on the decedent's intent, with the criminal characterization proceeding independently in the legal system.

## Undetermined

Undetermined is the manner classification when the evidence does not support either suicide or accident to reasonable medical certainty. The classification is appropriate when the case has ambiguous features (a suicidal decedent might have had an accident, or an accidental decedent might have had unrecognized suicidal intent) or when specific evidence is unavailable (an unwitnessed death with limited scene evidence). Undetermined manner is a professional determination reflecting the honest limits of the reasoning; it is not a failure but an appropriate use of the classification when specificity is not warranted.

## Alcohol-Related Motor Vehicle Fatalities

Alcohol-impaired driving fatalities represent a substantial fraction of alcohol-related mortality in most jurisdictions. The forensic pathology contribution in the driver fatality integrates the injury findings from the collision (mechanism developed in Chapter 5), the toxicological confirmation of alcohol impairment (with blood ethanol interpretation as developed in Chapter 17 including consideration of vitreous ethanol as a check on blood interpretation), and the case reasoning about the specific cause and manner. The manner determination is typically accident with the impairment identified as contributing; specific jurisdictions may prosecute the impaired driver criminally with the medical determination supporting the prosecution. The pathologist reasoning about a passenger or third-party fatality in a collision caused by an impaired driver documents the injury pattern with the same rigor as any traffic fatality; the manner determination reflects the third-party casualty pattern integrated with the case reasoning. Deaths of pedestrians struck by impaired drivers, cyclists, and other vulnerable road users are documented similarly.

## Wernicke Encephalopathy and Chronic Neurologic Sequelae

Wernicke encephalopathy — acute thiamine deficiency in chronic alcohol users with associated neurological syndrome — is a documented cause of death in individuals with chronic alcohol dependence. The classic triad of encephalopathy, ocular signs, and ataxia may not all be present, and the diagnosis is often clinical during life or established at autopsy. Autopsy findings include characteristic hemorrhages and necrosis in the mammillary bodies, hypothalamus, and other periventricular regions of the brain, with corresponding histologic changes on microscopy. Korsakoff syndrome represents the chronic sequelae in survivors of Wernicke encephalopathy. Deaths from Wernicke encephalopathy specifically occur when the acute syndrome produces cardiovascular collapse or when the encephalopathy is severe enough to produce fatal outcome despite thiamine treatment. The reasoning integrates the antecedent history of chronic alcohol use, the clinical presentation if available, and the autopsy findings.

## Postmortem CT in Drug-Related Death Cases

Postmortem CT integration in drug-related death cases has developed as a routine element in some offices and as a case-specific tool in others. Postmortem CT can identify: pulmonary edema of the character seen in opioid overdose; cerebral edema in overdose cases; gastrointestinal contents suggesting recent oral ingestion; ingested drug packets in body packing cases (developed in Chapter 17); and specific findings supporting alternative or contributing mechanisms. The technique complements but does not replace autopsy findings; postmortem CT identifies patterns that guide the autopsy examination and supports documentation, while the autopsy provides the tissue-level findings and specimen collection that PMCT cannot substitute for. Integration of PMCT with the drug death workflow reflects office resources and case volume; the specific use varies substantially among practices.

### The Chronic Pain Patient Death

The death of a decedent under active management for chronic pain is a specific case pattern with substantial nuance. The decedent may have died from prescribed medications used as directed with an adverse outcome, from prescribed medications combined with additional substances (alcohol, other prescriptions, illicit drugs), from intentional overdose using accumulated medication, or from unrelated cause with the chronic pain therapy incidental to the death. The reasoning integrates: the specific medications prescribed and their stability over recent history; the pattern of prescription refills and any evidence of accumulated medication; toxicological confirmation of prescribed medication levels and any other substances; scene evidence supporting or contradicting specific mechanisms; and the antecedent history including any documented concerns about the decedent's pain management. Deaths in the chronic pain patient population have been a focus of substantial public attention and policy response over the past decade, and the individual case reasoning contributes to the aggregate understanding.

### Alcoholic Ketoacidosis

Alcoholic ketoacidosis is a metabolic complication in chronic alcohol users, typically arising during a period of heavy drinking followed by cessation with associated poor nutritional intake. The syndrome involves ketosis without the hyperglycemia of diabetic ketoacidosis, and the pathogenesis reflects the depleted glycogen stores and impaired gluconeogenesis of the chronic alcohol user combined with the metabolic effects of ethanol clearance. Deaths from alcoholic ketoacidosis show ketosis on vitreous chemistry, may show hypoglycemia, and may show cardiovascular collapse from the metabolic derangement. The autopsy findings include the substrate of chronic alcohol-related disease and the acute metabolic pattern; the reasoning integrates the vitreous chemistry with the clinical history and with the exclusion of alternative causes. The syndrome is documented and identifiable when the differential includes it and appropriate ancillary studies are performed.

### Communication With Families in Drug-Related Deaths

The communication with families in drug-related deaths carries particular sensitivity. Families often carry substantial grief, some accompanied by feelings of guilt or self-blame for their inability to prevent the death. The stigma associated with substance use disorder may compound the family's difficulty. The office's communication addresses the specific findings with sensitivity to family circumstances, provides information about available grief and support resources, and, where applicable, provides information about naloxone access and about treatment resources for surviving family members with their own substance use concerns. Some offices have integrated peer support specialists (individuals with lived experience of substance use disorder and recovery) into the family communication process for drug-related deaths. The forensic pathology contribution to the aggregate response includes not only the case data but also the direct family engagement in many cases.

### Cannabis-Related Deaths

The forensic reasoning about cannabis-related deaths has evolved substantially with the changing legal landscape of cannabis in the United States. Acute cannabis intoxication is rarely directly fatal; the substance has a wide therapeutic window relative to other drugs of abuse and lethal cannabis intoxication in the isolated sense is essentially not documented in the peer-reviewed literature. However, cannabis-associated deaths do occur through several mechanisms: cannabinoid hyperemesis syndrome (a specific pattern in chronic heavy users producing severe vomiting with dehydration and electrolyte derangement, occasionally fatal); accidents while impaired (motor vehicle collisions, falls, drownings, similar patterns to alcohol impairment); adverse cardiovascular events in individuals with specific vulnerabilities (arrhythmia in decedents with cardiac substrate); and specific patterns from synthetic cannabinoid exposure (the K2/spice class with substantially different pharmacology from natural cannabis). The changing legal landscape has produced new access patterns and new product forms (edible cannabis products with delayed onset and greater risk of overdose, high-potency concentrates); the forensic pathology response evolves with these patterns.

### Kratom and Novel Recreational Substances

Kratom (Mitragyna speciosa) is a plant-derived substance with opioid receptor activity that has gained substantial recreational and quasi-therapeutic use in the United States. Its legal status varies by state, and it is sold widely as an unregulated product. Kratom-related deaths have been documented in polysubstance combinations more commonly than as a sole cause; the alkaloids mitragynine and 7-hydroxymitragynine are the primary active compounds and are identifiable on specific toxicological analysis when the exposure is suspected. Isolated kratom mortality is documented but less common than polysubstance kratom deaths. The reasoning about kratom-related cases parallels the reasoning about other opioid substances with specific attention to the analytical identification and to the interpretive framework. Other emerging recreational substances — including novel psychedelic-related products, dissociative agents, and various legal and quasi-legal preparations — present similar analytical and interpretive challenges.

### The Harm Reduction Context

The forensic pathology response to the drug crisis intersects with the broader harm reduction framework that has been increasingly adopted in public health approaches. Harm reduction elements include: naloxone distribution to individuals with opioid use disorder and to their households (with documented effectiveness in reducing overdose mortality); supervised consumption sites (established in some jurisdictions with documented reductions in overdose deaths in served populations); drug checking services allowing individuals to test drug supplies for fentanyl or other contaminants; and treatment access improvements including buprenorphine and methadone maintenance therapy. The individual case documentation supports the aggregate evidence base for these interventions. Forensic pathology deaths in which naloxone was available, was used, and did or did not affect the outcome contribute to the understanding of naloxone effectiveness in real-world use. Deaths in which specific harm reduction interventions might have made a difference support the aggregate evidence for expanded implementation of the interventions.

### Deaths Associated With Substance Use Treatment

Deaths that occur during or shortly after substance use disorder treatment present specific reasoning challenges. The immediate post-treatment window (the days to weeks following completion of residential or intensive outpatient treatment) is a documented high-risk period for opioid overdose due to loss of tolerance during abstinence; the case reasoning integrates this well-documented pattern. Deaths during medication-assisted treatment (with buprenorphine or methadone) may reflect the treatment medication (rare), concurrent use of other substances (more common), or unrelated cause. The reasoning about specific manner in these cases integrates the treatment history with the specific findings. The pattern of accidental overdose during the immediate post-treatment period has policy implications supporting extended naloxone availability, longer transitions between treatment intensities, and specific interventions to bridge the vulnerable window.

### The Aggregate Reporting Requirements

State and federal reporting requirements for drug-related deaths have specific data elements that guide the individual case documentation. The Centers for Disease Control and Prevention State Unintentional Drug Overdose Reporting System (SUDORS) captures detailed data on drug overdose deaths including the specific substances, the circumstances, the demographic pattern, and the case context. State reporting systems capture similar data with jurisdiction-specific elements. The forensic pathology contribution to this aggregate reporting is the specific documentation of substances involved, the specific mechanism, and the case circumstances. The individual case certification supports both the immediate legal and administrative purposes and the aggregate public health surveillance. Attention to complete and specific documentation supports both goals; abbreviated or vague documentation compromises the aggregate value.

### SCENE-TO-CERTIFICATION DECISION SYSTEM — Drug and Alcohol Death Determination Arcs

---

**The Framework and Aggregate Function:** Drug-related deaths in current American practice reach unprecedented levels. Each individual case certification contributes to aggregate epidemiological surveillance supporting the public health response. Specific documentation of substances involved and case context is essential; vague certifications limit both the individual case and the aggregate data.

**Opioid Overdose Recognition:** Opioid overdose is identified by the constellation of respiratory depression mechanism findings (foam cone, pulmonary edema, congestion), route-specific external findings, scene evidence, and toxicological confirmation. Fentanyl and fentanyl analogs dominate the current landscape, with unexpected contamination of other drug supplies a common pattern.

**Stimulant Death Mechanisms:** Stimulant overdose produces cardiovascular death from catecholamine excess (arrhythmia, hypertensive events, myocardial injury) or from hyperthermic crisis. Cocaine, methamphetamine, MDMA, and synthetic cathinones each have specific patterns integrated with the general framework.

**Alcohol-Related Death Categories:** Alcohol-related deaths span acute intoxication, chronic disease complications, withdrawal syndromes, and injury-related deaths with impairment. Each category has specific reasoning integrating toxicology, autopsy findings, and history. Chronic alcohol use disease is documented histologically and integrated with the case reasoning.

**The Manner Determination:** Manner classification (suicide, accident, homicide, undetermined) reflects transparent case reasoning. Accident dominates opioid overdose deaths in the current epidemic. Suicide requires evidence of intent. Homicide requires evidence of administration by another with intent. Undetermined is appropriate when specificity is not warranted by the evidence.

## Summary and Key Concepts

Drug-related deaths in the United States have reached unprecedented levels driven by the opioid epidemic and by the emergence of fentanyl and fentanyl analogs. Individual case certification contributes to aggregate public health surveillance supporting the response.

Opioid overdose is identified by the constellation of respiratory depression mechanism findings, route-specific external findings, scene evidence, and toxicological confirmation. Fentanyl and its analogs dominate the current epidemic and are frequently found as contamination of other drug supplies.

Stimulant overdose (cocaine, methamphetamine, MDMA, synthetic cathinones) produces cardiovascular death from catecholamine excess or hyperthermic crisis. Combined stimulant-opioid patterns are common in current cases.

Alcohol-related deaths span acute intoxication with fatal outcome, chronic disease complications (cirrhosis, cardiomyopathy, others), alcohol withdrawal syndromes, and injury-related deaths with alcohol impairment. Each category has specific reasoning.

Prescription medication deaths involve prescription opioids, benzodiazepines, antidepressants, antipsychotics, and other categories with specific mechanisms. Multi-drug patterns are common and require reasoning about interactive effects. Postmortem redistribution is a specific consideration for many prescription medications.

The manner determination in drug-related deaths (suicide, accident, homicide, undetermined) requires transparent reasoning. Accident dominates opioid overdose deaths in the current epidemic; suicide requires evidence of intent; homicide requires evidence of administration by another; undetermined reflects honest limits of certainty.

# CHAPTER 19: POSTMORTEM IMAGING (VIRTOPSY) AND RADIOLOGIC CORRELATION

**Learning Objectives**

1. Articulate the principles of postmortem imaging and its evolving role in forensic pathology practice.
2. Interpret postmortem computed tomography findings with attention to normal postmortem changes and to specific forensic applications.
3. Recognize the role of postmortem MRI in specific case types and articulate its complementary role to CT.
4. Perform and interpret postmortem radiography and skeletal survey with recognition of forensic-relevant findings.
5. Integrate postmortem imaging findings with autopsy findings for the aggregate case reasoning, and articulate the appropriate role of virtopsy in specific case categories.

## Principles of Postmortem Imaging

Postmortem imaging — the application of medical imaging techniques to decedents — has evolved from an occasional supplement to autopsy into a routine element of forensic pathology practice in many jurisdictions. The technique borrows from clinical radiology but applies to the specific context of the deceased body, with recognition of the postmortem changes that alter imaging findings and with specific attention to the forensic questions the imaging supports. The forensic pathologist working in an office with postmortem imaging capability integrates the imaging findings with the autopsy examination for the aggregate case reasoning.

The rationale for postmortem imaging includes multiple objectives. Imaging identifies findings not readily accessible to standard autopsy examination — gas patterns in the vasculature and cavities, foreign bodies including radiographic identification of retained projectiles, spatial relationships of internal injuries, and skeletal injuries not apparent on external examination. Imaging supports the reconstruction of injury mechanisms through documentation of the spatial pattern of injury. Imaging permits some non-invasive investigation in cases where family or religious concerns limit invasive autopsy. Imaging provides documentation preserving the internal state of the body in a form that supports later review and integrates with the aggregate documentation.

The limits of postmortem imaging are important. Imaging does not replace the tissue-level examination that autopsy provides; findings identified on imaging typically require autopsy correlation for full characterization. The interpretation of imaging findings requires attention to normal postmortem changes (gas from decomposition, blood pooling, temperature-related changes) that produce findings not present in life. The interpretation is best performed by radiologists with specific training in postmortem imaging; forensic pathologists interpreting the images benefit from formal or informal training in the specific interpretive framework. The integration of imaging into the office workflow requires investment in equipment, technologist time, and integration of the imaging into the case management.

### The Historical Development

Postmortem imaging has a substantial historical precedent — postmortem radiography has been used for over a century, particularly for identification of retained projectiles and for skeletal survey in child abuse cases — but the current era of comprehensive postmortem imaging developed with the adoption of computed tomography and magnetic resonance imaging in forensic contexts, beginning in the late 1990s and accelerating through the 2000s and 2010s. The Swiss Virtopsy project, based at the University of Bern, was influential in developing the concept of comprehensive non-invasive postmortem investigation using imaging as the primary examination. Current American practice varies substantially: some offices have integrated postmortem CT as a routine element of every case; others use imaging selectively based on case-specific indications; still others do not have imaging capability and refer complex cases to facilities with capability. The trend is toward increased use as equipment becomes more accessible and as the professional understanding of the interpretive framework develops.

## Postmortem CT: Applications and Interpretation

Postmortem CT is the most widely used postmortem imaging modality and has substantial forensic utility across multiple case types. The technique produces cross-sectional images of the entire body with high spatial resolution and good bone-air contrast, supporting identification of a wide range of findings relevant to forensic reasoning.

### Applications by Case Type

Postmortem CT has documented utility across multiple forensic case types. In trauma cases including gunshot wounds and blunt injury, CT identifies retained projectiles, fracture patterns, injury paths through the body, and internal injuries not readily identified from external examination. In pediatric death investigation, CT provides a comprehensive skeletal survey without the technical challenges of positioning small bodies for standard radiography. In sudden death cases, CT identifies findings supporting or excluding structural mechanisms (aortic dissection, hemopericardium, pulmonary embolism at some limits of sensitivity, other cardiovascular emergencies). In cases with decomposed or severely damaged bodies, CT identifies specific findings that guide the autopsy examination. In cases with religious or family objections to autopsy, CT provides a substantial fraction of the information autopsy would generate.

### Normal Postmortem Findings on CT

Interpretation of postmortem CT requires familiarity with the normal postmortem findings that are not seen on antemortem CT. Postmortem gas is a specific consideration: gas in the vasculature from decomposition (particularly in advanced postmortem interval), gas in the cardiac chambers, gas in the liver and other organs, and gas in the soft tissues can all appear as findings that mimic pathologic gas but that reflect decomposition rather than antemortem process. The distinction between decomposition gas and antemortem gas (from injury introducing atmospheric air, or from specific pathology) requires attention to the pattern, distribution, and consistency with other findings. Postmortem blood pooling in dependent vessels and cavities is another normal finding requiring recognition. Postmortem cooling produces some changes in tissue density; postmortem changes in specific organs alter their imaging appearance.

Figure 19.2: Postmortem Radiographic Skeletal Survey in Pediatric Case

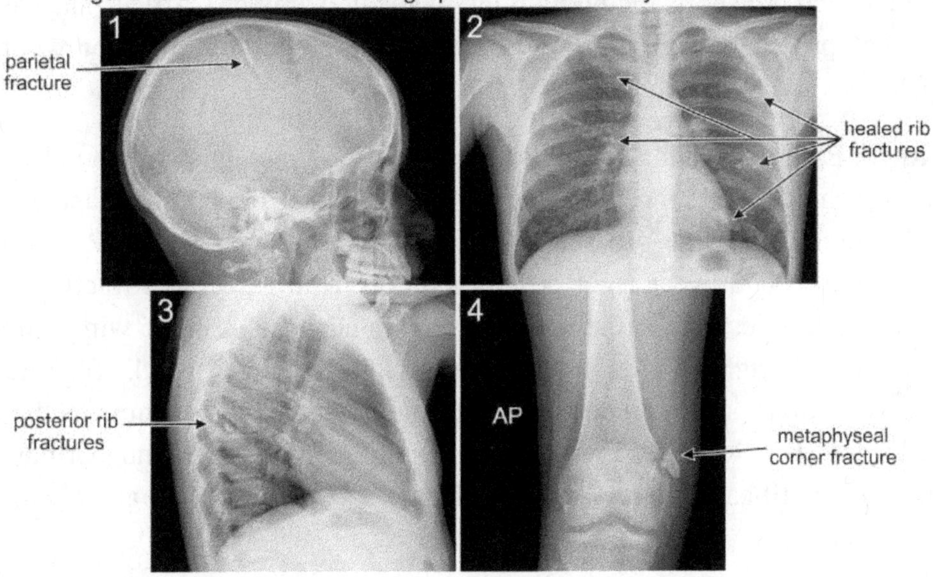


## Trauma Imaging: Specific Findings

Postmortem CT in trauma cases provides specific findings that substantially support the reasoning. Skull fractures are identified with high sensitivity, including subtle fractures that may be missed on external examination; three-dimensional reconstruction of the skull supports characterization of the fracture pattern for mechanism reasoning. Facial fractures are identified with the anatomical relationships preserved. Cervical spine fractures are documented with the specific level and morphology, supporting reasoning about mechanism (hyperflexion versus hyperextension versus direct impact). Long bone fractures are documented systematically. Retained projectiles are localized precisely in three-dimensional space, supporting reasoning about the wound track and the projectile behavior. Internal injuries — pulmonary contusion, hepatic and splenic lacerations, retroperitoneal hemorrhage, aortic transection — are identified with specific spatial characterization.

## Gunshot Wound Imaging

Postmortem CT has particular utility in gunshot wound cases. The retained projectile is localized in three-dimensional space, supporting reasoning about the wound track. Bone fragmentation along the wound track is documented with detail beyond what autopsy dissection can preserve; the fracture pattern supports reasoning about the specific projectile characteristics and the spatial relationships. Multiple projectiles are identified and localized. In cases with fragmentation of the projectile, individual fragments are localized and can be correlated with the wound path. Cases where autopsy dissection may lose spatial information (particularly complex intracranial wound tracks with dissection required for brain removal) benefit substantially from CT documentation before autopsy proceeds.

**SCENE-TO-CERTIFICATION DECISION SYSTEM — Postmortem CT Integration Arc**

**Presenting Death Scenario:** A 32-year-old man is found deceased with multiple gunshot wounds after a domestic dispute reported by neighbors. Emergency response confirms death at scene. Law enforcement documents the scene and transports the body to the medical examiner's office. The case is anticipated to proceed to criminal prosecution. The office's standard protocol for gunshot wound cases includes postmortem CT before autopsy dissection.

**Autopsy Signature:** External examination documents three distinct gunshot wounds: an entrance wound over the left anterior chest, an entrance wound over the right anterior abdomen, and an entrance wound at the left temporal region of the head. No exit wounds are identified externally. Postmortem CT identifies three retained projectiles: one in the right posterior thorax with associated fracture of the T6 vertebral body and posterior rib injuries; one in the retroperitoneum near the left iliac wing with associated pelvic hemorrhage; one in the right posterior cerebrum with associated skull fracture and intracranial hemorrhage. The three-dimensional reconstruction of the wound tracks documents the specific trajectory of each projectile. Internal examination confirms the imaging findings and permits recovery of each projectile for firearm identification. The wound tracks are documented photographically with the imaging as a reference.

**Cause Determination:** Multiple gunshot wounds to the chest, abdomen, and head.

**Manner Determination:** Homicide. The pattern of multiple gunshot wounds with wound tracks documented on both imaging and autopsy is consistent with the reported mechanism and supports the manner determination.

**Trap Logic:** The value of postmortem CT in gunshot wound cases is documented preservation of the spatial relationships of the wound tracks before dissection alters the tissue relationships. Without CT documentation, the dissection may not preserve the exact spatial relationships in the report; with CT documentation, the spatial pattern is preserved for later review by opposing experts, appellate reviewers, or aggregate analysis. The trap in not using imaging for these cases is the loss of documentation potential; the trap in relying only on imaging is missing findings that require tissue-level examination. The systematic integration uses both examinations.

**Certification Anchor:** Postmortem CT in gunshot wound cases documents wound tracks, retained projectiles, and associated injuries in three-dimensional detail supporting the reconstruction reasoning. The imaging supplements rather than replaces autopsy examination; the systematic integration produces the most complete case documentation.

## Postmortem MRI and Its Role

Postmortem magnetic resonance imaging has more limited application than CT in current forensic practice but has specific utility in defined case types. The technique produces high-resolution soft tissue imaging with contrast between different tissue types substantially better than CT provides.

### Applications

Postmortem MRI has particular value in pediatric death investigation where soft tissue contrast supports identification of injuries and pathology that may be less apparent on CT. Neuropathology assessment benefits from MRI's superior brain imaging contrast: subtle cerebral injury, ischemic changes, and specific structural findings are better characterized on MRI. Cardiac imaging on MRI can identify structural cardiac disease including cardiomyopathy morphology; the finding may be sufficient in some cases without invasive dissection. In cases where family or religious objection limits autopsy, MRI provides supplementary information beyond CT alone; some jurisdictions have developed protocols using combined CT and MRI as a virtopsy approach with limited or no invasive dissection.

### Limitations of Postmortem MRI

The limits of postmortem MRI include: substantially longer acquisition times than CT (limiting throughput for offices with high case volumes); technical challenges with imaging the postmortem body (positioning, temperature effects on tissue relaxation properties, artifact management); interpretive complexity requiring specialized expertise; and equipment cost and access constraints. The technique remains substantially less widely deployed than CT in current forensic practice but has developed specific applications where the additional information justifies the cost.

## Postmortem Radiography and Skeletal Survey

Standard radiography (plain film or digital radiography) has substantial ongoing role in forensic pathology despite the increasing use of CT. The technique is relatively inexpensive, widely available, and effective for specific applications.

### The Pediatric Skeletal Survey

The pediatric skeletal survey (developed in Chapter 12 in the SUID context and in Chapter 13 in the child abuse context) is one of the classic applications of postmortem radiography. Multiple views of the skull, spine, chest (with oblique views for posterior rib fracture identification), pelvis, and long bones identify occult and subtle fractures characteristic of infant abuse. The survey is performed by dedicated radiologic technologists with specific pediatric positioning technique; pediatric radiologist interpretation is standard for the findings. The pattern of injuries identified on the survey — metaphyseal corner fractures, posterior rib fractures, complex skull fractures, injuries at multiple stages of healing — supports the reasoning about inflicted mechanism when the pattern is present.

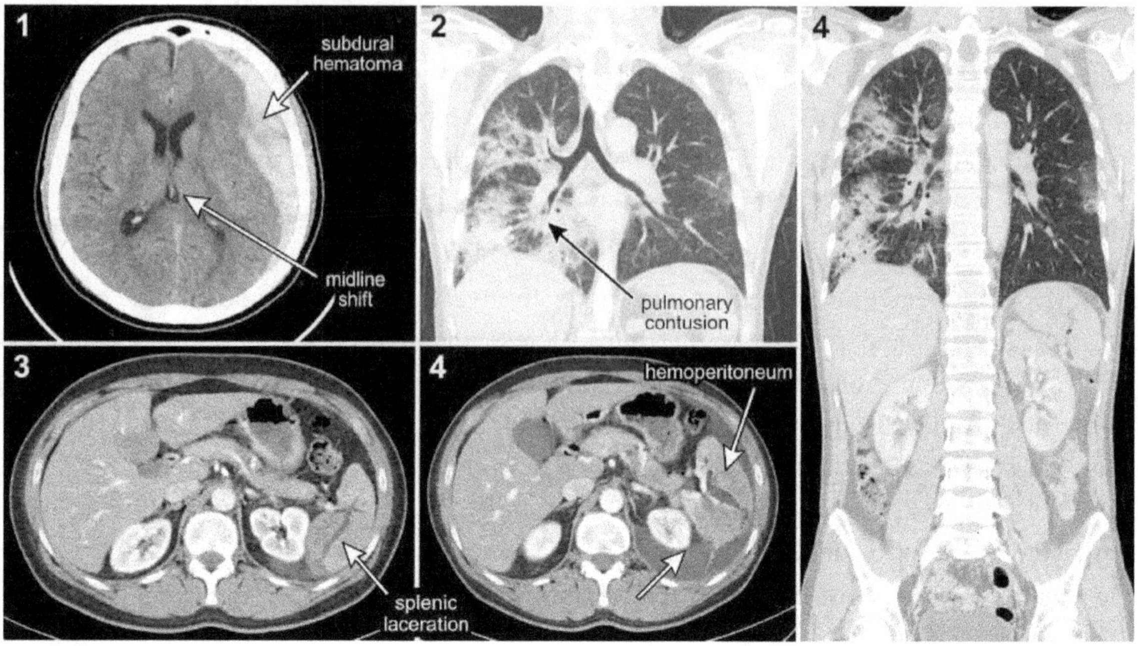


## Radiography for Retained Projectiles

Radiography is the traditional technique for identification and localization of retained projectiles. Plain film radiography identifies radiopaque projectiles with high sensitivity, characterizes their size and shape, and, with orthogonal views, localizes them in three dimensions. The technique remains useful even in offices with CT capability because it is quick and inexpensive; some offices use radiography as an initial screen with CT reserved for cases requiring more detail. The specific technique is well-established and produces images that are directly comparable across the historical record of forensic practice.

## Other Applications

Additional applications of radiography include: identification of surgical implants (with specific patterns that may support identification of the decedent); identification of osseous pathology (fractures old and new, arthritic changes, other skeletal disease); documentation of ingested foreign material (in body packing cases, though CT is more useful for this application); and general documentation of the internal state of the body for cases where CT is not available. The technique remains a foundational element of forensic radiographic practice.

## Integration With Autopsy Findings

The integration of imaging findings with autopsy findings is the pathologist's responsibility and reflects the overall case reasoning. The imaging is performed before or after autopsy depending on office practice; when performed before, imaging findings can guide the autopsy examination toward specific findings and can preserve documentation of features that dissection would disturb. When performed after, imaging may address specific questions arising from the autopsy examination.

### Documentation Standards

Documentation of imaging findings in the autopsy report describes the specific findings identified, their forensic significance, and the integration with autopsy findings. The imaging is preserved for later review; the images are typically retained in the office archive and copies are provided to reviewing parties on request. Photographic documentation may be created from specific imaging views for inclusion in the report and for use in testimony. The pathologist reasoning about imaging findings for the report typically consults with the radiologist who interpreted the images to ensure accurate representation of the findings and reasonable interpretation.

### Communication With the Radiologist

Effective use of postmortem imaging depends on communication between the pathologist and the radiologist. The pathologist provides the clinical context that guides the radiologic interpretation; the radiologist provides the imaging findings and their interpretation. In some offices, dedicated forensic radiologists are integrated into the case workflow; in others, general radiologists interpret postmortem images with case-specific consultation. The relationship benefits from ongoing communication about the specific interpretive framework for postmortem imaging, which differs from standard clinical radiology in important respects.

## Virtopsy: Non-Invasive Postmortem Investigation

The concept of virtopsy — virtual autopsy using imaging as the primary examination — has developed as a specific approach for cases where invasive autopsy is limited by family objection, religious concerns, or other considerations. The approach uses comprehensive imaging (CT, MRI, and often specialized techniques) to gather the information that autopsy would traditionally provide, with invasive procedures limited to specific specimen collection (blood, tissue biopsy under CT guidance) rather than complete evisceration.

### The Rationale and Scope

The rationale for virtopsy includes: family or religious objection to invasive autopsy (particularly in specific religious traditions with prohibitions against body invasion); preservation of the body for viewing and disposition; efficiency in high-volume settings; and, in some jurisdictions, deployment of forensic capability in resource-limited settings where invasive autopsy infrastructure is not available. The scope of virtopsy varies with the case: some cases can be adequately investigated with imaging alone; others require targeted invasive procedures for specific specimen collection; still others require full autopsy despite objections when the case involves criminal investigation. The forensic pathologist reasoning about a specific case identifies what the imaging can provide and what the specific case requires.

### Case Types Where Virtopsy Is Adequate

Virtopsy is generally adequate for specific case types: natural death cases where the imaging identifies structural cause (cardiovascular disease, cerebrovascular event, other structural natural death) and no specific concerns require tissue examination; injury cases where the imaging documents mechanism adequately (blunt trauma with obvious injury pattern, specific injury cases); and specific investigative contexts where the medical question is limited. The pathologist reasoning about a virtopsy adequate case documents the imaging findings, notes the specific case circumstances supporting the limited approach, and integrates with any collected biological specimens for toxicology or other analysis.

### SCENE-TO-CERTIFICATION DECISION SYSTEM — Virtopsy-Versus-Autopsy Decision Arc

**Presenting Death Scenario:** An 82-year-old woman with a documented history of severe congestive heart failure, chronic kidney disease, and mild dementia is found deceased in bed at her assisted living facility by staff. Documentation shows the decedent was in advanced end-stage cardiovascular disease with hospice discussions initiated but hospice enrollment not yet completed. The family has requested that the body not undergo invasive autopsy due to religious concerns. The medical examiner's office accepts jurisdiction on the unwitnessed death and reviews the specific circumstances.

**Autopsy Signature:** The pathologist reviews the case and determines that virtopsy approach is appropriate given the specific circumstances: elderly decedent with well-documented advanced cardiovascular disease; expected end-of-life trajectory; specific family religious objection to invasive procedures; and absence of any concerning features suggesting alternative cause. Postmortem CT is performed and documents: severe cardiomegaly with marked left ventricular hypertrophy consistent with hypertensive heart disease; enlarged left atrium consistent with chronic congestive heart failure; pulmonary edema; hepatomegaly consistent with chronic congestive changes; no acute pathology identified; no evidence of injury; no findings suggesting alternative cause. Peripheral blood is collected under image guidance for toxicological analysis. Toxicology shows expected levels of prescribed medications and no other substances.

**Cause Determination:** Congestive heart failure due to hypertensive and ischemic cardiovascular disease. The cause statement reflects the imaging findings integrated with the antecedent history documenting the specific medical trajectory.

**Manner Determination:** Natural.

**Trap Logic:** The virtopsy approach is appropriate for cases where the specific case circumstances support the limited investigation. The trap is applying virtopsy in cases where the specific findings would have been better identified by invasive examination — particularly cases with any suggestion of trauma, poisoning, or other non-natural mechanism. Systematic reasoning about the specific case before choosing the approach prevents inappropriate use of virtopsy in cases requiring full autopsy. In this case, the well-documented medical trajectory, the imaging findings supporting the natural mechanism, the family religious concerns, and the absence of any concerning features support the virtopsy approach as adequate for the case determination. Documentation of the reasoning in the report supports the transparency of the approach.

**Certification Anchor:** Virtopsy is an appropriate approach for specific case types where imaging can adequately support the case reasoning and where family, religious, or other considerations support limited invasive examination. The pathologist reasons about the specific case circumstances before choosing the approach; systematic evaluation supports the appropriate use of virtopsy without compromising cases that require full autopsy.

Figure 19.3: Postmortem CT Findings of Trauma: Retained Projectile and Wound Track

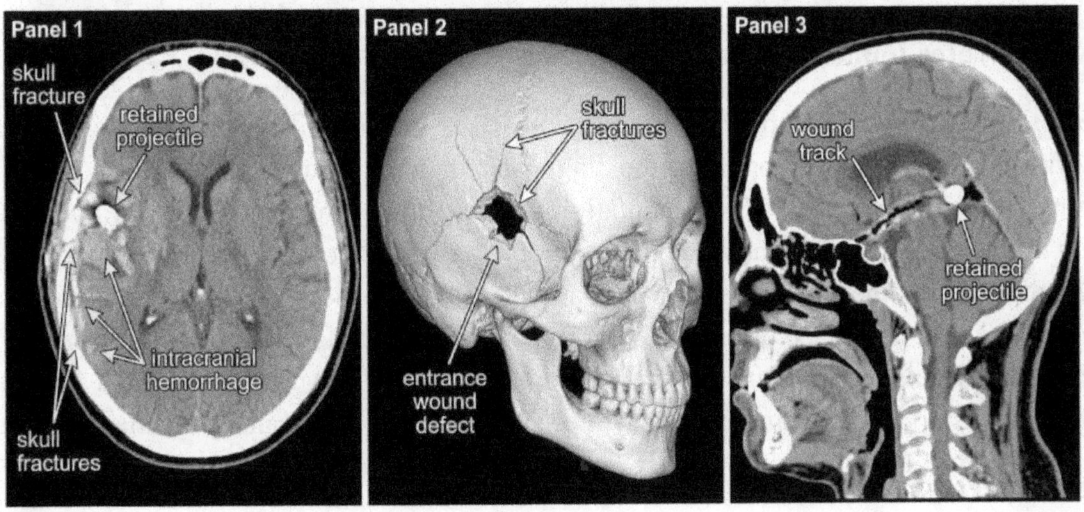


## Postmortem CT Angiography

Postmortem CT angiography is an advanced technique in which contrast material is introduced into the vascular system after death to visualize the vessels with the same detail achievable in living patients. The technique has particular utility for visualization of cardiovascular pathology (coronary arteries, aortic dissection, cerebral vasculature) that would otherwise require invasive dissection to characterize. Various protocols have been developed using different contrast delivery methods (pressurized injection through peripheral vessels or through central catheterization) and different contrast agents. The technique is not routinely available in most American forensic pathology offices due to equipment and technique requirements but is used in specialized centers including in Europe where forensic postmortem imaging has been developed to a more comprehensive level. The information generated approaches or in some cases exceeds what conventional autopsy provides for vascular pathology, and the technique represents the current frontier of postmortem imaging capability.

### Artifact Recognition on Postmortem CT

Recognition of postmortem imaging artifacts is central to accurate interpretation. Common artifacts on postmortem CT include: dependency artifacts from blood pooling and gas distribution that alter the expected appearance of organs; motion artifacts (uncommon in postmortem imaging but possible with unstable body positioning); artifacts from metal (dental fillings, surgical implants, retained projectiles) producing streak artifacts that can obscure adjacent anatomy; and artifacts from body bag material or other extraneous material in the imaging field. Beam hardening from dense structures produces characteristic streak patterns. Postmortem tissue changes (early autolysis in some organs, tissue temperature effects on density measurement) produce apparent findings that require distinction from true pathology. The interpreting radiologist maintains familiarity with the specific artifact patterns of postmortem imaging and integrates recognition into the interpretive framework.

### Drowning and Water Immersion Cases

Postmortem CT in drowning and water immersion cases has specific applications. Airway fluid is identified with high sensitivity, supporting the diagnosis when the character and volume of fluid matches the drowning medium. Sinus fluid documentation is straightforward on CT and provides evidence of antemortem drowning (sphenoid sinus fluid particularly characteristic). Pulmonary edema of the character seen in drowning is documented. In cases where autopsy findings may be difficult to interpret (advanced postmortem changes in immersed decedents, decomposition), CT can identify findings that autopsy might miss. The technique also documents any injuries the decedent may have sustained before or during immersion, supporting the reasoning about whether alternative or contributing mechanisms are present.

### Advanced 3D Reconstruction and Visualization

Modern postmortem CT can be reconstructed in three dimensions with substantial detail, supporting specific forensic applications. Skull reconstruction shows fracture patterns in a form that supports mechanism reasoning — a skull with multiple radiating fractures from a specific impact point demonstrates the mechanism more clearly than autopsy dissection typically preserves. Skeleton reconstruction supports identification cases where skeletal features are used. Vascular reconstruction (particularly with postmortem CT angiography) documents vessel pathology with three-dimensional detail. The reconstructions can be presented in court testimony as visual demonstrations of the case findings, supporting the jury's understanding of the reasoning. Some offices maintain the reconstructions as part of the case file with the imaging archive for later review.

### Quality Standards and Training

Quality standards for postmortem imaging have developed over recent years with professional society position statements and consensus documents providing guidance. The Radiological Society of North America, the International Society of Forensic Radiology and Imaging, and other professional bodies have contributed to the framework. Training in postmortem imaging is available through fellowship programs (particularly in Europe), through short courses at professional meetings, and through mentored practice within offices that have integrated the modality. Certification specifically in postmortem imaging is not yet established as a distinct credential in American practice, though many practitioners have developed substantial expertise through practice and continuing education.

### Cost, Benefit, and Office Integration

The decision to integrate postmortem imaging into an office's workflow involves substantial cost-benefit analysis. Equipment costs (dedicated postmortem CT scanner, or shared clinical equipment with appropriate time allocation) are substantial. Technologist time and radiologist interpretation costs add to the ongoing expense. The benefits include improved case documentation, support for specific case types, capability for virtopsy in family-objection cases, and educational and research applications. Some offices have integrated CT as a routine element of every case; others use imaging selectively; still others have limited or no imaging capability with referral to other facilities when needed. The specific approach reflects office resources, case volume, and the specific case types the office handles. The trend across American practice is toward increased integration, but the pace of adoption has been uneven.

### International Variations in Practice

The integration of postmortem imaging into forensic pathology practice varies substantially across international jurisdictions. Switzerland and Germany have been leaders in comprehensive postmortem imaging including the Virtopsy Project at the University of Bern; several Scandinavian countries and the Netherlands have similarly integrated advanced imaging. Japan has developed postmortem CT capacity as a substantial element of forensic practice. The United Kingdom, Australia, and Canada have integrated postmortem imaging in variable patterns across jurisdictions. The United States shows the most heterogeneous practice with substantial variation among individual offices. The international literature contributes substantially to the developing understanding of postmortem imaging capability and to the evidence base for specific applications; American practice benefits from engagement with the international literature and from participation in international collaborative research.

### Future Directions in Postmortem Imaging

The future directions for postmortem imaging include continued technical development (advanced CT and MRI capabilities, integration with novel imaging modalities including optical coherence tomography and ultrasound), expansion of applications (particularly in virtopsy contexts where reduced-invasive investigation becomes appropriate for wider case types), integration with digital pathology (with imaging and histology combined in aggregated case documentation), and development of specific artificial intelligence applications for image interpretation. The technology continues to evolve and the professional practice adapts to the developing capability. The forensic pathologist entering practice today can reasonably anticipate continued evolution of the imaging component of the specialty over the career period ahead.

## Imaging of Decomposed Bodies

Postmortem imaging has substantial specific value in cases of decomposed bodies where autopsy examination is limited by tissue changes. CT can identify skeletal features, retained projectiles, surgical implants (supporting identification), and specific pathologic findings that persist through decomposition. Skull and facial imaging supports identification through dental correlation and through morphologic features. Skeletal survey identifies fractures old and new, supporting reasoning about mechanism when soft tissue findings are compromised. In severely decomposed cases where autopsy dissection may yield limited information, imaging may provide the primary means of investigation and may support the identification and cause of death determination when tissue examination cannot. The specific value in decomposition contexts has driven substantial adoption of imaging in offices handling significant numbers of decomposed cases.

## Dental Identification and Postmortem Imaging

Dental identification is a specific forensic application supported by postmortem imaging. Dental radiographs — either standard panoramic and periapical views or CT-based dental imaging — document the dental features of the decedent for comparison with antemortem dental records. The distinctive nature of dental features (fillings, extractions, restorations, natural variations in tooth morphology) supports identification with high specificity when antemortem dental records are available. In cases where visual identification is not possible (severely damaged remains, severely decomposed cases, cases involving fire or other destructive processes), dental identification is often the definitive means of confirming decedent identity. The forensic odontologist provides the interpretation and comparison; the pathologist facilitates the imaging and the integration of the identification into the case documentation. The topic is developed further in Chapter 20 in the specific identification context.

## Postmortem Ultrasound

Postmortem ultrasound has limited but specific application in forensic practice. The technique has been explored for guided specimen collection (particularly for targeted tissue biopsy in virtopsy contexts) and for specific findings that ultrasound characterizes well (fluid collections, some cardiovascular findings). The limits of postmortem ultrasound include the loss of standard antemortem physiological signals that support ultrasound interpretation (blood flow patterns, respiratory motion, cardiac motion), the changes in tissue acoustic properties postmortem, and the general dominance of CT and MRI for most postmortem imaging applications. Ultrasound remains a niche application in current practice but has specific value where the modality fits the case reasoning.

## Postmortem MRI Applications Extended

The specific applications of postmortem MRI beyond those already described include: detailed cardiac morphology assessment supporting characterization of cardiomyopathies without invasive dissection; detailed brain examination supporting identification of subtle neurologic pathology that autopsy dissection may not preserve equivalently; detailed soft tissue injury characterization in specific cases; and imaging of specific body regions where MRI provides advantages over CT. The role of MRI in pediatric death investigation deserves particular note — the superior soft tissue contrast of MRI is well suited to the small structures of infant and pediatric bodies, and MRI has been used systematically in some centers as a complement or partial substitute for standard autopsy in pediatric cases. The specific case types where MRI adds substantial value support its integration in offices with the capability.

### The Legal and Administrative Framework

The legal and administrative framework for postmortem imaging varies by jurisdiction. Some jurisdictions have specific statutes or regulations addressing imaging in medicolegal death investigation; others incorporate imaging under general autopsy authority. The pathologist working with imaging maintains familiarity with the specific jurisdictional framework. Chain of custody for imaging data (digital images stored in imaging archives) follows similar principles to chain of custody for physical evidence, with attention to secure storage, controlled access, and documented transfers. Discoverability of imaging in legal proceedings is generally similar to autopsy documentation — the images become part of the case record and may be reviewed by opposing experts and by the court. The pathologist prepares the imaging documentation with attention to the potential legal use, integrates the interpretation with the autopsy report, and archives the images for the office's retention period.

### Research and Publication

The scientific literature on postmortem imaging has developed substantially over recent decades with contributions from both radiology and forensic pathology researchers. Peer-reviewed journals including Forensic Science International, the American Journal of Forensic Medicine and Pathology, the Journal of Forensic Sciences, and specialized radiology journals publish substantial content on postmortem imaging applications and interpretation. Academic institutions and forensic pathology offices contribute case series, comparison studies (imaging findings against autopsy findings), and studies of specific technical developments. The forensic pathologist maintaining familiarity with current literature engages with this developing evidence base and integrates the findings with practice. Contribution to the literature through case reports and case series from individual practice supports the aggregate development of the specialty knowledge.

### SCENE-TO-CERTIFICATION DECISION SYSTEM — Postmortem Imaging Determination Arcs

**The Framework:** Postmortem imaging is a routine element of forensic pathology practice in many jurisdictions and has specific applications where the imaging provides information beyond what autopsy alone can capture. The imaging complements rather than replaces the tissue-level examination that autopsy provides.

**Postmortem CT Applications:** PMCT has documented utility in trauma cases (fracture patterns, retained projectiles, wound tracks), pediatric death investigation (skeletal survey), sudden death cases (structural causes), and virtopsy contexts. Recognition of normal postmortem findings on CT (decomposition gas, blood pooling) supports accurate interpretation.

**Postmortem MRI Role:** PMMRI has specific application in pediatric death investigation with superior soft tissue contrast, in neuropathology assessment, and in virtopsy contexts where MRI adds to the CT information. Longer acquisition times and interpretive complexity limit routine deployment.

**Postmortem Radiography:** Standard radiography continues to have foundational role including the pediatric skeletal survey for suspected abuse, identification and localization of retained projectiles, and general documentation. Some applications transition to CT in offices with capability; others continue with radiography for efficiency.

**Virtopsy Approach:** Virtopsy as non-invasive postmortem investigation is appropriate for specific case types where imaging can adequately support the case reasoning and where family, religious, or other considerations support limited invasive examination. Systematic reasoning about the specific case prevents inappropriate use in cases requiring full autopsy.

## Summary and Key Concepts

Postmortem imaging has evolved into a routine element of forensic pathology practice in many jurisdictions. The technique complements rather than replaces autopsy examination and requires attention to normal postmortem findings that alter imaging interpretation.

Postmortem CT has broad forensic utility including trauma imaging (fracture patterns, retained projectiles, wound tracks), pediatric skeletal survey, sudden death cases (structural causes), and virtopsy contexts. Recognition of decomposition gas and other normal postmortem findings supports accurate interpretation.

Postmortem MRI has specific applications in pediatric death investigation, neuropathology assessment, and virtopsy contexts. Longer acquisition times and interpretive complexity limit routine deployment but the technique adds value in specific cases.

Standard radiography continues to have foundational role including the pediatric skeletal survey, projectile identification, and general documentation. Some applications transition to CT while others continue with radiography for efficiency and cost.

Integration of imaging with autopsy findings is the pathologist's responsibility and reflects the overall case reasoning. Communication between the pathologist and the radiologist supports effective use of the imaging.

Virtopsy as non-invasive postmortem investigation is appropriate for specific case types where imaging can adequately support the case reasoning and where family, religious, or other considerations support the limited approach.

# CHAPTER 20: HUMAN IDENTIFICATION, SKELETAL REMAINS, AND ODONTOLOGY

**Learning Objectives**

1. Articulate the framework for human identification in forensic pathology and distinguish presumptive from scientific identification methods.
2. Recognize the primary scientific identification methods (fingerprint, DNA, forensic odontology) and articulate their appropriate applications.
3. Perform systematic examination of skeletal remains with recognition of the specific findings that support biological profile estimation.
4. Interpret the biological profile (sex, age, ancestry, stature) developed from skeletal analysis and articulate the interpretive limits of each element.
5. Recognize the framework for mass disaster identification and articulate the coordination required across forensic and non-forensic agencies.

## Principles of Human Identification

Human identification — the confirmation that a specific decedent is a specific named individual — is one of the foundational tasks of forensic pathology practice. The identification supports the family's need to know that their loved one has been located, supports the legal system's need to attribute a death to a specific person for estate, insurance, and criminal purposes, and supports the aggregate epidemiology by connecting the case to the individual who was the subject of it. The forensic pathology framework distinguishes presumptive identification (based on circumstantial evidence including visual recognition and personal effects) from scientific identification (based on comparison of biometric features with antemortem records), with different case types requiring different approaches.

The framework recognizes that most decedents are identified presumptively in the routine caseload. A decedent found in his own residence with recognizable features and personal identification is typically identified through the aggregate of these circumstantial elements without requiring scientific comparison. The scientific identification methods are reserved for cases where presumptive identification is inadequate: decedents in mass casualty events, decedents with severe injury or decomposition that limits visual identification, decedents found without personal effects, decedents whose identity is disputed, and specific cases where the legal proceedings require heightened certainty about identity.

The forensic pathology contribution to identification is one element of a multidisciplinary process. Fingerprint identification is conducted by fingerprint examiners with specific training and credentialing. DNA identification is conducted by forensic biology laboratories. Forensic odontology is conducted by forensic odontologists with specific credentials. Forensic anthropology is conducted by forensic anthropologists. The pathologist coordinates with each of these specialists as case circumstances require and integrates their findings with the aggregate case documentation.

### The Reasonable Certainty Standard

Identification in the forensic pathology framework requires reasonable certainty rather than absolute certainty. The standard is not that no alternative identity could conceivably be correct but that the evidence supports the specific identification to a level consistent with the practical purposes served. Presumptive identification through the aggregate of circumstantial elements is often adequate for routine cases; scientific identification through fingerprint, DNA, or odontology comparison provides substantially higher certainty and is used when the case circumstances warrant. The pathologist reasoning about the appropriate identification approach considers the specific case features and applies the level of certainty required.

**KEY POINT:** Human identification requires reasonable certainty appropriate to the case purpose. Presumptive identification through circumstantial evidence supports routine cases; scientific identification through fingerprint, DNA, or odontology comparison is used when case circumstances require heightened certainty. The pathologist reasons about the appropriate method for the specific case.

## Presumptive Identification Methods

Presumptive identification methods draw on the aggregate of circumstantial evidence supporting the identification of a specific decedent as a specific named individual. Multiple elements combine to support the identification, and no single element is typically definitive on its own.

### Visual Recognition

Visual recognition by family members remains a substantial element of routine identification. A family member viewing the decedent and recognizing the specific features (facial features, distinctive markings, unique physical characteristics) supports the identification. The reliability of visual recognition depends on the condition of the body (severe injury, decomposition, or thermal damage reduces reliability), on the family member's familiarity with the decedent, and on the specific circumstances of the viewing. Modern practice often uses photographic identification (with photographs taken at the medical examiner's office and reviewed by the family) rather than in-person viewing when circumstances permit, both for efficiency and to reduce the family's exposure to the scene of the death.

### Personal Effects and Documentation

Personal effects found on or with the decedent frequently support identification. Government-issued identification (driver's license, passport, state identification card) provides strong evidence when present and undisputed. Wallet contents, phone contents, and other personal materials support the identification pattern. Vehicle identification when the decedent was in a vehicle at the time of death. Clothing and jewelry with distinctive features. The aggregate of personal effects supports the identification when consistent, but each element has interpretive limits (personal effects can be transferred between individuals, borrowed, or otherwise not conclusive on their own).

### Circumstantial Identification

The circumstances of the discovery support identification through the aggregate of contextual evidence. A decedent found in his own residence with his own personal effects, with no witnesses to contradict identification, is presumptively identified through the aggregate. A decedent found in a location known to be frequented by a specific missing person supports the identification pattern. The circumstantial evidence combines with other elements to support the aggregate identification when scientific confirmation is not required.

## Scientific Identification: Fingerprint, DNA, and Odontology

The three primary scientific identification methods — fingerprint, DNA, and forensic odontology — provide biometric comparison between the decedent and antemortem records with substantially higher certainty than presumptive methods. Each method has specific applications and interpretive frameworks.

### Fingerprint Identification

Fingerprint identification relies on the individual specificity of the friction ridge patterns on the fingertips (and, less commonly, palms and soles). The technique requires that the decedent has usable fingerprints (which may be limited in cases of severe fire damage, extensive decomposition, or extensive skin damage from other mechanisms) and that antemortem fingerprint records are available for comparison. Fingerprint records are commonly available for individuals with prior arrests (through the Automated Fingerprint Identification System), for military service members, for individuals in specific occupations requiring background checks, and, in some cases, through direct comparison with items known to have been handled by the missing person. The fingerprint examiner performs the comparison using standardized techniques (typically requiring identification of multiple matching characteristics with no unexplainable differences); the result is reported as identification, exclusion, or inconclusive. The technique has been the foundation of scientific identification for over a century and continues to be widely used.

### DNA Identification

DNA identification has transformed forensic identification over the past three decades. The technique compares the DNA profile from the decedent (obtained from blood, tissue, or bone specimens) with reference samples (from known personal effects of the missing person, from relatives providing kinship comparison, or from prior DNA records). Multiple DNA analysis techniques are used: short tandem repeat (STR) analysis for standard comparison, mitochondrial DNA analysis for degraded specimens or maternal-line comparison, and Y-chromosome analysis for paternal-line comparison. The technique has substantial power for identification when reference material is available, and the exclusion power is essentially absolute for unrelated individuals. The technique has specific applications for mass disaster identification, for identification of severely damaged remains, and for identification of missing persons where relative reference samples can be obtained.

DNA identification requires reference material for comparison. Direct reference samples include personal effects (toothbrush, hairbrush, other items known to have been used by the missing person) and prior clinical or forensic DNA samples if the individual had these on record. Kinship reference samples are obtained from close relatives (typically parents, siblings, and children); statistical analysis of kinship DNA supports the identification with quantifiable probability calculations. The chain of custody for reference samples is essential to preserve the identification evidence.

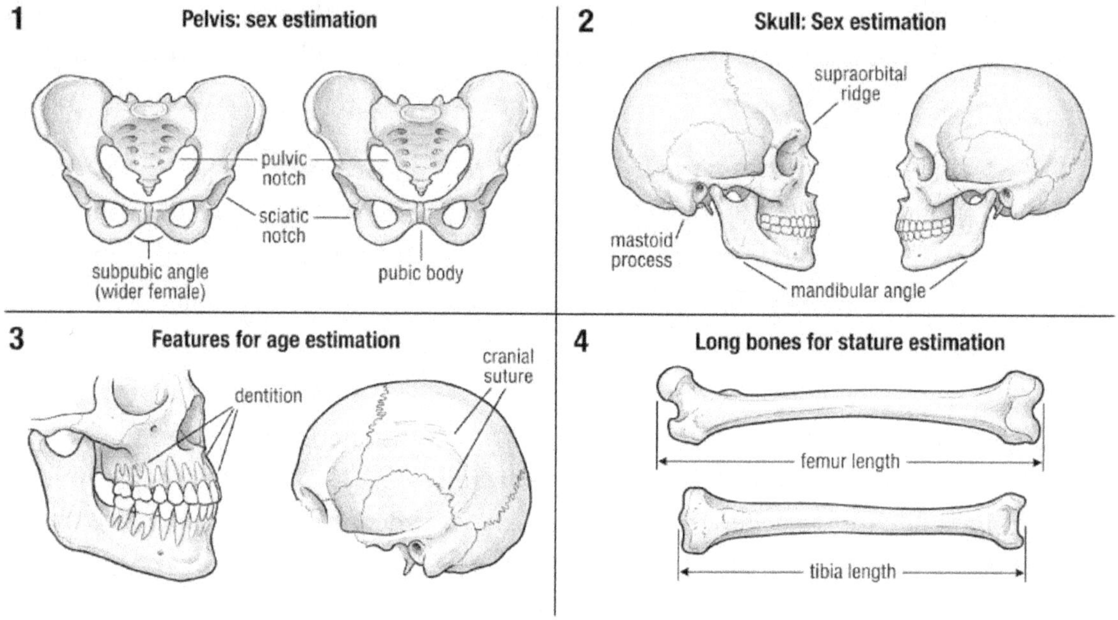


## Forensic Odontology

Forensic odontology uses dental features for identification through comparison of antemortem and postmortem dental records. The technique exploits the substantial individuality of dental features including tooth positions, restorations, extractions, orthodontic work, distinctive morphologic variations, and specific dental pathology. Dental features have specific advantages for identification: teeth are among the most durable elements of the body, surviving conditions that destroy soft tissue including severe fire exposure and extended postmortem interval; dental records are commonly maintained for individuals who have received dental care; and the comparison is relatively straightforward for a trained forensic odontologist. The technique has been particularly valuable in mass disaster identification, in identification of severely damaged remains, and in cases where other biometric identification is not available.

The forensic odontologist obtains postmortem dental documentation (visual examination, dental radiographs, and photographs of the dentition) and compares with antemortem records obtained from the presumed decedent's dentist. The comparison identifies matching features and any unexplainable differences. Identification requires sufficient matching features to support the aggregate identification. The specific standards for identification vary across professional guidance and reflect the reasonable-certainty standard applied to the specific case.

**SCENE-TO-CERTIFICATION DECISION SYSTEM — Presumptive-Versus-Scientific-Identification Arc**

**Presenting Death Scenario:** A decedent is recovered from a residential fire that consumed the home. The decedent is severely burned throughout the body with essentially no soft tissue remaining in identifiable form. The residence was known to be occupied by a single individual who has been reported missing since the fire. Family members have provided prior dental records from the missing individual's dentist and are prepared to provide DNA reference samples if needed. The medical examiner's office accepts jurisdiction and coordinates the identification approach.

**Autopsy Signature:** External examination documents extensive fourth-degree burn injury throughout the body with severely damaged soft tissue precluding visual identification. Postmortem radiography documents the dentition (which remains largely intact despite the surrounding tissue damage), and reveals distinctive dental features including multiple restorations, a distinctive orthodontic pattern, and a specific missing tooth pattern. Postmortem dental examination by the forensic odontologist and comparison with antemortem records provided by the family's dentist confirms multiple matching features supporting identification. DNA is also collected from femoral bone for confirmatory analysis. Toxicology on peripheral blood confirms carboxyhemoglobin above 60 percent, consistent with antemortem fire exposure. Layered anterior neck dissection performed as standard for fire cases shows no evidence of alternative mechanism.

**Cause Determination:** Smoke inhalation and thermal injury from residential fire, with confirmatory identification of the decedent as the reported missing occupant based on forensic odontology comparison.

**Manner Determination:** Accident (in the absence of evidence of alternative mechanism); fire investigation may modify the manner determination if intentional fire setting or other homicide mechanism is identified.

**Trap Logic:** The trap in fire death identification is either to accept presumptive identification based on circumstances alone (the fire consumed the residence occupied by a specific individual) without scientific confirmation, or to rely on any single scientific method without adequate integration. The systematic approach in this case combines: the circumstantial context supporting the presumptive identification; the postmortem odontology comparison with antemortem records providing scientific confirmation; and the DNA confirmation providing additional support. The multiple lines of evidence support the identification to reasonable medical certainty. The certification is prepared with documentation of the identification reasoning transparent in the report.

**Certification Anchor:** Identification in severely damaged remains cases requires scientific comparison beyond circumstantial evidence. Forensic odontology, DNA analysis, and fingerprint identification each have specific applications; the appropriate method or combination depends on the specific case circumstances and on the available reference material. The identification is documented in the report with the specific method used and the reasoning supporting the identification.

## Skeletal Remains: Recovery, Analysis, and Reconstruction

Skeletal remains — decedents whose soft tissue has been substantially or completely lost through decomposition, animal activity, or other processes — present specific investigation challenges. The forensic pathology response typically involves close coordination with forensic anthropology and, where the case circumstances warrant, with law enforcement search and recovery teams.

### Recovery From the Scene

Recovery of skeletal remains from a scene is a specialized process typically involving forensic anthropologists, archaeologists, or specifically trained recovery personnel. The scene is documented systematically before disturbance: the position and distribution of skeletal elements, the associated materials (clothing, personal effects, environmental materials), the ground conditions, and the specific location details. Recovery proceeds systematically to preserve the spatial relationships that support the reconstruction. Small bones (hand and foot bones, cranial fragments) are commonly recovered separately using screening and archeological techniques. The distribution of skeletal elements at the scene provides evidence about scavenger activity, environmental disturbance, and any specific processes affecting the remains. The recovery documentation supports subsequent analysis.

### Inventory and Documentation

Skeletal remains are inventoried systematically upon receipt at the office. Each bone is cataloged, cleaned as needed to permit examination without loss of specimen material, and documented photographically. The completeness of the inventory supports the assessment of what analysis can be performed — some analyses require specific bones or complete elements. Missing bones are documented as missing rather than assumed. The inventory serves as the foundation for the subsequent biological profile analysis and, where applicable, for identification comparison.

### Time Since Death From Skeletal Remains

Estimation of time since death from skeletal remains is generally imprecise but the general framework identifies broad categories. Fresh skeletal remains with some tissue remnants and specific soft tissue changes suggest weeks to months. Skeletal remains without soft tissue but with residual grease and organic material in the bone suggest months to a few years. Bare bone without residual organic material suggests years. Bone showing weathering, cortical erosion, and specific environmental effects suggests a longer period. The estimation is broad because the rate of tissue loss depends heavily on environmental conditions (temperature, humidity, soil chemistry, animal activity), and specific quantitative dating is generally not available. The pathologist reports the time frame in broad ranges consistent with the interpretive limits.

## Forensic Anthropology and the Biological Profile

The biological profile developed from skeletal analysis includes the four primary elements of sex, age, ancestry, and stature. Each element has specific analytical approaches, specific reliability limits, and specific implications for identification investigation.

### Sex Estimation

Sex estimation from skeletal features exploits the sexual dimorphism of the human skeleton. The pelvis is the single most reliable region for sex estimation with multiple diagnostic features: the subpubic angle (wider in females); the sciatic notch (wider in females); the pubic body morphology; and the ventral arc of the pubic symphysis. The skull provides multiple features (supraorbital ridge, mastoid process, mandible angle, temporal ridge, occipital protuberance) that are more prominent and rugged in males. Long bones provide some features (larger overall size and joint dimensions in males). Adult sex estimation from a complete skeleton with pelvis and skull is generally reliable; estimation from a partial skeleton or from juvenile remains has substantially greater interpretive limits.

### Age Estimation

Age estimation from skeletal features uses developmental features in juveniles and degenerative features in adults. In juvenile remains, dental development (eruption and calcification of teeth) is the primary indicator, with specific stages corresponding to specific age ranges with high precision. Epiphyseal fusion of long bones and other skeletal elements provides secondary indicators in adolescents and young adults. In adult remains, degenerative changes provide estimates with less precision: the pubic symphysis and the auricular surface of the ilium show characteristic morphologic changes across the adult age range that support broad estimation; cranial suture closure provides supplementary information with substantial interpretive limits; dental attrition provides some information but is affected by dietary and behavioral factors. Adult age estimation is reported in broad ranges (typically 10 to 20 year windows for older adults) consistent with the interpretive limits.

### Ancestry Estimation

Ancestry estimation from skeletal features is one of the more contested elements of the biological profile. The classical framework identifies specific cranial and dental features that vary across broadly defined ancestral groups; contemporary understanding recognizes that human variation is continuous rather than categorical and that individual features vary within and across groups. Current forensic anthropology practice increasingly uses quantitative morphometric analysis with statistical comparison to reference populations rather than categorical classification. The estimate is reported as a probability distribution across ancestral groups rather than as a categorical identification. The interpretation is calibrated to the specific case context and to the specific comparative reference populations available.

## Stature Estimation

Stature estimation from skeletal features uses long bone length measurements applied to regression equations derived from reference populations. The femur and tibia (weight-bearing lower extremity bones) provide the most reliable estimates. The equations differ by sex and by ancestral group, reflecting different body proportions across populations. Stature estimates are reported with confidence intervals consistent with the interpretive limits of the regression approach; single-point estimates are typically not reliable without the associated statistical range. The estimate supports identification when antemortem stature is known for the missing person; the specific comparison uses appropriate statistical framework.

Figure 20.2: Dental Comparison for Forensic Odontology Identification

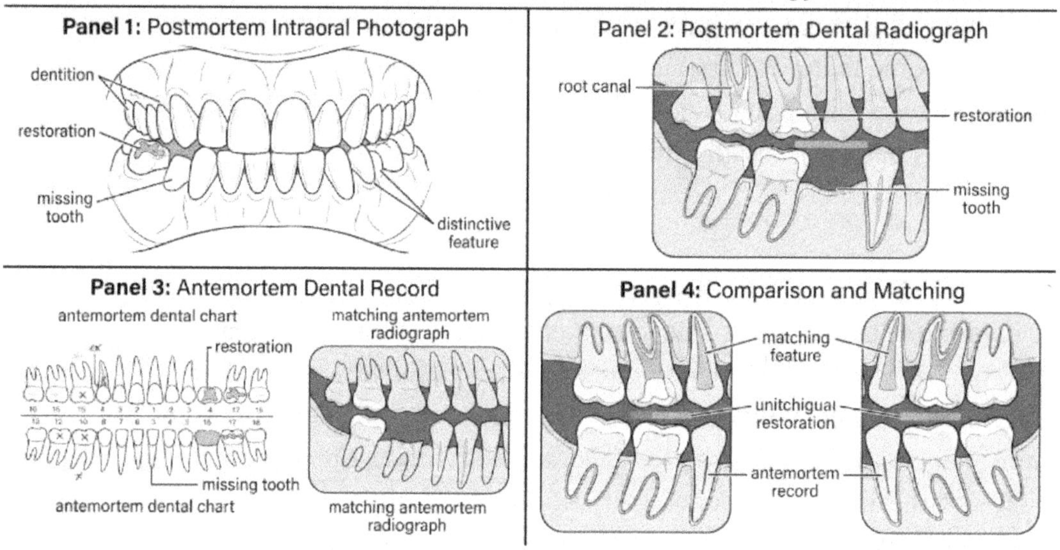


## SCENE-TO-CERTIFICATION DECISION SYSTEM — Skeletal Remains Reconstruction Arc

**Presenting Death Scenario:** Skeletal remains are recovered from a wooded area by hikers. Law enforcement responds to the scene and secures the area. A forensic anthropology team performs the recovery with archaeological technique documenting the spatial distribution of the elements. Approximately 85 percent of the skeleton is recovered including complete cranium, pelvis, and long bones; some hand and foot bones are missing and consistent with scavenger activity. Environmental context suggests exposure of approximately 6 to 18 months. No identification is available at scene.

**Autopsy Signature:** Skeletal inventory documents 85 percent completeness. Biological profile analysis by forensic anthropology consultation identifies: female sex (based on pelvis and skull morphology, high confidence); age approximately 25 to 40 years (based on pubic symphysis and auricular surface morphology, moderate confidence); stature approximately 160 to 168 centimeters (based on femur length regression, moderate confidence); ancestral estimation consistent with mixed European and African ancestry probability. The skull shows evidence of blunt injury with three depressed fractures in the parietal and temporal regions consistent with impacts by a heavy blunt object. DNA is extracted from femoral bone and submitted for analysis. Comparison with missing person databases in the region is initiated.

Dental radiographs are compared with dental records of missing persons whose profiles match the biological profile.

**Cause Determination:** Blunt force injury to the head, with pattern of multiple depressed fractures consistent with assault by a heavy blunt object. The determination reflects the physical evidence identified on skeletal examination.

**Manner Determination:** Homicide. The multiple blunt injury pattern to the head is inconsistent with accidental mechanism and supports homicidal mechanism. Identification proceedings continue with the biological profile and physical evidence supporting integration with the missing person database.

**Trap Logic:** The trap in skeletal remains cases is either to overinterpret the specific findings (biological profile elements are reported with appropriate confidence intervals; specific categorical claims exceed the interpretive framework) or to underinterpret and miss identifiable findings (specific injury patterns, distinctive features, and biological profile characteristics that support the aggregate reasoning). The systematic approach uses forensic anthropology consultation for the biological profile with appropriate confidence intervals, documents the injury pattern with reference to the interpretive framework for skeletal injury, and coordinates with law enforcement for identification investigation and with DNA analysis for confirmation when reference material becomes available.

**Certification Anchor:** Skeletal remains cases require systematic examination of biological profile with appropriate confidence intervals and reasoning about identifiable injury patterns. Certification of cause of death is possible when the skeletal findings support a specific mechanism; manner determination requires integration with the injury pattern and case context. Identification proceeds through comparison with available records and reference materials as case investigation develops.

## Mass Disaster Identification

Mass disaster identification — the identification of multiple decedents from mass casualty events including aviation disasters, natural disasters, terrorism, industrial accidents, and mass shootings — requires coordinated multidisciplinary response. The topic is developed in detail in Chapter 21; this section provides the general framework as it applies to individual case identification within the mass casualty context.

### The Aggregate Framework

The aggregate framework for mass disaster identification integrates individual case work with coordinated overall response. Each decedent receives individual documentation — external examination, photographic documentation, biological profile assessment for cases requiring identification, and specimen collection for scientific comparison. The individual case work supports the aggregate identification response. The Disaster Mortuary Operational Response Teams (DMORT) system in the United States, coordinated through the National Disaster Medical System, provides trained personnel to support local jurisdictions during mass casualty events. International mass casualty events have developed similar coordinated response mechanisms.

### Surgical Implants and Medical Devices as Identification Aids

Surgical implants and medical devices provide substantial identification support when present. Orthopedic implants (hip prostheses, knee prostheses, spine hardware, fracture fixation devices) typically carry manufacturer information, model numbers, and serial numbers that can be traced back to the specific patient through manufacturer databases and hospital records. Cardiac devices (pacemakers, implantable cardioverter defibrillators) carry electronic identification that can be interrogated with device programmers to obtain the patient identifier. Cochlear implants, spinal cord stimulators, and other medical devices carry similar identifying information. The pathologist encountering these devices at autopsy documents them systematically, photographs the identifying markers, and coordinates with the manufacturer or with the treating hospital to complete the identification when relevant. Serial number tracking through these devices has resolved numerous identification cases where other biometric methods were unavailable.

### Facial Reconstruction and Approximation

Facial reconstruction (also termed facial approximation) is a specialized technique used in cases of unidentified skeletal remains where no reference material is available for scientific comparison. The technique reconstructs the probable facial appearance from the skull morphology using either traditional clay-modeling approaches or computer-based digital reconstruction. The reconstructed face is then disseminated through media, missing person databases, and other channels in the hope that someone recognizes the individual and provides identification leads. The technique has limitations: soft tissue features (skin color, hair color and style, weight, facial expression) are inferred rather than determined from the skull, and the reconstruction is a probability rather than a specific individual match. Nonetheless, the technique has produced identification successes when other methods have failed and remains a valuable component of the identification toolkit for otherwise unidentified remains.

### Isotope Analysis and Geographic Origin

Stable isotope analysis of bone, hair, and tooth material can support inference about geographic origin and life history of unidentified decedents. Specific isotopes (oxygen, strontium, sulfur, others) vary geographically due to local water sources, geology, and dietary patterns. The isotope signature of tissues incorporated during life reflects the geographic locations where the individual lived. Tooth enamel formed during childhood retains the isotope signature of the childhood geographic location; hair reflects the most recent months; bone reflects a longer averaging window. Isotope analysis has supported identification investigation in cases where the decedent's geographic origin is unclear, particularly in undocumented migrant deaths, in cases of persons from distant regions who died away from home, and in specific missing person contexts. The analysis is specialized and typically requires collaboration with academic or specialized commercial laboratories.

### Missing Person Databases and Case Integration

The identification investigation of unidentified decedents integrates with missing person databases at multiple levels. The National Missing and Unidentified Persons System (NamUs) in the United States provides a searchable database combining missing person records with unidentified remains records; matching of the biological profile and other case features supports investigation. State and local missing person systems provide additional records. International databases including Interpol's missing person system support cross-border investigation. The forensic pathology contribution to these systems is the documentation of specific case features (biological profile, distinctive markings, dental features, medical device information, DNA profile) that supports database matching. The individual case investigation contributes to the aggregate database function while the aggregate function supports the individual case.

### Undocumented Migrant Deaths

Undocumented migrant deaths present specific identification challenges. Decedents are frequently found in remote environments (border crossing regions, desert or mountainous areas) with no personal identification and often with severe environmental degradation of remains. Family reference material for DNA comparison is often not available in the local jurisdiction because families may be in other countries and reluctant to engage authorities. The identification investigation requires cross-border coordination with source-country authorities, family associations, and non-governmental organizations that specifically support migrant identification. Isotope analysis for geographic origin, dental features characteristic of specific regional dental care patterns, and other specialized approaches support these investigations. The identification of undocumented migrant decedents has become a substantial subspecialty of forensic identification practice in border regions, with specific expertise developed for the pattern.

### Historical and Prosecutorial Identification

Historical identification investigation (of remains from historical events, previously unsolved cases, or long-cold missing person investigations) has developed as a specific practice area over recent decades. Advances in DNA technology have enabled identification of remains from decades earlier when reference material becomes available through familial DNA analysis. Investigation of remains from military conflicts (including the Defense POW/MIA Accounting Agency work on identifying remains from historical conflicts) has developed substantial specialized practice. Prosecutorial identification of remains related to specific criminal investigations (particularly serial killer cases and long-term missing person cases) has been advanced through specific investigation. Each of these contexts applies the general identification framework with adaptations for the specific case type.

### The Chain of Custody for Identification Evidence

The chain of custody for identification evidence follows the same rigorous standards as any forensic evidence chain. Reference material collected from families (DNA reference samples, personal effects for comparison) is documented at collection with signed forms establishing the source, the collection location, and the transfer to the analytical facility. Postmortem specimens are documented similarly. Analytical results and comparison findings are documented in laboratory reports that become part of the case file. The chain preservation supports the subsequent legal use of the identification evidence, whether in probate matters, insurance proceedings, or criminal prosecution. The pathologist coordinates the chain preservation as part of the case management.

### Family Communication About Identification

Communication with families about identification carries substantial emotional weight. Confirmation that an unidentified decedent has been identified as a family member's missing person completes an investigation that families may have been living with for weeks, months, or years. Failure to identify remains after extensive investigation is also a specific communication challenge. The office's communication is calibrated to family circumstances, typically integrated with support services, and provides clear information about the identification method and the specific findings. Some offices have developed specific protocols for these communications, including family engagement specialists who work with families through the identification process. The forensic pathology contribution includes not only the case work but also the compassionate communication that supports the family through the process.

### The Forensic Anthropology Consultation

Formal forensic anthropology consultation is standard practice for cases involving substantial skeletal analysis. Forensic anthropologists are typically doctoral-level specialists with specific training in human osteology, biological anthropology, and forensic applications. They serve as consultants to medical examiner offices, providing the biological profile assessment, injury pattern analysis on skeletal remains, and reconstruction assistance for identification investigation. In offices without full-time forensic anthropology staffing, consultation with academic anthropologists or with specialized forensic anthropology services is arranged for specific cases. The consultation report becomes part of the case file and is integrated into the aggregate case documentation. Coordination between the pathologist and the anthropologist ensures that the analytical work supports the case reasoning and that findings are integrated appropriately.

### Taphonomy and Postmortem Environmental Effects

Taphonomy is the study of postmortem changes to remains including decomposition, scavenger activity, environmental disturbance, and other processes that alter the state of remains from the antemortem body. Understanding taphonomic processes supports the reasoning about skeletal remains cases: which processes account for the observed state of the remains, what environmental conditions produced the observed pattern, what time frame is consistent with the observed changes, and whether specific alterations (fractures during scavenger activity, dispersal by carnivores, environmental transport) can be distinguished from antemortem or perimortem events. Taphonomic analysis is a specialized area within forensic anthropology; the pathologist encountering complex skeletal cases coordinates with anthropology consultants for the specific interpretation. The Body Farm at the University of Tennessee and similar research facilities have developed substantial evidence base for taphonomic interpretation of skeletal cases.

### Subadult Identification and Analysis

Subadult remains (juvenile decedents, infants) present specific analytical challenges. Sex estimation from subadult skeletal remains is substantially more limited than adult estimation because the pelvic and cranial features supporting adult sex assessment are not fully developed in juveniles; DNA analysis provides the primary means of sex determination in subadult remains. Age estimation in subadults uses dental development (which is highly reliable in this age range) and skeletal development (epiphyseal centers, long bone length, specific ossification patterns) with substantial precision, particularly in the younger age ranges. Ancestry estimation is limited in subadults and is not typically attempted. Identification of subadult decedents may proceed through dental features when comparison records exist, through DNA when reference material is available, and through other methods as the specific case allows. Missing children investigations coordinate with specific child-focused missing person systems and family reference DNA programs.

### Identification Errors and Their Prevention

Misidentification of decedents has occurred with substantial consequences — family members receiving remains of a different person, families being informed of the death of a person who was still living, and legal consequences arising from mistaken identification. Prevention of misidentification requires systematic approach: use of scientific identification methods when circumstances warrant rather than reliance on presumptive identification alone; independent verification when identification is doubtful; clear communication of identification confidence in the case documentation; and organizational safeguards including specimen tracking, case documentation, and quality assurance systems. The reasonable certainty standard is not absolute certainty, but the aggregate approach to reduce misidentification requires systematic attention to the identification process at each step. When an identification is later challenged or found to be incorrect, systematic review supports both the individual case correction and the aggregate improvement of the practice.

### The Public Health Function of Identification

Identification of decedents supports substantial public health functions beyond the immediate case. Death certificate completion with accurate identification supports vital statistics that inform public health policy, epidemiological research, and resource allocation. Family completion of grief supports mental health and social functioning of surviving relatives. Legal proceedings including estate administration and insurance claims depend on identification. In mass casualty events, identification supports both the individual families and the aggregate response to the event. The forensic pathology contribution to identification is not only the technical case work but also the aggregate public health function it supports. Attention to systematic identification practices in individual cases supports both the immediate case purpose and the broader public health function.

**SCENE-TO-CERTIFICATION DECISION SYSTEM — Identification Determination Arcs**

**The Framework:** Human identification distinguishes presumptive from scientific methods. Presumptive identification through visual recognition, personal effects, and circumstantial evidence supports routine cases. Scientific identification through fingerprint, DNA, or odontology comparison provides higher certainty for cases where circumstances warrant.

**Scientific Identification Methods:** The three primary scientific identification methods each have specific applications. Fingerprint identification requires usable fingerprints and antemortem records. DNA identification requires reference material either directly or through kinship comparison. Forensic odontology uses dental features with substantial durability through severe damage and decomposition.

**Skeletal Remains Analysis:** Skeletal remains investigation includes systematic recovery, inventory, and analysis with close coordination with forensic anthropology. Time since death estimation is broad and reflects the environmental context. Injury identification on skeletal remains supports mechanism reasoning within the specific interpretive framework.

**The Biological Profile:** The biological profile developed from skeletal analysis includes sex, age, ancestry, and stature estimation, each with specific analytical approaches and interpretive limits. Sex estimation from the pelvis is generally reliable in complete adult remains; age estimation from degenerative features is reported in broad ranges; ancestry estimation increasingly uses quantitative morphometric approaches; stature estimation uses regression from long bone length.

**Mass Disaster Framework:** Mass disaster identification integrates individual case work with coordinated multidisciplinary response. Individual documentation supports aggregate identification through comparison with missing person profiles and with reference materials. Coordinated response mechanisms including the DMORT system in the United States support jurisdictions during mass casualty events.

## Summary and Key Concepts

Human identification distinguishes presumptive methods (visual recognition, personal effects, circumstantial evidence) from scientific methods (fingerprint, DNA, forensic odontology). The reasonable certainty standard guides the choice of method for the specific case circumstances.

Fingerprint identification, DNA identification, and forensic odontology are the three primary scientific identification methods. Each has specific applications and interpretive limits. The forensic pathology contribution to scientific identification integrates the pathologist's case documentation with the specialist examiners' technical work.

Skeletal remains investigation includes systematic recovery from the scene, careful inventory and documentation, and analysis with forensic anthropology consultation. Time since death estimation is broad and reflects environmental context; specific quantitative dating is generally not available.

The biological profile developed from skeletal analysis includes sex, age, ancestry, and stature. Each element has specific analytical approaches and interpretive limits, and reporting uses appropriate confidence intervals consistent with the analytical framework.

Injury identification on skeletal remains supports mechanism reasoning when specific findings are present. Skeletal injury patterns require interpretation within the specific framework for skeletal analysis, integrated with case context and with any available identification.

Mass disaster identification integrates individual case work with coordinated multidisciplinary response. The topic is developed in Chapter 21.

# CHAPTER 21: MASS FATALITY AND DISASTER VICTIM IDENTIFICATION

**Learning Objectives**

1. Articulate the framework for mass fatality response including the coordination structures that support multi-agency response.
2. Recognize the role of the Disaster Mortuary Operational Response Team (DMORT) system and other coordinated response mechanisms.
3. Understand the function of the Family Assistance Center in mass fatality events.
4. Apply the systematic identification approach in mass casualty contexts with attention to prioritization, throughput, and scientific rigor.
5. Recognize the specific reconstruction considerations for aircraft mass casualty events, natural disasters, terrorism, and other event categories.

## The Mass Fatality Framework

Mass fatality events — incidents involving multiple decedents that exceed the routine capacity of a local jurisdiction — represent one of the most demanding categories of forensic pathology practice. The events include aircraft disasters, natural disasters (hurricanes, floods, earthquakes, wildfires), terrorism, mass shootings, industrial disasters, transportation disasters (train and bus collisions), and pandemic contexts producing surge mortality. Each event category has specific reconstruction requirements, but the general framework for response applies across categories.

The mass fatality framework recognizes that the individual case work of forensic pathology must be scaled substantially to address multi-decedent events. The routine autopsy process — designed for individual case work at a rate consistent with the office's daily capacity — does not scale directly to events involving dozens, hundreds, or in extreme cases thousands of decedents in a single event. The framework provides coordinated response mechanisms, deployment of resources beyond the local jurisdiction, and specific process modifications that support the aggregate response.

The forensic pathology response is one element of the broader emergency response framework. Emergency management coordinates the overall response including scene management, casualty transport, medical response for survivors, family notification, and, in some cases, criminal investigation. The forensic pathology component focuses on the decedents: examination, identification, cause and manner determination for each decedent, and coordination with families for release of remains. The response requires substantial coordination across disciplines and across levels of government.

### Scale and Complexity Factors

Several factors determine the specific response required for a mass fatality event: the number of decedents, which determines the scale of resources required; the condition of the remains, which determines the identification approach; the geographic scope, which determines the coordination challenges; the type of event, which determines specific reconstruction requirements; the criminal or terrorism component if any, which determines evidence handling requirements; and the international dimension if the decedents include citizens of multiple countries. Small mass fatality events (typically fewer than 20 decedents) may be manageable within local resources; larger events require external support through the coordinated response mechanisms developed for this purpose.

**KEY POINT:** Mass fatality response requires coordinated multi-agency response beyond the routine capacity of local jurisdictions. The framework provides deployed personnel, mobile equipment, and process modifications that support aggregate response. The forensic pathology component focuses on decedent examination and identification within the broader emergency response framework.

## Response Coordination and Personnel Deployment

The coordinated response for mass fatality events in the United States is organized through the National Disaster Medical System (NDMS), a federal program administered by the Department of Health and Human Services with support from other federal agencies. Within NDMS, the Disaster Mortuary Operational Response Team (DMORT) system provides the specific mass fatality response capability.

### The DMORT System

DMORT teams are regional teams composed of forensic pathologists, forensic anthropologists, forensic odontologists, fingerprint examiners, DNA analysts, medicolegal death investigators, funeral directors, mental health providers, and administrative and support personnel. Team members are federal employees when activated but are typically volunteers from local forensic and medical practice during non-deployment periods. Multiple teams cover different regions of the country. When a mass fatality event exceeds local capacity, the affected jurisdiction requests DMORT deployment through the emergency management coordination process, and the appropriate team is deployed to support the local response.

The DMORT deployment includes not only personnel but also mobile equipment: portable morgue units, refrigerated storage, portable examination equipment, imaging equipment, and information technology to support the case management. The mobile Disaster Portable Morgue Unit (DPMU) can be transported to the affected region and set up as a functional forensic pathology operation supporting the response. Multiple DPMU capacity has been deployed for major events including hurricane response, the September 11 attacks, and other large-scale incidents.

### International Coordination

International mass fatality events — involving decedents from multiple countries or events occurring outside American jurisdiction — require additional coordination beyond domestic mechanisms. Interpol's Disaster Victim Identification (DVI) capability provides an international coordination framework. Individual countries provide DVI expertise to the international response through their national forensic organizations. Aircraft mass casualty events typically involve international coordination because passengers commonly include citizens of multiple countries. Terrorism events with international dimensions similarly require the international coordination framework.

### State and Local Emergency Management Integration

Within American practice, state and local emergency management structures integrate with the federal response. The state Medical Examiner or Chief Coroner coordinates the state-level mortuary response and interfaces with federal DMORT deployment. Local medical examiner offices work with state coordination for events that exceed local capacity but do not require federal-level response. The specific coordination arrangements vary by state, and forensic pathology offices maintain familiarity with their state's emergency response framework.

### SCENE-TO-CERTIFICATION DECISION SYSTEM — Mass Fatality Response Coordination Arc

---

**Presenting Death Scenario:** A commercial airliner crashes shortly after takeoff, producing a substantial mass casualty event with approximately 180 decedents anticipated. The crash occurred in a rural area of a mid-sized state, exceeding the local medical examiner's office capacity by orders of magnitude. Emergency management activates the state and federal response. The local medical examiner coordinates with the state emergency management, requests DMORT deployment, and works to establish the temporary morgue and processing operation. The National Transportation Safety Board coordinates the aviation investigation; the Federal Bureau of Investigation coordinates the criminal investigation ruling out terrorism as a factor.

**Autopsy Signature:** The temporary morgue operation is established at a suitable local facility (typically a warehouse or aircraft hangar) with the deployed DPMU providing functional forensic capacity. Each decedent receives systematic documentation: initial reception with body bag identification, external examination with photographic documentation, imaging (typically postmortem CT if equipment is available or radiography), specimen collection for DNA analysis, dental documentation, fingerprint collection where possible, and preliminary cause of death determination. Identification proceeds through parallel analytical streams: fingerprint identification when antemortem records exist; dental identification through comparison with antemortem records collected from family dentists; DNA identification through kinship comparison with family reference samples collected at the Family Assistance Center. Cause of death for aviation mass casualty is typically blunt force injury from the impact; the systematic documentation supports the aggregate case work rather than requiring individualized investigation for each decedent.

**Cause Determination:** For each decedent: blunt force injury of the specific mechanism identified. The general aviation mass casualty cause pattern applies with individual variation reflecting the specific position of the decedent relative to the impact forces.

**Manner Determination:** For each decedent: accident (in the absence of evidence of alternative mechanism). If subsequent investigation identifies specific criminal component (bombing, deliberate crash), the manner may be modified for the individual cases affected.

**Trap Logic:** The trap in mass fatality response is either to attempt individual case work at the routine pace (producing inability to complete the case work within reasonable time frames) or to reduce case rigor below the required standard (producing identification errors and inadequate documentation). The systematic approach: adopts specific mass fatality protocols that maintain identification rigor while scaling processing capability; uses parallel analytical streams for identification (fingerprint, dental, DNA) so that identification proceeds efficiently; establishes clear coordination among the multiple agencies involved so that no critical function is missed; and maintains family communication throughout the process. The framework is developed specifically to preserve rigor at scale.

**Certification Anchor:** Mass fatality response uses coordinated multi-agency mechanisms with specific process modifications supporting aggregate case work. The systematic approach preserves identification rigor and case documentation quality while scaling to the event demands. Federal DMORT and NDMS deployment support jurisdictions when local capacity is exceeded.

## The Family Assistance Center

The Family Assistance Center is a coordinated response element that supports families of the deceased throughout the mass fatality event. The center provides information about the response, collects information supporting identification (antemortem descriptions, dental records, DNA reference samples), communicates identification results to families, coordinates family services (grief support, financial assistance information, logistical support for family members traveling to the region), and maintains contact throughout the ongoing response.

### Antemortem Data Collection

Antemortem data collection at the Family Assistance Center is systematic. Families provide detailed descriptions of the missing family member: physical characteristics (height, weight, hair color, eye color, distinctive features including tattoos and scars), medical history (surgical implants, dental work, distinctive medical conditions), personal effects (typical clothing, jewelry, documents), and specific circumstances of the incident. Standardized forms (developed for this purpose by DMORT and by Interpol DVI) capture the data in a form that supports systematic comparison with postmortem findings. DNA reference samples are collected from close relatives (typically parents, siblings, or children of the missing person) using standardized protocols preserving chain of custody. Dental records are obtained from the missing person's dentist. The antemortem data forms one side of the identification comparison; the postmortem data collected at the morgue operation forms the other side.

**Figure 21.1: Mass Fatality Response Workflow: Coordinated Operations**

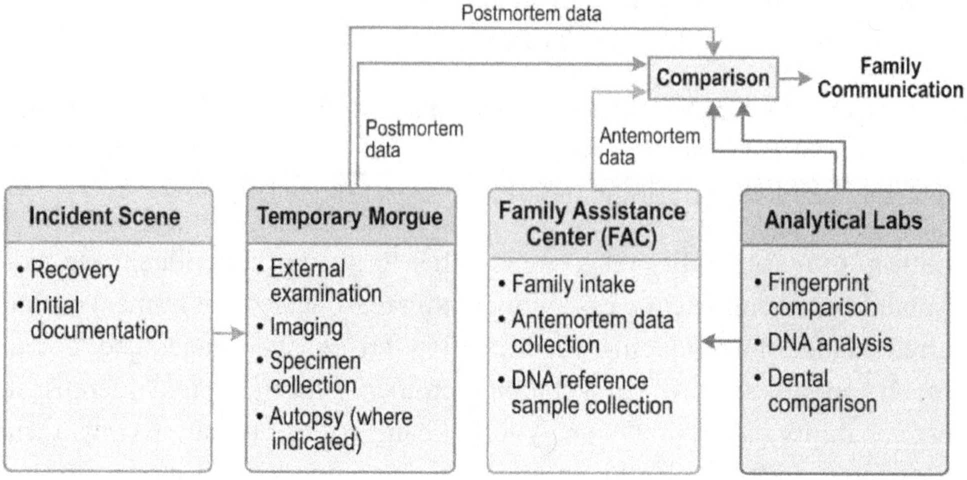


### Family Communication During the Response

Communication with families during the ongoing response is a critical function of the Family Assistance Center. Families in the immediate aftermath of a mass fatality event are in acute grief and are often overwhelmed by media attention, logistical challenges, and uncertainty about the fate of their family member. The center provides accurate information about the response progress, communicates identification results as they become available, coordinates release of remains when identification is complete, and supports the transition from acute response to longer-term family support. Trained mental health providers, family engagement specialists, and, in many cases, religious support are integrated into the center's functions.

## Identification Approaches in Mass Casualty Events

Identification in mass casualty events uses the same scientific methods developed in Chapter 20 (fingerprint, DNA, forensic odontology) with specific process modifications supporting the aggregate scale. The primary identification methods are used in parallel to maximize the efficiency of the aggregate response.

### Primary and Secondary Identification Categories

The Interpol DVI framework categorizes identification methods as primary (fingerprint, DNA, dental) and secondary (medical devices, personal effects, distinguishing features, circumstantial evidence). Primary identification methods provide the scientific basis for identification; secondary methods provide supporting evidence. Standard practice requires positive identification through at least one primary method, with secondary methods providing supporting evidence rather than serving as the sole basis for identification. In cases where primary methods are unavailable (severely destroyed remains where fingerprint, dental, and DNA are all unavailable), the aggregate secondary evidence may support identification in specific circumstances, but the identification is documented as reflecting the aggregate evidence with the specific limits.

**Prioritization in High-Volume Events**

In events with substantial fatality numbers, prioritization of case processing considers several factors. Family concerns about specific missing individuals may accelerate work on the associated remains. Investigative priorities may accelerate work on remains associated with specific investigation questions. Preservation concerns (early identification of remains at risk of further deterioration during storage) may accelerate specific cases. The prioritization is balanced against the overall response requirement that all decedents receive appropriate identification and documentation; some events involve reprioritization as the response evolves and as the specific case circumstances become clearer.

**SCENE-TO-CERTIFICATION DECISION SYSTEM — Identification Prioritization Arc**

---

**Presenting Death Scenario:** A natural disaster (major hurricane with substantial storm surge) has produced approximately 400 confirmed deaths across a coastal region, with additional decedents still being recovered. The state emergency management has requested DMORT deployment, which is in progress. The temporary morgue operation is receiving decedents from multiple recovery sites over an extended time period (recovery continues for weeks after the initial event). Case workload substantially exceeds normal capacity even with DMORT deployment.

**Autopsy Signature:** Each decedent receives systematic documentation using mass fatality protocols. External examination documents cause-of-death-relevant findings (drowning findings, blunt trauma from structural damage, environmental exposure findings). Imaging (portable radiography and, where feasible, portable CT) documents skeletal findings and retained foreign material. Fingerprints are collected when the condition of the hands permits. Dental documentation and specimen collection for DNA proceed for every decedent. Cause of death is typically drowning or environmental exposure with contributing conditions; individual cases with specific alternative causes (structural collapse, injury from wind-thrown debris, indirect deaths from lack of medical care) are documented as such. Identification proceeds through parallel analytical streams with prioritization reflecting the family requests, investigative priorities, and preservation concerns.

**Cause Determination:** For each decedent: the specific mechanism identified (drowning, blunt injury, environmental exposure, etc.), with the disaster context noted.

**Manner Determination:** For most decedents: accident (natural disaster). Specific cases may receive alternative manner determinations if evidence supports (homicide during the chaos of the disaster, suicide, natural death not related to the disaster).

**Trap Logic:** The trap in prolonged mass fatality events is either the maintenance of routine processing pace (producing case backlogs that extend response for months or years) or excessive processing acceleration (producing quality problems in identification or case documentation). The systematic approach: maintains identification rigor while scaling processing throughput; uses prioritization framework transparently so families understand the basis for the sequence; preserves families' access to remains and to accurate information throughout the response; and coordinates with state and federal authorities for the sustained resource commitment. The response to major natural disasters may extend over weeks to months of active case work with ongoing coordination requirements.

**Certification Anchor:** Mass fatality response in natural disaster contexts requires sustained multi-agency coordination with prioritization framework, scaled processing throughput, and maintained identification rigor. The individual case work supports both the immediate response and the aggregate documentation of the disaster event.

## Aircraft and Vehicle Mass Casualty Events

Aircraft mass casualty events have specific characteristics affecting the forensic response. The event typically involves multiple decedents in a defined location (the crash site), with the National Transportation Safety Board coordinating the aviation investigation and the Federal Bureau of Investigation coordinating any criminal investigation. The decedents are typically substantially damaged by the crash forces, with the identification challenge often requiring scientific methods rather than visual identification. International passenger lists may involve multiple countries requiring the international coordination framework.

### The Aviation Response Framework

The Federal Aviation Administration and the National Transportation Safety Board coordinate the aviation-specific response. The Family Assistance Act of 1996 established specific requirements for airline response to families of victims, including the provision of family assistance centers with government coordination. The forensic pathology response works within this framework, with specific coordination requirements for the aviation investigation elements (identification of crew versus passengers, correlation of decedents with specific aircraft locations for the reconstruction, integration with the aviation investigation timeline). The framework has been developed through experience with major aviation events over recent decades and represents mature coordination practice.

### Reconstruction of the Aviation Event

Forensic pathology contribution to aviation event reconstruction integrates the individual case findings with the aggregate reconstruction of the event. Position of decedents within the aircraft at the moment of impact (identified by seat assignment matched with the specific injuries and their patterns) supports the reconstruction of the event. Specific findings (evidence of survivable impact versus immediate fatal impact, evidence of specific mechanisms including bombing versus mechanical failure versus other causes) support the aviation investigation. Individual case autopsy of the crew members (particularly the flight crew) may involve additional analysis including toxicology and medical history relevant to the aviation investigation. The forensic pathology work supports the aggregate aviation investigation with the individual case work integrated into the overall reconstruction.

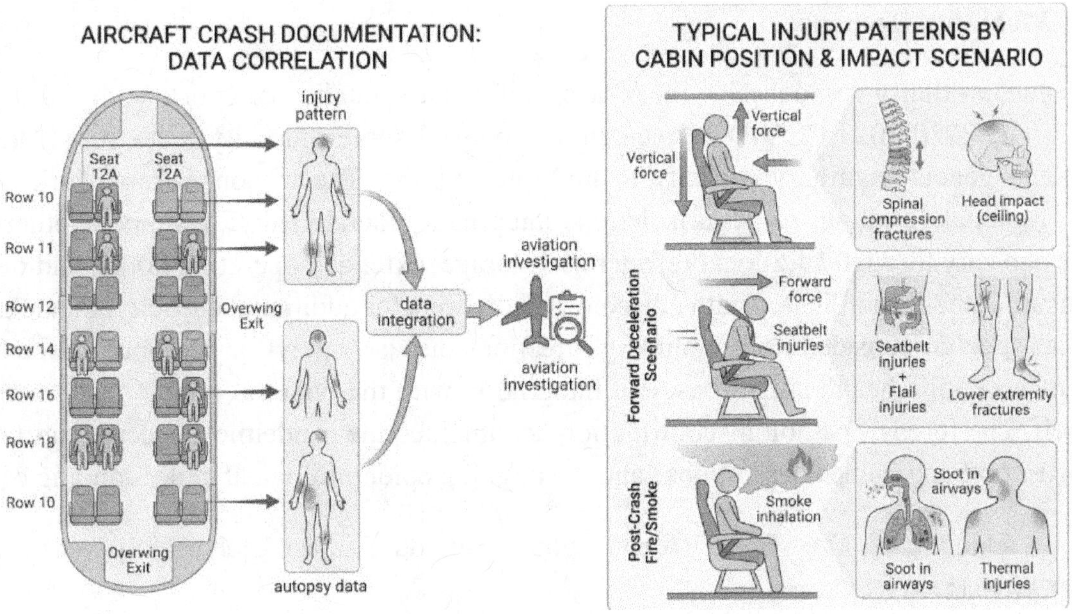


## Terrorism, Natural Disaster, and Other Mass Casualty Types

The specific mass casualty event categories each have particular reconstruction considerations.

### Terrorism Events

Terrorism events (bombings, mass shootings with terrorism motivation, chemical or biological attacks, other terrorism categories) require specific coordination with law enforcement, particularly the FBI in the American context. The forensic pathology contribution to terrorism cases integrates the individual case work with the criminal investigation. Evidence collection for the criminal case is a specific priority: retained fragments from bombings supporting device reconstruction; specific evidence of chemical or biological agent exposure supporting the attack characterization; specific injury patterns supporting the reconstruction of the specific event. Coordination with the criminal investigation team throughout the response is central. Cases involving international coordination (foreign national victims or foreign national perpetrators) integrate the international framework.

### Natural Disaster Response

Natural disaster mass casualty response varies with the specific disaster type. Hurricane response involves drowning, blunt injury, and environmental exposure predominantly, with the timeline typically extending over weeks as decedents are recovered from flood areas, from collapsed structures, and from environmental exposure locations. Earthquake response involves crush injury and structural collapse deaths. Wildfire response involves thermal and inhalation injury. Tornado response involves blunt injury from wind-thrown debris and structural collapse. Each disaster type has its specific reconstruction requirements, and the response framework adapts to the specific circumstances.

## Pandemic Mortality Response

The pandemic mortality response has been a specific mass fatality category with substantial recent experience. The 2020-2023 COVID-19 pandemic produced surge mortality that overwhelmed forensic pathology and general mortuary capacity in multiple regions. The response framework adapted with substantial regional variation: some jurisdictions integrated federal DMORT support; others developed local surge capacity through additional refrigerated storage, extended operating hours, and modified case processing; still others coordinated with adjacent jurisdictions for additional capacity. Pandemic mortality response has specific considerations including infectious disease safety for personnel, specific reporting requirements to public health authorities, and integration with the ongoing public health response to the disease itself. The forensic pathology contribution documented the pandemic's specific mortality patterns and supported both the immediate response and the ongoing epidemiological understanding of the disease.

Figure 21.3: Mass Fatality Identification Methods: Parallel Analytical Streams

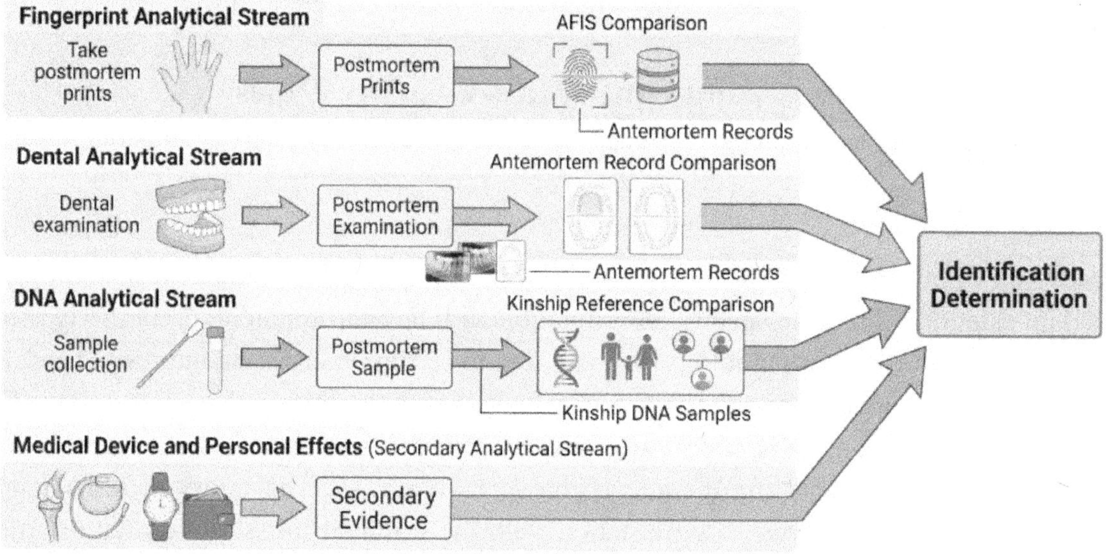


## Industrial and Transportation Disasters

Industrial disasters (chemical release, refinery explosions, mining accidents) and transportation disasters (train derailments, bus crashes, marine casualties) each have specific characteristics affecting the response. Industrial disaster response involves coordination with occupational safety authorities and with the specific industry response mechanisms. Transportation disaster response involves the specific transportation regulator (National Transportation Safety Board for domestic events, Federal Railroad Administration for railroad events, others). Each event category benefits from specific expertise in the response mechanism, and mature response practice draws on precedent from previous events in the same category. The specific reconstruction considerations for each category are integrated with the general mass fatality framework.

### Remains Commingling and Its Resolution

Remains commingling — the mixing together of body parts and remains from multiple decedents — is a specific challenge in mass fatality events with substantial impact forces. Aviation crashes, terrorism events with explosive components, and specific natural disasters produce commingled remains that require systematic sorting into individual decedents before identification can proceed. The sorting process uses several approaches: gross anatomical matching (matching body parts by anatomical fit, continuity of injury patterns, and other physical features); DNA analysis of individual specimens with comparison to establish which specimens are from the same decedent; and imaging correlation. Commingling adds substantially to the identification challenge because each individual decedent may be represented by multiple specimens that must be reunited, and because incomplete remains reduce the identification information available. Specialized expertise in commingled remains resolution has developed with experience from major events including the September 11 attacks and specific aviation events. The specific resolution approach reflects the event characteristics and the resources available.

### Incident Command Structure

The Incident Command System (ICS) is the standardized emergency management structure used in the United States and adopted internationally for coordinated response. Mass fatality response operates within the ICS framework with specific functional units. The Mortuary Affairs Branch typically operates within the Medical Group of the Operations Section, though the specific placement varies with the event structure. The forensic pathology leadership integrates with the ICS structure providing information on the mortuary operations status, resource needs, and coordination requirements. Understanding the ICS framework supports effective participation in the coordinated response; forensic pathology offices participating in mass fatality response should have familiarity with ICS training and structure. Formal ICS training is available through federal emergency management courses and is a professional development standard for forensic pathology leadership.

### Personnel Safety and Support During Response

Personnel safety in mass fatality response encompasses multiple dimensions. Physical safety includes ergonomic considerations for extended case processing, personal protective equipment for infectious disease or hazardous material contexts, and general safety in the temporary morgue environment. Psychological support addresses the specific stresses of mass fatality work: exposure to significant numbers of decedents, work in emotionally intense circumstances, family contact under difficult conditions, and the sustained response over extended periods. Deployed personnel typically receive briefings on psychological support resources, access to mental health services during and after deployment, and structured debriefing sessions to support processing of the experience. Attention to personnel welfare supports both individual well-being and sustained response capability; personnel who experience significant psychological injury from response work may be unable to continue in the specialty.

**CAUTION:** Mass fatality response involves substantial physical and psychological demands on responding personnel. Attention to personnel welfare through structured support, appropriate work-rest cycles, and access to mental health resources supports both individual well-being and sustained response capability. Personnel experiencing significant response-related stress warrant specific support and, where indicated, temporary or permanent removal from the deployment.

### Historical Mass Fatality Events and Lessons Learned

The forensic pathology response to major historical mass fatality events has contributed substantially to the development of current practice. The September 11, 2001 attacks in New York, at the Pentagon, and in Pennsylvania produced substantial mass casualty response experience including specific challenges of commingled remains, identification of severely damaged remains, and sustained response over years for the victims of the World Trade Center attacks where identification work continued far beyond the immediate response period. Hurricane Katrina in 2005 produced substantial natural disaster mass casualty response with lessons about pre-event preparation, coordinated federal support, and sustained state and local response. Aviation events including the disappearance of Malaysia Airlines Flight 370 and specific major aviation crashes have contributed to aviation mass casualty response practice. Terrorism events including bombings and mass shootings have contributed to terrorism-specific response practice. Each event produces after-action review and lessons-learned documentation that informs the developing practice; the professional community integrates these lessons into training and preparation.

### International Cooperation and DVI

International mass fatality events require cooperation across national forensic organizations. Interpol's Disaster Victim Identification standing committee provides framework for international coordination including standardized forms for antemortem and postmortem data, protocols for information exchange, and coordination during specific events. Individual countries provide DVI teams that can be deployed to support international response. The 2004 Indian Ocean tsunami produced substantial international DVI response with multiple national teams supporting the affected countries. Aviation events with international passenger complements typically require international coordination. The professional relationships developed through international training exercises and through participation in international response support effective coordination when major events occur.

### Media Coordination During Mass Fatality Response

Media coordination during mass fatality response is a specific function requiring attention. Media attention on major events is intense and can affect the response if not managed appropriately. The forensic pathology office coordinates with the broader Public Information Officer function within the Incident Command Structure to provide accurate information about the response while protecting family privacy and preserving the integrity of ongoing investigations. Common information provided publicly includes the response status (number of decedents processed, general timeline for identification), the coordinated response structure, and information supporting the aggregate response. Specific case information is not shared publicly until identification is complete and family notification has occurred. Individual case details supporting criminal investigations are typically not shared to preserve the investigation. Effective media coordination supports public understanding of the response while protecting the individual cases and the response process.

**Post-Response Documentation and Analysis**

After the immediate response concludes, mass fatality events produce substantial documentation that supports subsequent analysis, legal proceedings, and future response improvement. Case files for each decedent are integrated with the aggregate documentation of the event. Statistical analysis of the event mortality patterns supports public health and policy understanding. Lessons learned reports from the response support the developing practice. Legal proceedings arising from the event may draw on the case documentation for years or decades. The forensic pathology contribution to the post-response phase includes maintaining accessible case documentation, supporting legal proceedings when required, and contributing to lessons-learned analysis for the professional community.

**Preparation and Readiness**

Preparation and readiness for mass fatality events is a specific responsibility of forensic pathology offices and jurisdictions. Elements of preparation include: mass fatality response plans developed and periodically updated with specific role designations; personnel training including ICS training, mass fatality-specific training, and general disaster preparedness; participation in exercises testing response capability; coordination with local, state, and federal emergency management for role clarification; and resource identification including surge capacity, mutual aid agreements, and coordination with DMORT deployment mechanisms. Offices that maintain active preparation and readiness respond more effectively when events occur; offices without preparation may face substantial challenges during actual response. Investment in preparation is a specific professional responsibility of forensic pathology leadership.

**Evidence Preservation in Mass Casualty Contexts**

Evidence preservation in mass casualty events requires attention beyond routine autopsy practice because of the potential for criminal investigation, civil litigation, and international proceedings arising from the event. Physical evidence recovered from decedents (fragments of the causative device in bombing cases, projectiles in shooting events, retained material in specific mechanisms) is documented, secured, and transferred with chain of custody preservation. Photographic documentation includes overall documentation of each decedent, specific injury documentation, and documentation of retained materials. Biological specimens for toxicology, DNA, and other analyses are preserved with appropriate chain of custody. The systematic approach preserves evidence quality for the potentially wide range of legal proceedings that may arise from the event, including proceedings occurring years or decades after the event. Terrorism prosecutions, aviation litigation, product liability cases, and other proceedings may depend on the evidence preserved during the initial mass fatality response.

### Remains Disposition and Family Preferences

Remains disposition after mass fatality events involves specific considerations. Individual family preferences vary substantially: some families request full return of all identified remains for private disposition; others accept partial return with the understanding that not all fragments may be recovered or identified; still others request disposition through the disaster response mechanism. The Family Assistance Center supports families through these decisions with information about the disposition options and coordination of the specific arrangements. In some mass fatality events with substantial commingling and incomplete identification, communal memorial disposition may be arranged for unidentified or unassigned remains with appropriate ceremony and family involvement. The disposition arrangements reflect the specific event circumstances, the specific religious and cultural preferences of the affected families, and the coordination with the broader response mechanism.

### Legal and Insurance Aftermath

The legal and insurance aftermath of mass fatality events extends over years to decades after the immediate response. Death certificates for the individual decedents support the immediate legal purposes: estate administration, insurance claims, and other proceedings depending on documented death. Civil litigation arising from the event (aviation crashes producing airline and manufacturer litigation, terrorism producing state-sponsor litigation, industrial disasters producing employer and manufacturer litigation) may proceed for years with the forensic pathology documentation supporting the litigation. Criminal proceedings for terrorism and other criminal-component events may proceed similarly. The office maintains the case documentation accessible for these proceedings and may provide expert testimony as required. Attention to the legal aftermath during the initial response supports the subsequent proceedings; abbreviated documentation or preserved chain of custody problems can compromise the aftermath work substantially.

### Technology Integration in Mass Fatality Response

Technology integration in mass fatality response has developed substantially over recent decades. Information technology supporting case management (specialized databases coordinating antemortem and postmortem data, tracking case status through the response, coordinating identification comparison across multiple analytical streams) is essential for large events. Communication technology supporting coordination among distributed personnel is central. Imaging technology (portable CT, digital radiography) supports rapid case documentation. Analytical technology (automated fingerprint comparison, DNA analytical platforms with high throughput, specific mass fatality identification software) supports the aggregate identification workflow. Preparation for future events includes technology infrastructure investment; the specific capabilities needed depend on the anticipated event types and the resources available.

### Professional Development and Community

The forensic pathology community engaged in mass fatality response maintains active professional networks supporting preparation and response. The American Academy of Forensic Sciences, the National Association of Medical Examiners, and the American College of Forensic Sciences each address mass fatality response through committees, professional development programs, and periodic conferences. International professional organizations including the International Association of Forensic Sciences engage similarly. Individual professional development in mass fatality response includes formal training courses, participation in exercises and drills, engagement with the professional literature on response practice, and, ideally, direct experience with response events under mentored supervision. The community that develops through these engagements supports both individual professional development and the aggregate response capability.

### SCENE-TO-CERTIFICATION DECISION SYSTEM — Mass Fatality Determination Arcs

**The Framework:** Mass fatality response requires coordinated multi-agency response beyond routine local capacity. The National Disaster Medical System and the DMORT program provide federal support for large events; state and local structures provide the initial response and coordination. The framework preserves identification rigor and case documentation quality while scaling to event demands.

**Family Assistance Center Function:** The Family Assistance Center is the central coordination point for family communication during mass fatality response. Antemortem data collection (descriptions, medical records, dental records, DNA reference samples) supports identification. Family communication throughout the response supports both the immediate need and the transition to longer-term family support.

**Identification in Mass Casualty:** Identification uses fingerprint, DNA, and forensic odontology as primary methods with secondary methods (medical devices, personal effects, distinguishing features) providing supporting evidence. Parallel analytical streams maximize efficiency. Prioritization framework balances family concerns, investigative priorities, and preservation considerations.

**Specific Event Categories:** Aviation, terrorism, natural disaster, pandemic, industrial, and transportation mass casualty events each have specific reconstruction considerations integrated with the general framework. Aviation events involve NTSB coordination; terrorism involves FBI coordination; natural disasters involve emergency management coordination; each category has specific expertise and precedent.

**Coordination Discipline:** The forensic pathology role in mass fatality response is one element of the broader emergency response framework. Effective response depends on coordination across agencies, disciplines, and jurisdictions. The individual case work supports both the immediate response and the aggregate documentation of the event.

## Summary and Key Concepts

Mass fatality events exceeding routine local jurisdiction capacity require coordinated multi-agency response. The National Disaster Medical System and the DMORT program provide federal support; state and local structures provide initial response and ongoing coordination.

DMORT teams include forensic pathologists, forensic anthropologists, forensic odontologists, fingerprint examiners, DNA analysts, medicolegal death investigators, and support personnel. Mobile equipment including the Disaster Portable Morgue Unit provides functional forensic capability at the event site.

The Family Assistance Center supports families through the response, collects antemortem data supporting identification, and communicates identification results and other case information. Trained mental health providers, family engagement specialists, and religious support are integrated into center functions.

Identification uses fingerprint, DNA, and forensic odontology as primary scientific methods with secondary methods providing supporting evidence. Parallel analytical streams maximize efficiency. Prioritization framework balances multiple considerations.

Aircraft mass casualty response works within the aviation investigation framework with NTSB and FBI coordination. Forensic contribution to aviation event reconstruction integrates individual case findings with the aggregate event reconstruction.

Terrorism, natural disaster, pandemic, industrial, and transportation mass casualty events each have specific reconstruction considerations integrated with the general framework. Coordination discipline is central to effective response across categories.

# CHAPTER 22: DEATH CERTIFICATION

**Learning Objectives**

1. Articulate the purpose and structure of the death certificate in American practice and its role in vital statistics.
2. Apply the cause of death framework distinguishing immediate cause, intermediate causes, and underlying cause with the specific cascade reasoning.
3. Apply the five manner of death categories (natural, accident, suicide, homicide, undetermined) with attention to the specific reasoning framework for each.
4. Recognize the special certification considerations including presumptive certification, delayed certification pending workup, and specific case patterns.
5. Perform certificate amendment and correction when subsequent findings warrant, and articulate the aggregate function of death certification for vital statistics and public health.

## The Death Certificate: Purpose and Structure

The death certificate is the official legal document recording a death, and it serves multiple substantial functions: it establishes the legal fact of the death for probate, insurance, and administrative purposes; it provides the medical certification of cause and manner of death that supports both the individual case and the aggregate vital statistics; it enables burial, cremation, or other disposition of remains through the required legal documentation; and it contributes to public health surveillance through the aggregate data on mortality patterns. The forensic pathologist certifying a case addresses each of these functions simultaneously through the specific documentation on the certificate.

The structure of the death certificate in American practice follows the Standard Certificate of Death promulgated by the National Center for Health Statistics, with state-specific variations. The document is divided into demographic and administrative sections (completed by the funeral director or other administrative personnel) and medical certification sections (completed by the certifying physician or medicolegal death investigator). The medical certification includes cause of death (with the specific cascade structure discussed below), manner of death (one of the five categories), specific event circumstances, and any other information relevant to the certification. The signed certificate is filed with the state vital records office and becomes the official record.

The forensic pathologist certifying cases falling under medical examiner or coroner jurisdiction has specific responsibility for the medical certification. The certification reflects the systematic case reasoning developed through the autopsy examination, the specimen analysis (toxicology, histology, other laboratory studies), the scene evidence, and the antecedent history. The certificate summarizes the aggregate case reasoning in a form suitable for the official record; the full case documentation exists separately in the autopsy report and the case file. The certificate and the report are complementary elements of the case documentation.

### Medical Examiner and Coroner Jurisdiction

The jurisdiction of the medical examiner or coroner over a specific death is defined by state statute and covers deaths that meet specified categories: sudden and unexpected deaths, deaths from injury or violence, deaths in custody, suspicious deaths, deaths without a treating physician, deaths of persons unidentified at the time of death, and other categories varying by state. Deaths not falling within medicolegal jurisdiction are certified by the treating physician (typically the last physician who managed the decedent's care). The forensic pathologist certifying medicolegal cases follows the state framework for jurisdiction and applies the certification approach appropriate to the medicolegal context.

**KEY POINT:** The death certificate serves both immediate legal and administrative functions and aggregate public health surveillance. The medical certification by the forensic pathologist summarizes the systematic case reasoning in a form suitable for the official record. The certificate and the autopsy report are complementary elements of the case documentation.

## Cause of Death: The Framework

The cause of death framework in American practice distinguishes the immediate cause of death, intermediate causes, and the underlying cause with a specific cascade structure. Part I of the certificate lists the sequential causes leading to death; Part II lists conditions contributing to death but not part of the direct causal chain. Understanding the cascade structure is essential for accurate certification.

### The Immediate Cause of Death

The immediate cause of death — listed on line (a) of Part I — is the specific physiological event that produced death at the moment it occurred. Examples include acute myocardial infarction, pulmonary embolism, hemorrhage, respiratory failure, or specific mechanistic entities. The immediate cause is typically the physiological event closest to death in time and directly producing the moment of death. In some cases the immediate cause is not further characterized ("cardiopulmonary arrest" or "multiorgan failure" are examples of terminal events that are not adequate immediate causes for certification purposes because they do not identify the specific mechanism producing the event).

### Intermediate Causes

Intermediate causes — listed on lines (b), (c), and where needed (d) of Part I — identify the intermediate mechanisms in the causal cascade from the underlying cause to the immediate cause. For example, an acute myocardial infarction (immediate cause) may result from a specific coronary artery thrombosis (intermediate cause) resulting from underlying coronary atherosclerosis (underlying cause). Each intermediate cause is documented on a separate line with the temporal cascade preserved: line (b) causes line (a); line (c) causes line (b); and so forth. The cascade may include one, two, or three intermediate causes depending on the specific case.

## The Underlying Cause of Death

The underlying cause of death — listed on the lowest line of Part I filled — is the disease or injury that initiated the cascade of events leading to death. The underlying cause is the primary target of vital statistics coding and the primary focus of aggregate mortality surveillance. In natural death cases, the underlying cause is typically the specific disease that eventually produced death (coronary atherosclerosis, hypertensive heart disease, specific malignancy, etc.). In injury and violence cases, the underlying cause is the specific injury or the specific event mechanism (gunshot wound, motor vehicle collision, drug overdose). The specific underlying cause identification is central to the certification's aggregate value.

## Part II: Contributing Conditions

Part II of the certificate lists significant conditions contributing to death but not part of the direct causal cascade. These conditions affected the decedent's overall vulnerability but are not identified as specific elements of the causal chain producing the moment of death. Examples include: chronic pulmonary disease in a decedent whose direct cause of death was myocardial infarction; diabetes mellitus contributing to overall vulnerability but not directly producing the immediate mechanism; alcohol use disorder contributing to overall risk pattern; and other specific conditions. Part II is important for the aggregate documentation of the decedent's clinical context even when the specific conditions are not the direct cause.

Figure 22.1: The Death Certificate Cause-of-Death Structure

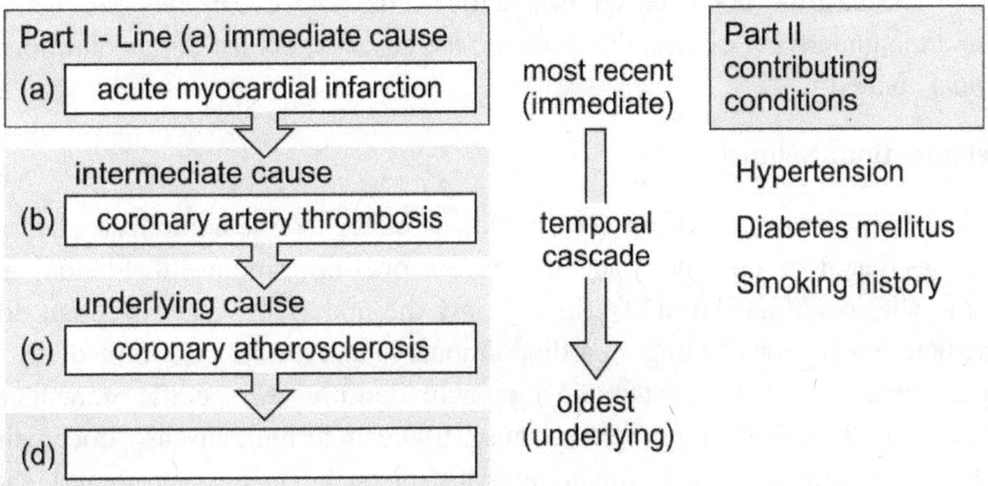


## The Time Interval Column

Each cause-of-death line has an associated time interval column indicating the approximate duration of the specific condition. For chronic conditions the interval may be measured in years (chronic coronary atherosclerosis: 20 years); for acute events the interval may be minutes to hours (acute myocardial infarction: minutes). The time intervals support the aggregate documentation of the disease trajectory and provide clinical context for the certification. Interval documentation is approximate and reflects the best available information from the case reasoning rather than precise measurement.

**Presenting Death Scenario:** A 68-year-old man is found deceased at home by his wife. He had a well-documented history of type 2 diabetes mellitus for approximately 15 years, hypertension for 20 years, and prior myocardial infarction 4 years earlier with subsequent coronary artery bypass grafting. He had complained of chest pain for approximately one hour before collapse. Emergency response confirms death at scene. The medical examiner's office accepts jurisdiction based on the sudden death and coordinates the certification approach.

**Autopsy Signature:** External examination is unremarkable. Internal examination shows severe atherosclerotic disease of the coronary vessels with occlusive thrombus in the left anterior descending artery at a location distal to the prior bypass graft insertion; the bypass graft to that vessel shows patency but the native distal circulation is compromised. Acute infarct of characteristic pattern is present in the anterior wall of the left ventricle. Left ventricular hypertrophy and diffuse atherosclerotic changes throughout the coronary tree. Other findings include diabetic nephropathy and hypertensive vascular disease. Toxicology is negative for drugs of abuse and confirms therapeutic levels of the prescribed medications. Vitreous chemistry supports antemortem hyperglycemia.

**Cause Determination:** Cause of death cascade: Part I(a) Acute myocardial infarction (interval: minutes); (b) Coronary artery thrombosis (interval: hours); (c) Coronary atherosclerosis (interval: 20 years). Part II Contributing conditions: type 2 diabetes mellitus (15 years); hypertension (20 years); prior coronary artery bypass grafting. The cascade documents the specific immediate event, the intermediate mechanism producing it, and the underlying disease that initiated the cascade; contributing conditions document the aggregate clinical context.

**Manner Determination:** Natural.

**Trap Logic:** The trap in cause-of-death certification is either to overcomplicate the cascade (adding intermediate causes that are not distinctly separate events, or listing findings that belong in Part II as part of the causal cascade) or to undersimplify (listing only the underlying cause without documenting the specific immediate event, or writing "cardiopulmonary arrest" as an immediate cause without characterizing the mechanism). The systematic approach: identifies the specific immediate physiological event; traces backward through the intermediate causes to the underlying disease; documents contributing conditions in Part II; and includes approximate intervals for each. The cascade should read as a coherent narrative of the specific events producing this death, with the certification reader able to understand from the certificate alone what specifically happened.

**Certification Anchor:** The cause-of-death cascade documents the specific immediate physiological event, the intermediate mechanisms leading to it, and the underlying disease or injury that initiated the sequence. Part II documents contributing conditions supporting the aggregate clinical context. The certification is the summary; the autopsy report provides the full case documentation.

## Manner of Death: The Five Categories

Manner of death is classified into one of five categories: natural, accident, suicide, homicide, and undetermined. Each category has specific reasoning framework, and the choice among categories reflects the systematic case analysis. Understanding each category and the specific reasoning for its application is central to accurate certification.

### Natural

Natural manner is applied when death results entirely from disease or age-related processes without contribution from injury, poisoning, or other external factors. The specific disease may be acute (acute myocardial infarction, pulmonary embolism, cerebrovascular event) or chronic in its terminal presentation (metastatic cancer, end-stage heart failure, end-stage renal disease). Natural manner requires the case reasoning to have identified the specific disease and to have excluded contribution from external factors that would move the case to another manner category. Deaths in individuals with substance use disorder where the terminal event is a natural disease process (not the substance use itself) may be classified as natural depending on the specific reasoning; the framework applies systematic analysis rather than categorical rules.

### Accident

Accident manner is applied when death results from unintentional injury or exposure that was not deliberately sought by any party. The category covers motor vehicle collisions without intentional cause, falls, drownings without intent, most drug overdose deaths in individuals using substances for personal effect rather than to die, unintentional injuries in workplace or recreational contexts, and other injury deaths without intentional cause. Accident manner requires evidence supporting unintentional mechanism; the specific reasoning documents the accidental nature and excludes suicide or homicide contribution.

### Suicide

Suicide manner is applied when death results from injury or exposure that the decedent inflicted or accepted with intent to die. The determination requires evidence supporting intent: a note or documented prior communication of intent; a discrete pattern consistent with intentional self-inflicted mechanism; scene evidence supporting the intent (weapon positioning consistent with self-infliction, arrangement of pill bottles suggesting intentional overdose, other specific scene evidence); and, in the aggregate, a case reasoning that supports suicide over accident. The specific evidence supporting intent varies by mechanism, and the reasoning uses systematic evaluation rather than categorical rules. Suicide requires evidence rather than absence of alternative explanation — a death from an unexplained overdose is not classified as suicide without evidence supporting intent.

### Homicide

Homicide manner is applied when death results from the action of another person that caused the death, whether by direct injury (assault, gunshot wound, stabbing) or by other mechanism (poisoning, deprivation). The determination is a medical classification based on the case findings supporting external causation; it is not a legal determination of criminal responsibility, which is decided by the criminal justice system. The homicide determination indicates that another person's action caused the death; the legal characterization of whether that action was criminal, and if so what specific crime, proceeds independently. Justifiable homicide (self-defense, law enforcement action within lawful authority) still receives homicide manner from the medical certification even when no criminal proceeding results.

### Undetermined

Undetermined manner is applied when the evidence does not support any of the other four categories to reasonable medical certainty. The classification is appropriate when: the death has both natural and non-natural features and the specific contribution cannot be determined; the injury pattern is inconsistent with any specific manner without additional evidence; the case has ambiguous features that could support either accident or suicide; or the specific case circumstances are unclear and additional investigation cannot resolve them. Undetermined manner is a professional determination reflecting the honest limits of the case reasoning; it is not a failure but an appropriate use of the classification when specificity is not warranted. Overreliance on undetermined manner across a caseload can suggest inadequate case work, but appropriate use in genuinely ambiguous cases is a mark of professional integrity.

**SCENE-TO-CERTIFICATION DECISION SYSTEM — Manner-of-Death Determination Arc**

**Presenting Death Scenario:** A 35-year-old woman is found deceased in her apartment by her sister. She had a documented history of major depression with a prior suicide attempt approximately 8 months earlier, and had been managing her illness with prescription antidepressants and periodic therapy. Recent mental health notes describe her as "stable but concerning". Scene evidence shows an empty prescription bottle for amitriptyline (recently filled), an empty wine bottle, and a note written to family members with themes suggesting ending of pain. Emergency response confirms death at scene.

**Autopsy Signature:** External examination shows no evidence of trauma. Internal examination is unremarkable structurally with no acute pathology identified adequate to independently explain death. Toxicology on peripheral blood: amitriptyline 1,200 nanograms per milliliter (well above the therapeutic range of 50-300 nanograms per milliliter and consistent with a fatal overdose); nortriptyline (metabolite) 300 nanograms per milliliter; ethanol 0.19 grams per deciliter (consistent with the empty wine bottle at scene); other drugs negative. Cardiac disease is absent; no alternative structural cause.

**Cause Determination:** Cause of death cascade: Part I(a) Acute amitriptyline intoxication with alcohol (interval: hours); (b) Ingestion of amitriptyline and alcohol. Part II Contributing conditions: major depressive disorder (documented history).

**Manner Determination:** Suicide. The determination reflects: the discrete pattern of ingestion of a substantial dose of the prescription antidepressant combined with alcohol; the note communicating intent to family; the recent prescription refill providing the means; the documented history of major depression with prior suicide attempt; and the aggregate pattern consistent with intentional overdose. The evidence supporting intent is systematic and integrated across multiple elements of the case.

**Trap Logic:** The trap in manner determination is either to overinterpret ambiguous evidence as suicide (or to underinterpret clear evidence as accident when suicide evidence is present), or to fail to recognize the specific patterns that distinguish suicide from accident from natural. Systematic evaluation integrates the toxicological pattern (level well above therapeutic range with substantial ingestion), the scene evidence (note, pattern of drug availability), the antecedent history (major depression, prior attempt), and the aggregate reasoning. The suicide determination in this case reflects the integrated evidence supporting intent. Alternative determinations — accident (unintentional overdose), undetermined (unclear intent) — are considered systematically and rejected in favor of the specific determination that fits the evidence.

**Certification Anchor:** Manner of death is determined through systematic reasoning integrating the case findings. Each manner category has specific reasoning framework; the determination reflects the aggregate evidence rather than a single element. Documentation of the reasoning in the autopsy report supports transparency and enables review of the determination if needed.

## Special Certification Considerations

Beyond the standard cause and manner determinations, several special certification considerations apply in specific case circumstances.

### Presumptive and Amended Certification

Presumptive certification at initial autopsy with amendment when subsequent workup is complete is common practice for cases with pending toxicology or other analyses. The initial certificate documents the findings available at autopsy with pending items noted; the amended certificate documents the final findings when workup is complete. The practice supports timely release of the body and support of family needs while preserving certification accuracy. Amendment procedures vary by state; the pathologist follows the specific procedure required by the vital records office. Amendment is a routine element of forensic pathology practice, not an admission of error, and reflects the natural workflow of case investigation.

### Delayed Certification

Certification may be delayed pending workup in cases where initial findings are inadequate to support the specific determination. Complex neuropathology cases pending neuropathology consultation, pediatric cases pending metabolic workup, and cases with unusual toxicological questions may require delayed final certification. Provisional certification may be used to permit disposition of the body while final workup continues; specific state procedures vary.

### In-Hospital Deaths

Deaths occurring during hospitalization or shortly after hospital discharge require specific consideration for certification. Deaths from natural progression of the underlying illness are typically certified by the treating physician; deaths from medical intervention, procedural complications, or specific circumstances may fall under medical examiner jurisdiction. The specific determination depends on state statute and on the specific case circumstances. Deaths that begin as one manner but that involve medical intervention (a homicide victim who dies days later from complications of surgical treatment for gunshot wounds; a drug overdose victim who survives initial resuscitation but dies later from anoxic brain injury) are typically certified with the manner reflecting the original event (homicide, accident) even when the terminal event is a natural complication of the medical care.

**Figure 22.2: Manner of Death Determination Framework: Reasoning Cascade**

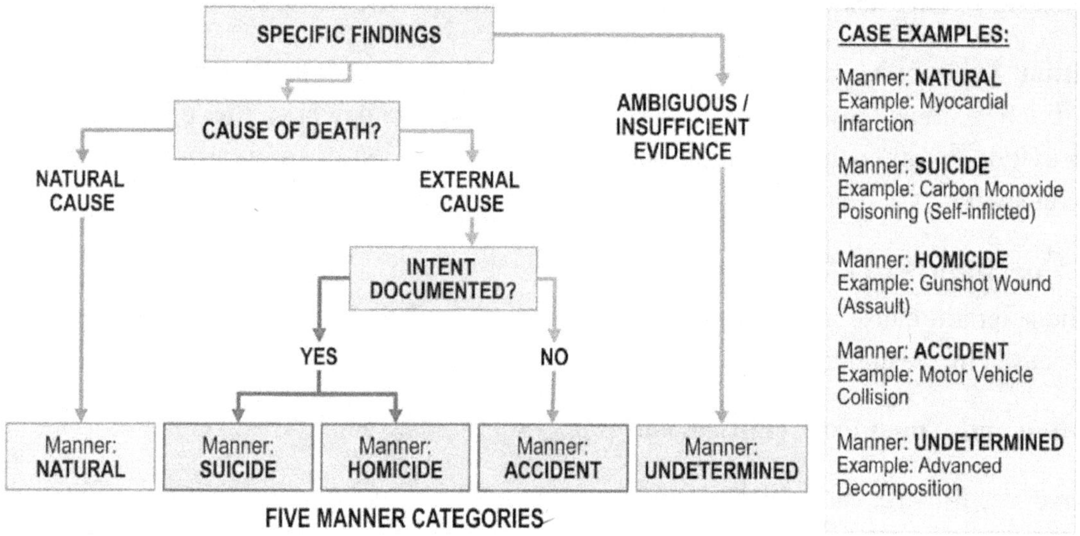


### Sequelae of Remote Injury

Deaths from sequelae of injury sustained months, years, or decades earlier present specific reasoning. A decedent who dies from complications of paraplegia sustained in a motor vehicle collision 15 years earlier may be certified with the manner reflecting the original event (accident) if the case reasoning supports the direct causal chain from the injury to the terminal event. Similarly, a decedent who dies decades after a gunshot wound from complications directly attributable to the injury may be certified as homicide. The reasoning requires the specific causal chain to be traceable from the original event to the terminal event without intervening independent cause; the interval alone does not preclude the determination when the causal chain is intact.

## Certificate Amendment and Correction

Amendment and correction of the death certificate follows specific procedures established by state vital records offices. Amendment is used when new information becomes available (toxicology completion, additional case findings, subsequent investigation revealing specific circumstances); correction is used when errors are identified in the original certificate.

### Amendment Procedures

Amendment procedures typically require submission of an amended certificate through the state vital records office with documentation of the specific changes. Some states require specific forms for amendment; others accept an amended certificate with the changes noted. The pathologist follows the specific procedure required by the state. Common amendment scenarios include: change of cause of death from presumptive to confirmed based on toxicology; addition of contributing conditions identified in subsequent workup; change of manner based on subsequent investigation findings; and correction of factual errors in the original certificate. Amendment is a routine part of the certification process and is used whenever the case findings warrant.

### The Case Review Process

Case review — systematic review of certifications for quality assurance — is standard practice in many offices. Peer review of specific cases (particularly complex cases, homicides, or cases with substantial community interest) supports the aggregate quality of certifications. Regular review of the office's aggregate certification patterns identifies potential systematic issues (excessive undetermined manner, specific cause categories that may be over- or under-used, patterns suggesting training needs). The review process supports both individual case quality and the aggregate office practice.

## Aggregate Function of Death Certification

The aggregate function of death certification supports substantial public health and policy activity. The individual case certifications, integrated across jurisdictions and time, form the mortality data that supports vital statistics, epidemiological research, and public health surveillance.

### Vital Statistics and Public Health Surveillance

State and federal vital statistics compile the death certificate data into aggregate mortality patterns. The National Center for Health Statistics maintains the national mortality data; state and local departments maintain jurisdiction-level data. The data supports: identification of mortality trends (increasing or decreasing rates of specific causes); identification of health disparities across demographic groups; monitoring of specific public health concerns (drug overdose deaths, injury patterns, disease-specific mortality); and evaluation of public health interventions. The forensic pathology contribution to this aggregate function is substantial — medicolegal case certifications provide the specific documentation of injury and violence deaths that would otherwise not be adequately documented in the aggregate data.

### Epidemiological Research

Epidemiological research draws extensively on death certificate data. Studies of mortality patterns, disease trajectories, injury risk, and specific public health questions use the certification data as a primary information source. The research supports policy development, clinical practice, and public health intervention. Individual case certifications contribute to this aggregate research base; attention to accuracy and completeness in individual certifications supports the aggregate research quality.

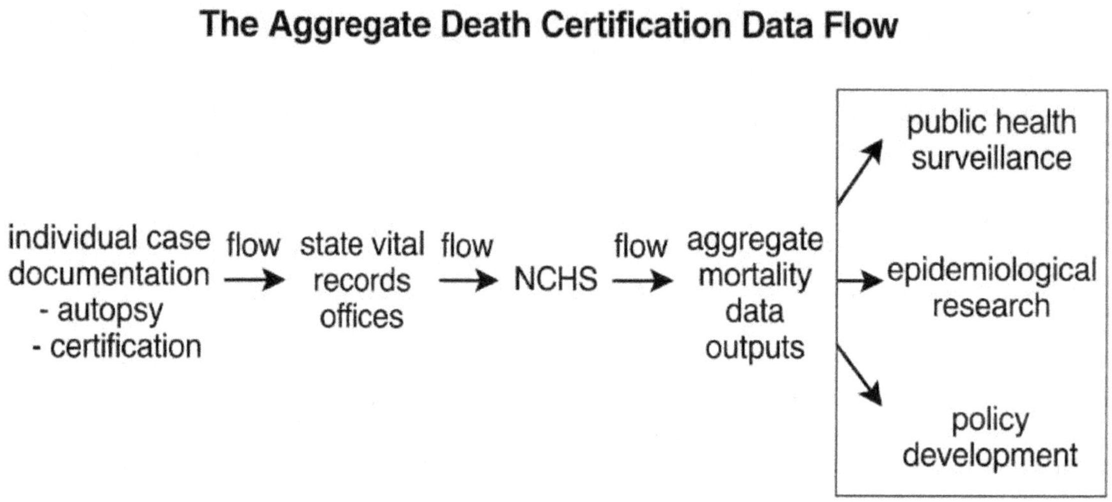


**Figure 22.3** 'The Aggregate Death Certification Data Flow'

### The Coder and the Underlying Cause

Vital statistics coders at the state and federal level review the individual death certificates and assign specific ICD codes to the causes documented. The coding follows international standards (currently ICD-10 for cause of death coding in most American practice) and assigns a single underlying cause code to each death. The specific underlying cause identified by the coder may not always match the pathologist's intent — the coder applies coding rules that may lead to selection of a different line in the cascade as the underlying cause. Familiarity with the coding process supports certification that will code as intended by the pathologist; clear documentation of the cascade with specific, distinct causes at each level supports accurate coding. Communication with the state vital records office when specific coding questions arise is appropriate.

### The Individual and Aggregate Contribution

Each individual certification contributes to both the immediate case purposes (family, legal, administrative) and the aggregate purposes (vital statistics, epidemiological research, public health surveillance). The forensic pathologist certifying cases recognizes both functions and attends to the specificity and accuracy that supports both. Vague or generic certifications limit the aggregate value; specific and accurate certifications support both functions. The professional responsibility of the certifying pathologist extends beyond the individual case to the aggregate contribution to public health understanding.

### Certification of Deaths With Unidentified Decedents

Deaths of unidentified decedents present specific certification considerations. The certificate typically identifies the decedent as "John Doe" or "Jane Doe" with an assigned case number, provides the demographic information available from the examination (estimated age, sex, biological profile), and provides the medical certification of cause and manner as determined from the examination. Subsequent identification through fingerprint, DNA, dental, or other means supports amendment of the certificate with the correct decedent identity. The pattern of certification in unidentified cases supports the ongoing identification investigation while providing the necessary legal documentation of the death. Some jurisdictions require specific procedures for certification of unidentified decedents; the pathologist follows the state framework.

### The Certifier as Witness in Legal Proceedings

The certifying pathologist may be called as a witness in legal proceedings arising from the death: criminal prosecution in homicide cases; civil litigation including wrongful death actions and insurance disputes; probate proceedings involving contested wills; and administrative proceedings. The certification and the underlying autopsy report typically form the primary evidence of the medical findings. Preparation for testimony draws on the systematic documentation developed during the case; the pathologist reviews the case documentation, refreshes recall of specific findings, and prepares to explain the reasoning supporting the certification. Expert testimony is developed in detail in Chapter 24; the certification is the summary document that anchors the testimony.

### Pandemic Certification Considerations

The 2020-2023 COVID-19 pandemic produced substantial certification-specific considerations that remain relevant for future infectious disease events. Death certificates for COVID-19-related deaths required specific coding to support the aggregate pandemic mortality tracking; guidance from the National Center for Health Statistics and from the World Health Organization was provided on certification for pandemic-related deaths. Distinguishing deaths from COVID-19 (where the disease was the direct cause) from deaths with COVID-19 (where the disease was present but not the direct cause) required specific reasoning; the certification framework accommodated both patterns. Contributing conditions in Part II were used to document COVID-19 status in cases where the disease contributed to the terminal event but was not the primary cause. Similar frameworks would apply to future pandemic events; the professional community developed substantial practical experience during the COVID pandemic that informs ongoing preparation.

## International Death Certification Systems

Death certification systems in other countries follow similar general principles with specific national variations. The World Health Organization's International Classification of Diseases (currently ICD-11 in adoption, with ICD-10 still in widespread use) provides the international framework for cause of death coding. National vital statistics systems compile data using ICD codes with cross-national comparability supported through the standardized coding. Individual countries have specific manner of death categories (some using categories different from the five American categories) and specific certification procedures. International comparisons of mortality data draw on the standardized coding while acknowledging the specific procedural variations. American forensic pathologists working internationally or engaging with international mortality data develop familiarity with the specific system variations.

## Data Quality in Death Certification

Data quality in the aggregate death certification system depends on the quality of individual certifications. Studies of death certificate accuracy have identified specific quality issues: vague or non-specific cause of death entries ("cardiac arrest," "respiratory failure" without further specification); underuse of contributing conditions in Part II; incorrect coding based on inadequate information in the certification; and specific miscoding patterns across certain cause categories. Improvement in data quality requires attention at both the individual certification level and the aggregate coding level. Some jurisdictions have implemented specific quality improvement programs targeting certification accuracy; the National Association of Medical Examiners has published guidance on certification practices supporting data quality. Continued attention to certification accuracy supports both individual case documentation and aggregate data quality.

## Specific Certification Guidance From Professional Organizations

Professional organizations provide specific certification guidance for challenging case types. The National Association of Medical Examiners has published guidance on certification of drug-related deaths, sudden cardiac death cases, deaths in custody, deaths of infants, and other specific case categories. The College of American Pathologists provides guidance relevant to specific case types. State medical examiner and coroner organizations provide state-specific guidance. Familiarity with the current published guidance supports certifications aligned with the professional consensus practices. Guidance evolves with advancing evidence and practice; the pathologist maintains current familiarity with published guidance in areas of active certification decision-making.

## Communication With the Vital Records Office

The relationship between the medical examiner's office and the state vital records office supports both individual case certification and aggregate data quality. Direct communication when specific coding questions arise supports accurate representation of the pathologist's intent in the aggregate coding. Periodic coordination between the offices on aggregate patterns, systematic issues, and quality improvement supports both parties. The vital records office provides the aggregate coding function and interfaces with the National Center for Health Statistics for federal-level compilation; the medical examiner's office provides the individual case documentation. Effective coordination between these functions is central to the aggregate quality of the mortality data.

### The Historical Development of Death Certification

Death certification has a substantial historical development that informs current practice. Systematic recording of deaths for public health purposes developed in the 17th century with the Bills of Mortality in London providing early aggregate mortality documentation. The systematic use of medical certification for cause of death developed through the 19th century with increasing standardization. The International Classification of Diseases originated in the 1890s and has evolved through successive revisions to the current framework. American vital statistics developed through state-based systems that were gradually coordinated at the federal level; the National Vital Statistics System with its current structure developed through the 20th century. Understanding this historical context supports appreciation of the specific choices in current certification frameworks and the ongoing evolution of the practice.

### Electronic Death Registration and Digital Certification

Electronic Death Registration Systems (EDRS) have progressively replaced paper-based certification systems in most American jurisdictions. The systems support electronic filing of death certificates by physicians and by medical examiners, with real-time integration with the state vital records office. Benefits include reduced administrative burden, faster certificate processing (supporting more timely release of remains and completion of family administrative needs), improved data quality through built-in validation, and integration with the aggregate coding process. Adoption has been uneven across states, and paper-based backup systems remain necessary for specific circumstances. The pathologist working with EDRS develops facility with the specific state system; changes in EDRS platforms occur periodically and require adaptation. Integration between EDRS and the medical examiner's case management system supports efficient workflow when properly implemented.

### Jurisdictional Variation in Certification Authority

Jurisdictional variation in certification authority produces substantial variation across states. Medical examiner states (where the office is directed by a physician with forensic pathology expertise) and coroner states (where the office is directed by an elected official who may not be a physician) approach certification differently. Within coroner states, the certification may be performed by the coroner personally, by a designated deputy, or by a physician consultant. State statutes define specific jurisdiction over cases; the specific categories and thresholds vary substantially. Mixed systems (with some jurisdictions using medical examiners and others using coroners within the same state) exist in several states. The pathologist working across jurisdictional boundaries or consulting on cases from other jurisdictions develops familiarity with the specific frameworks. Efforts to standardize American death investigation have proceeded through several decades of professional advocacy but substantial variation persists.

## Certification of Deaths in Custody and Deaths During Law Enforcement Encounters

Deaths in custody and deaths during law enforcement encounters (developed in Chapter 16) require specific certification consideration. Manner determinations in these cases carry substantial public interest and are often contested. Homicide manner in officer-involved fatalities is applied when the specific case reasoning supports the action of the officer as the cause of death, even when the action was legally justified; the manner reflects the medical determination of cause rather than the legal determination of justification. Deaths of individuals in custody from natural causes (heart disease during custody, complications of medical conditions) are certified as natural. Deaths from other mechanisms during custody or law enforcement encounters are certified according to the systematic reasoning. Public interest in these cases makes clear and defensible certification particularly important; the reasoning is documented transparently in the autopsy report.

## Complex Cases Requiring Consultation

Complex certification cases benefit from consultation with colleagues. Cases with unusual pathology, unusual mechanism, competing possible causes, or specific case circumstances warrant discussion. Peer consultation within the office, formal consultation with regional experts, and case discussion through professional networks provide support for challenging determinations. National Association of Medical Examiners peer review and case discussion opportunities support difficult determinations. The pathologist recognizing that a specific case exceeds their comfort level in certification is exercising appropriate professional judgment by seeking consultation; the certification reflects the aggregate expertise brought to the reasoning. Documentation of the consultation in the case file supports transparency about the reasoning process.

## The Certification as a Professional Product

The death certification is a professional product that reflects the pathologist's systematic case work. Attention to specificity, accuracy, and completeness in each certification supports the individual case, the aggregate function, and the professional standing of the pathologist. Certifications that will be reviewed by families, by attorneys, by insurance representatives, by public health officials, and by other pathologists benefit from care in preparation. The specific language on the certificate should be clear to a lay reader while precise for professional interpretation. Explanatory documentation in the autopsy report supports the certification and provides the reasoning behind the specific language. The certification is the visible product of the case work; the report provides the reasoning supporting it.

**The Certification Function:** The death certificate serves both immediate legal and administrative functions and aggregate public health surveillance. The forensic pathologist certifying medicolegal cases summarizes the systematic case reasoning in a form suitable for the official record. The certificate and the autopsy report are complementary elements of the case documentation.

**Cause of Death Cascade:** The cause of death cascade documents the immediate cause (the specific physiological event producing death), the intermediate causes (the mechanisms leading from underlying cause to immediate cause), and the underlying cause (the disease or injury initiating the cascade). Part II documents contributing conditions supporting aggregate clinical context. The cascade reads as a coherent narrative of the specific events producing this death.

**The Five Manner Categories:** Natural, accident, suicide, homicide, and undetermined are the five manner categories. Each has specific reasoning framework: natural requires disease process without external contribution; accident requires unintentional external cause; suicide requires evidence of intent to die; homicide requires action of another person causing death; undetermined reflects honest limits of the reasoning when specificity is not warranted.

**Special Considerations:** Presumptive certification with subsequent amendment, delayed certification pending workup, and specific case patterns including in-hospital deaths and sequelae of remote injury each have specific certification approaches. Amendment and correction procedures follow state vital records office requirements.

**Aggregate Function:** The aggregate function of death certification supports vital statistics, epidemiological research, and public health surveillance. Individual certifications contribute to aggregate mortality data through the coding process. Specific and accurate certifications support both individual case and aggregate purposes.

## Summary and Key Concepts

The death certificate is the official legal document recording death and serves both immediate legal and administrative functions and aggregate public health surveillance. The forensic pathologist certifying medicolegal cases has specific responsibility for the medical certification.

The cause of death cascade in Part I documents the immediate cause, intermediate causes, and underlying cause; Part II documents contributing conditions. The cascade reads as a coherent narrative of the specific events producing death.

The five manner of death categories — natural, accident, suicide, homicide, and undetermined — each have specific reasoning framework. The determination reflects systematic case reasoning integrating findings across autopsy, toxicology, scene, and history.

Special certification considerations include presumptive certification with amendment when workup completes, delayed certification pending analysis, in-hospital deaths, and sequelae of remote injury. Amendment and correction follow state vital records procedures.

The aggregate function of death certification supports vital statistics, epidemiological research, and public health surveillance. Specific and accurate individual certifications support both immediate case purposes and aggregate public health understanding.

The professional responsibility of the certifying pathologist extends beyond the individual case to the aggregate contribution. Vague certifications limit the aggregate value; specific certifications support both functions.

# CHAPTER 23: AUTOPSY REPORT AND MEDICOLEGAL DOCUMENTATION

**Learning Objectives**

1. Articulate the purpose and structure of the forensic autopsy report and its relationship to the death certificate.
2. Perform systematic external and internal examination documentation supporting both individual case reasoning and subsequent review.
3. Apply photographic documentation standards preserving spatial relationships, scale, and clinical detail.
4. Document special case elements including specific injury patterns, toxicological workups, ancillary studies, and consulting specialist findings.
5. Maintain the case file with appropriate preservation, access controls, and quality assurance for subsequent review, legal proceedings, and aggregate function.

## The Autopsy Report: Purpose and Structure

The autopsy report is the comprehensive documentation of the forensic autopsy examination and the associated case investigation. Where the death certificate serves as the summary official document, the autopsy report provides the complete underlying documentation supporting the certification. The report serves multiple substantial functions: it preserves the systematic case reasoning in a form supporting later review; it provides the primary evidence in legal proceedings arising from the death; it supports quality assurance and peer review within the forensic pathology practice; and it contributes to the aggregate documentation of specific case patterns for professional education and research. Attention to report quality supports each of these functions.

The structure of the autopsy report varies across offices and jurisdictions but follows general principles reflecting the systematic case investigation. Most reports include: administrative sections identifying the case and the participants; a case history section describing the circumstances leading to the examination; a documentation of the external examination; a documentation of the internal examination organized systematically; specific documentation of injuries, ancillary studies, and consulting specialist findings; a summary of findings with correlation to cause and manner determination; and appropriate identification of the pathologist and other personnel involved. The specific format and structure follow office practice with attention to consistency across the practice.

The forensic pathologist preparing the report develops it as an integrated document that supports both the immediate case documentation and the range of subsequent uses. The language is precise and defensible, the organization supports the systematic reasoning, and the level of detail provides adequate documentation without excessive length. Reports that are too abbreviated fail to support the range of uses; reports that are excessively long may obscure the specific findings and reasoning. The professional standard develops through practice and mentorship, and offices typically maintain internal templates and quality standards that support consistent reporting.

### The Relationship Between the Report and the Certificate

The relationship between the autopsy report and the death certificate is complementary. The certificate provides the summary official documentation for administrative and vital statistics purposes; the report provides the underlying case documentation supporting the certification and available for detailed review. In most cases, the report is not routinely distributed with the certificate — the certificate is the public-facing document while the report is available on specific request through appropriate legal or administrative process. The relationship supports both the routine administrative flow and the specific documentation available when the case requires deeper examination.

**KEY POINT:** The autopsy report provides comprehensive documentation of the forensic examination supporting the death certificate summary. The report serves individual case documentation, legal proceedings, quality assurance, and aggregate professional function. Attention to report quality supports each of these functions.

## External and Internal Examination Documentation

The examination documentation is the substantive core of the autopsy report and provides the systematic record of findings identified during the physical examination.

### External Examination

External examination documentation includes: demographic and identifying information about the decedent (apparent age, sex, ancestry, general condition of the body); overall body measurements (height, weight, and specific measurements where relevant); documentation of clothing and personal effects as received (with attention to any relevant findings on the clothing including damage patterns and biological material); systematic description of external features (hair, eyes, teeth, general body configuration); documentation of postmortem changes (rigor mortis, livor mortis, decomposition status, environmental exposure findings) supporting the time-of-death reasoning; documentation of distinguishing features (tattoos, scars, birthmarks, surgical scars) supporting identification; and systematic documentation of external injuries with attention to specific patterns. The description proceeds systematically from head to feet, with the specific level of detail reflecting the case circumstances.

### Internal Examination

Internal examination documentation follows the systematic organ-by-organ approach with each organ described in terms of weight, size, external appearance, cut surface, and any specific findings. The examination proceeds through the standard cavities (thorax, abdomen, cranium) with each cavity described systematically. Specific systems (cardiovascular, respiratory, gastrointestinal, genitourinary, endocrine, hematolymphoid, nervous) are documented with attention to system-specific findings.

### Negative Findings

Documentation of negative findings — features that were examined and found to be absent or normal — is as important as documentation of positive findings. Absence of specific findings supports the case reasoning in specific ways: absence of trauma in a natural death case documents the systematic exclusion of trauma; absence of specific findings in a suspicious death case documents the systematic evaluation. Standardized statements such as "The brain shows no evidence of trauma, hemorrhage, or acute pathology" document the systematic examination of the specific organ with the negative finding. The specific pattern of positive and negative findings supports the aggregate case reasoning and demonstrates the systematic approach to the examination.

Figure 23.1: The Autopsy Report Structure and Information Flow

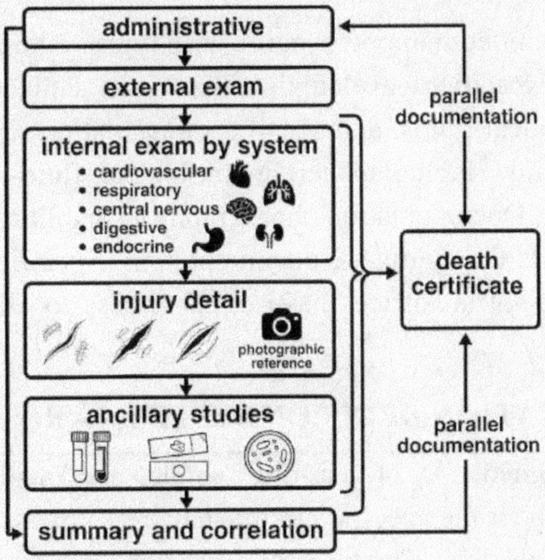


## Photographic Documentation Standards

Photographic documentation is central to modern forensic pathology practice. Photographs preserve specific findings in a form that supports later review, provides visual evidence for legal proceedings, and integrates with the aggregate case documentation.

### Systematic Photography

Systematic photography follows established protocols. Overall documentation photographs establish the general state of the body at reception and at various points during the examination. Regional documentation photographs capture specific anatomical regions with the relationships to surrounding structures. Detail photographs capture specific findings with attention to close-focus and appropriate scale. Photographs of injuries follow specific standards: overall photograph showing the injury in relation to the body region; medium-distance photograph documenting the injury with adjacent anatomy; close-up photograph with scale (ruler or standardized reference) documenting the injury detail. The systematic approach ensures adequate documentation of each finding at multiple levels of detail.

### Scale, Lighting, and Standardization

Scale reference in photographs supports subsequent measurement and comparison. Standardized rulers or scales positioned adjacent to findings during photography provide dimensional reference. Consistent lighting supports comparison across photographs; direct lighting typically works for detail photography with color-neutral illumination preferred. Consistent background (typically neutral gray or blue autopsy tables) supports the visual documentation. Photographic technique standardization across the practice supports consistency; new pathologists learn the specific office standards during training. Modern digital photography with high resolution and appropriate processing supports both immediate and long-term documentation.

### Special Photographic Techniques

Special photographic techniques support specific case types. Alternative light source photography (using ultraviolet, infrared, or specific wavelength filters) can enhance visualization of specific findings including bruising, biological fluids, and specific injury patterns. Fluorescence photography documents specific fluorescent findings including certain biological fluids. Macrophotography with specialized lenses captures fine detail. Documentation photography of ancillary studies (histology slides, radiographs, imaging findings) supports the aggregate documentation. Specific technique training supports effective use of these approaches; not all offices have equal access to all techniques, and practice varies with available equipment.

### SCENE-TO-CERTIFICATION DECISION SYSTEM — Report Structure Reasoning Arc

**Presenting Death Scenario:** A 24-year-old woman is found deceased in her apartment. Initial investigation is unclear about the specific circumstances — the scene is not overtly violent but includes some findings that raise questions. The medical examiner's office accepts jurisdiction and coordinates the case investigation. The pathologist recognizes that this case may involve subsequent legal proceedings (possible criminal prosecution or civil litigation) and prepares the case documentation accordingly.

**Autopsy Signature:** The case examination proceeds systematically. External examination documents the decedent's features, absence of overt trauma, and specific findings that require careful documentation including subtle bruising at the neck, possibly consistent with recent restraint. Photographs document each finding at multiple levels of detail with scale reference. Internal examination proceeds systematically with each organ documented; specific findings including subtle intracranial hemorrhage, subtle petechial hemorrhages consistent with asphyxial mechanism, and specific soft tissue findings are documented with photographs. Ancillary studies include comprehensive toxicology, sexual assault evidence collection given the circumstances, and specific consultative studies. The report is prepared with attention to the specific findings, the reasoning supporting each, and the aggregate case reasoning integrating the systematic evaluation.

**Cause Determination:** Cause of death is determined based on the aggregate findings identifying asphyxial mechanism consistent with strangulation.

**Manner Determination:** Homicide.

**Trap Logic:** The trap in case documentation for cases that will involve substantial legal review is either underdocumentation (missing specific findings that later prove important, or failing to document the reasoning transparently) or overdocumentation (excessive detail that obscures the specific findings and reasoning). Systematic reporting: documents each finding at appropriate level of detail; provides photographic support for specific findings; documents both positive and negative findings supporting the aggregate reasoning; and integrates the findings into a coherent case reconstruction. The report supports subsequent review by opposing experts, by prosecutors, by defense counsel, and by appellate courts; attention to quality at the initial preparation supports each of these later functions.

**Certification Anchor:** The autopsy report is the primary case documentation supporting the death certificate. Attention to systematic documentation, photographic support, negative finding documentation, and aggregate reasoning integration supports both individual case function and subsequent legal proceedings.

## Special Documentation: Injuries, Toxicology, Ancillary Studies

Beyond the general examination documentation, several special documentation elements deserve specific attention.

### Injury Documentation

Injury documentation follows specific standards reflecting the forensic significance of injuries in many cases. Each injury is documented with: anatomical location (specific reference to body region and relationship to landmarks); dimensions (with measurement); character (contusion, abrasion, laceration, incised wound, stab wound, gunshot wound); direction and orientation where applicable; specific features (patterned features suggesting a specific mechanism, presence of foreign material, healing status); and photographic documentation. The systematic approach supports the injury reconstruction and provides the specific documentation required for the case reasoning. Multiple injuries are documented in a systematic sequence (top-down, or by region) with each individually characterized.

### Toxicology and Analytical Documentation

Toxicology and analytical study documentation integrates the analytical results into the case documentation. The autopsy report typically includes: the specimens collected (with specific collection sites and volumes); the specific analyses ordered; the results as reported by the analytical laboratory; and the pathologist's interpretation of the results in the case context. The specific quantitative results are documented; interpretive comments explain the significance in the case reasoning. The relationship between the autopsy report and the toxicology report is clarified — the toxicology report is the primary analytical documentation while the autopsy report incorporates the interpretation.

### Consulting Specialist Integration

Consulting specialist findings are integrated into the aggregate case documentation. Forensic anthropology consultation results, forensic odontology examination results, neuropathology consultation results, cardiac pathology consultation results, and other specialist input are documented in the report with reference to the consulting specialist and the specific findings. The individual consulting reports are typically included in the case file; the autopsy report incorporates the key findings and integrates them into the aggregate case reasoning. This approach preserves the specialist's specific documentation while providing the integrated case reasoning.

Figure 23.2: Photographic Documentation Approach: Multiple Levels of Detail

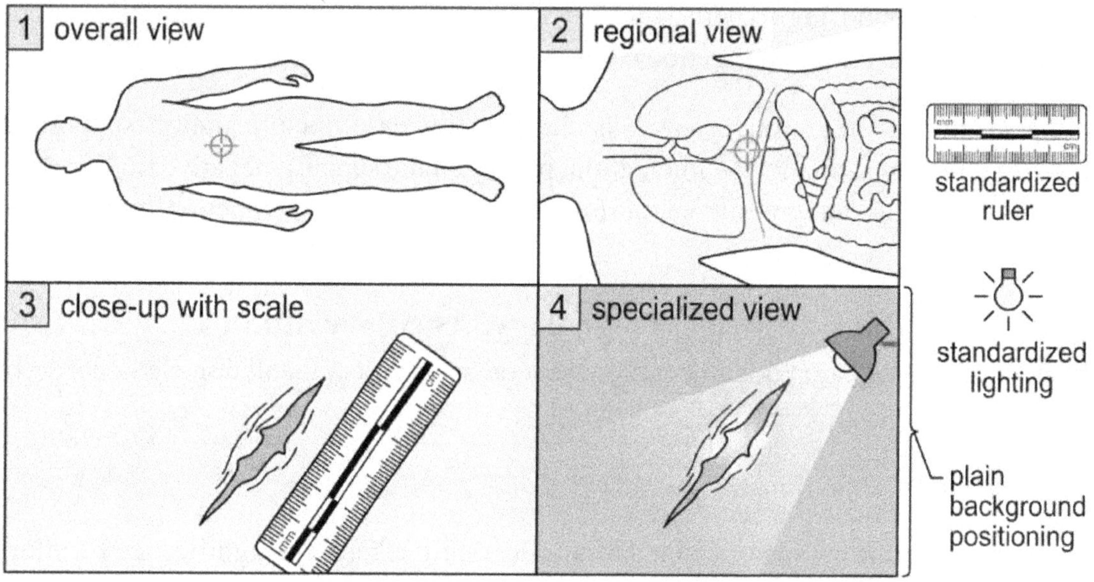


## The Case File and Its Preservation

The case file encompasses the complete documentation of the case: the autopsy report and its associated materials, the specimens and their tracking, the photographs, the ancillary study reports, the consulting specialist reports, the scene documentation received from law enforcement, and any other case-specific materials.

### Case File Organization

Case file organization follows office practice with attention to systematic organization supporting later retrieval and review. Standard elements include: administrative documentation identifying the case; the autopsy report and its amendments; photographs (typically organized systematically with reference to the report); ancillary study reports; consulting specialist reports; specimen tracking documentation; scene documentation; and any correspondence or communication related to the case. Digital case files typically use structured folders with standardized naming; paper case files use standard filing structures. The systematic organization supports efficient retrieval when subsequent review is required.

### Retention and Preservation

Retention periods for forensic case files vary by state statute and office policy but are typically substantial — many jurisdictions require retention of medical examiner case files for the decedent's life plus a specified period, or indefinitely for specific case categories. Preservation of physical specimens (blocks, slides, other tissue) follows specific protocols; specimens supporting cases in active investigation or with pending legal proceedings are preserved indefinitely, while other specimens follow standard retention. Photographs are preserved digitally with backup systems supporting long-term retention. The retention approach supports both individual case function and the potential for subsequent review, legal proceedings, or research use.

### Access Control and Confidentiality

Access control for case files preserves confidentiality of sensitive case information while enabling appropriate access for legitimate purposes. Family members typically have access to the autopsy report through specific request procedures; law enforcement has access through the investigation process; opposing counsel in legal proceedings has access through discovery; and other authorized parties have access through appropriate procedures. Unauthorized access is prevented through office security procedures. Public release of case information typically requires specific authorization and is restricted to non-sensitive summary information in most jurisdictions. The specific access control framework varies by state and reflects the balance between transparency and confidentiality.

### SCENE-TO-CERTIFICATION DECISION SYSTEM — Documentation Chain Integrity Arc

**Presenting Death Scenario:** A homicide case from three years earlier is being prepared for trial. The case involved substantial forensic pathology examination with multiple injuries requiring documentation, specific ancillary studies, and consulting specialist input. Defense counsel has requested access to the complete case file for review. The prosecutor requests the pathologist to review the file for trial preparation and to prepare for expert testimony. The case file must support both parties' needs while preserving the systematic reasoning documented at the original examination.

**Autopsy Signature:** The case file is retrieved from the office archive. The autopsy report documents the systematic examination: external documentation of the multiple injuries with specific characterization; internal examination documentation showing the injury pattern and associated findings; ancillary study integration including toxicology and specific studies; and photographic documentation supporting each finding. The photograph archive is intact with the specific images referenced in the report. The consulting specialist reports (neuropathology, forensic anthropology assessment of specific findings) are present. The systematic case reasoning is documented transparently. Preparation for testimony draws on the systematic documentation to refresh the pathologist's recall and to prepare for specific questions.

**Cause Determination:** The cause of death originally certified is confirmed through review of the systematic documentation.

**Manner Determination:** Homicide (as originally certified).

**Trap Logic:** The value of the case file preserved with attention to systematic documentation is evident when subsequent proceedings require access. A case file with abbreviated documentation, missing photographs, unrecorded reasoning, or inadequate consulting integration may not adequately support subsequent review. The trap is expected: cases from years earlier require the reasoning to be documented at the time of the examination because subsequent recall alone is inadequate. Attention to systematic documentation at case preparation supports the range of subsequent functions the case file must serve. The specific proceedings arising from this case demonstrate the value of the initial documentation quality.

**Certification Anchor:** The case file with systematic documentation supports the range of subsequent functions including legal proceedings, family requests, quality review, and aggregate professional function. Attention to documentation quality at case preparation supports each of these subsequent functions.

## Report Quality Standards and Peer Review

Quality standards for autopsy reports have developed through professional consensus and are documented in specific guidance from professional organizations.

### Professional Guidance

The National Association of Medical Examiners has published inspection and accreditation standards that include specific requirements for autopsy reports. The College of American Pathologists provides guidance on documentation standards. State medical examiner and coroner offices typically have specific standards reflecting the state framework. Individual office standards typically incorporate these external standards with office-specific requirements. Familiarity with current professional standards supports report preparation aligned with the consensus practices.

### Peer Review Systems

Peer review of autopsy reports supports quality assurance through systematic evaluation of specific cases. Common approaches include: initial peer review of specific case categories (homicides, complex cases, cases with specific concerns) supporting the specific case quality; ongoing case review of a sample of cases supporting aggregate quality assessment; and formal peer review through professional organizations or academic consultation for specific challenging cases. The peer review process is confidential to preserve the review function while supporting the aggregate quality. Documentation of the review process is maintained as part of the office quality assurance program.

## Continuous Quality Improvement

Continuous quality improvement in forensic pathology practice integrates individual case review with aggregate practice improvement. Common quality improvement approaches include: analysis of specific case categories for systematic issues; review of amendments and corrections identifying patterns suggesting training needs; evaluation of specific report elements for quality trends; and integration of professional guidance updates into practice. The office quality improvement program supports both individual practitioner development and aggregate practice improvement.

Figure 23.3: The Case File Archive: Organization and Access

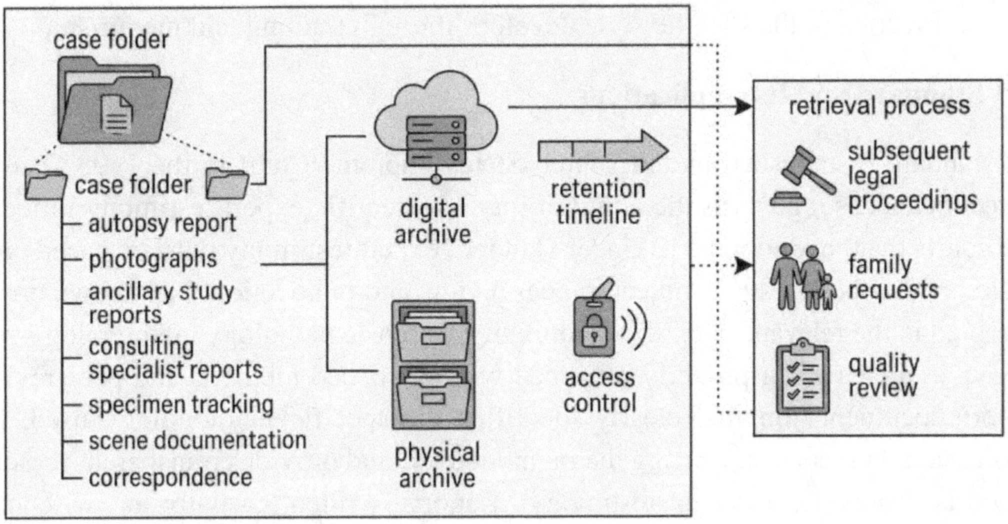


## Accreditation and External Review

Accreditation of forensic pathology offices through the National Association of Medical Examiners inspection program provides external review of practice standards. The inspection reviews facility standards, personnel qualifications, case management, report quality, and specific practice elements. Accreditation supports professional recognition and provides external validation of practice quality. Non-accredited offices may follow similar internal standards without the external validation; accreditation is not universally achievable due to resource constraints in smaller offices but represents the professional standard where feasible.

## The Report as Professional Product

The autopsy report, like the death certificate, is a professional product that reflects the pathologist's systematic case work and supports the range of subsequent functions the case documentation serves. Attention to quality at report preparation — including systematic organization, appropriate detail, defensible language, and integration of the aggregate case reasoning — supports each of the subsequent uses. Reports that will be reviewed by opposing counsel, appellate courts, professional peers, and public health researchers benefit from careful preparation. The report is the visible product of the case work and reflects the professional standing of the pathologist.

### Report Writing Style and Voice

Report writing style in forensic pathology has developed specific conventions that support clarity, defensibility, and consistency. The report is typically written in a formal, third-person voice describing observed findings rather than in narrative first-person. Specific findings are described with precise language: "There is a linear abrasion measuring 3.2 centimeters," rather than "I saw a scratch." Anatomical location uses precise reference to landmarks. Measurements are provided with appropriate units and precision. Interpretive language is distinguished from descriptive language — the description states what was observed; interpretive statements identify the pathologist's reasoning about the significance of what was observed. This distinction supports both the descriptive rigor and the interpretive transparency of the aggregate report. Practice of the specific style develops through training and mentorship.

### The Daubert Standard and Its Implications

The Daubert standard (established by the United States Supreme Court in the 1993 Daubert v. Merrell Dow Pharmaceuticals case) governs the admissibility of scientific expert testimony in federal court and in many state courts that have adopted it. Under Daubert, expert testimony must be based on methodology that is: testable and has been tested; subject to peer review and publication; has known error rates; and is generally accepted in the relevant scientific community. Forensic pathology methodology generally meets the Daubert requirements when properly practiced with published methods and peer-reviewed research support. Report documentation that clearly identifies the specific methodology used, references the aggregate professional practice supporting the methodology, and provides transparent reasoning about the findings supports Daubert-compliant testimony. Reports written casually or without attention to methodology transparency may compromise subsequent testimony admissibility.

### Documentation of Consultation and Second Opinions

Documentation of consultation with colleagues, second opinions, and peer input is a specific report element that supports transparency. When the case reasoning includes consultation with a colleague on specific findings, the consultation is documented with reference to the specific input received. When a second opinion is sought on specific findings, the second opinion source and content are documented. When the pathologist changes an initial impression based on subsequent findings or input, the change is documented rather than obscured. This transparency supports both the professional integrity of the reasoning and the aggregate case documentation. Consultation is a strength of forensic practice, not a weakness; documentation of consultation demonstrates professional engagement with the case reasoning.

### International Variation in Report Structure

International variation in autopsy report structure reflects national frameworks. European forensic pathology traditions have developed specific reporting conventions that differ from American practice in specific elements: some European reports separate the descriptive documentation from the interpretive summary more explicitly; some include specific legal or administrative elements not standard in American reports; some use different systematic organization approaches. British Commonwealth countries follow related but distinct patterns. Understanding international variation supports both engagement with international cases (deaths involving decedents of foreign nationality with potential foreign legal proceedings) and the professional understanding of the broader forensic pathology framework.

**Specific Report Elements for Different Case Types**

Different case types have specific report element considerations. Homicide cases require particular attention to injury documentation, chain of custody documentation for physical evidence, and thorough documentation of reasoning supporting the specific manner determination. Suicide cases require documentation of the specific evidence supporting intent. Accident cases require documentation of the specific mechanism and the reasoning excluding alternative causes. Natural death cases require systematic documentation of the disease process supporting the cause determination. Pediatric cases require particular attention to specific findings supporting or excluding non-accidental mechanism. Drug-related deaths require systematic toxicological interpretation integration. Each case type benefits from attention to the specific elements most relevant to the case reasoning.

**Family Communication Documentation**

Family communication during and after the case is a specific element that benefits from documentation. When families receive information about the case findings from the office, the specific communication is typically documented in the case file. When families have specific questions about the case, the questions and the responses are documented. When family concerns arise about the findings or the process, the concerns and the response are documented. This documentation supports both the family relationship and the aggregate case record. Some offices have integrated family engagement specialists into the communication function; others have the pathologist directly involved in specific family communications. The specific approach reflects office practice.

**Aggregate Reporting for Research and Public Health**

Aggregate reporting from forensic pathology practice supports research and public health function beyond the individual case. De-identified case data from series of cases can be aggregated for research purposes with appropriate ethical oversight. Aggregate mortality data for specific case categories (drug overdose deaths, homicides, specific injury patterns) supports public health surveillance and policy development. The aggregate function is served by attention to consistency and completeness in individual case documentation; cases documented with attention to systematic detail contribute to aggregate research and surveillance in a form that supports meaningful analysis. Individual case authorship of research using de-identified case data has produced substantial forensic pathology literature through case series publications.

**Report Translation and Cross-Border Cases**

Some cases involve deaths of foreign nationals whose bodies are returned to their country of origin, or deaths that will involve foreign legal proceedings. In these cases, the autopsy report may require translation into the language of the receiving country and may need to conform to the reporting expectations of that jurisdiction. Working with translation services with forensic pathology familiarity supports accurate translation. Documentation prepared with attention to potential international use benefits from clarity of language and systematic organization that supports translation. In some cases, communication with the foreign forensic pathology authorities during case preparation supports the aggregate documentation.

### The Case Summary and Diagnosis Statements

The case summary at the end of the autopsy report integrates the specific findings into the aggregate case reasoning supporting the cause and manner determinations. The summary typically provides a narrative synthesis of the case: the presenting circumstances, the specific findings identified through the examination, the interpretation of those findings, and the specific reasoning supporting the certifications. A concise final diagnosis statement lists the specific pathologic diagnoses identified through the case work. The summary and diagnosis statements together provide the interpretive integration that transforms the descriptive documentation into the actionable case reasoning. Attention to clarity and precision in these final sections supports both the immediate case function and the subsequent uses of the report.

### Technology Integration in Report Preparation

Technology integration in report preparation has developed substantially over recent decades. Voice recognition software supports dictation of autopsy findings during examination. Case management systems integrate photographs, ancillary study results, and consulting reports with the aggregate case documentation. Digital signature systems support formal authentication of reports. Cross-reference systems support integration between related documents. Reporting templates support consistency across the practice and reduce administrative burden. The specific technology in use varies by office; the general trend is toward increased integration and reduced administrative time per case. Investment in technology infrastructure supports both case quality and office throughput.

### Training in Report Writing

Training in autopsy report writing is a substantial component of forensic pathology fellowship and early practice. Fellows work with senior pathologists reviewing initial reports, receiving feedback on style, organization, and specific content elements, and progressively developing individual reporting practice. The mentored development supports gradual acquisition of the specific reporting standards and the professional judgment required for effective reports. Continued professional development throughout practice includes engagement with reporting standards updates, participation in peer review, and reflection on personal reporting practice. Reporting quality is not fixed at fellowship completion; ongoing practice development refines the specific reporting approach through experience with the full range of case types and subsequent uses.

## Electronic Medical Record Integration

Integration of forensic pathology case documentation with broader electronic medical record systems has developed with mixed patterns. Some hospital-based medical examiner offices have integrated case management with the hospital electronic medical record; independent medical examiner offices typically maintain separate case management systems. Direct integration supports efficient exchange of clinical history and hospital records that inform case reasoning; separate systems require specific data exchange for the equivalent information transfer. Interoperability standards for exchange of forensic pathology data with clinical and public health systems have developed to varying degrees. The specific integration approach reflects the specific office context and available technology.

## Discovery and Legal Access to the Case File

Discovery and legal access to the case file follows specific procedures in criminal and civil proceedings. In criminal cases, the prosecution has access to the case file through the normal medical examiner-prosecutor working relationship; the defense obtains access through discovery under the specific rules of criminal procedure. In civil cases, parties obtain access through civil discovery mechanisms. The case file components typically produced in discovery include the autopsy report, photographs, ancillary study reports, consulting specialist reports, and related documentation. Some elements may be withheld under specific privilege claims (personal notes, peer review documentation in some jurisdictions). Attention to the potential discoverability of case file elements during case preparation supports both the systematic documentation and the appropriate handling of specific content categories.

## Quality Metrics for Reporting Practice

Quality metrics for reporting practice support both individual practitioner improvement and aggregate office quality assessment. Common metrics include: time from autopsy to report completion (with attention to timeliness for family and administrative purposes); report length and completeness measures; consistency in specific report elements; amendment and correction rates (with attention to systematic patterns suggesting training needs); and feedback from case reviewers, prosecutors, and other users. Systematic tracking of quality metrics supports continuous improvement in reporting practice. Some metrics are amenable to automated measurement through case management systems; others require manual review. The specific metrics used reflect office priorities and available measurement approach.

## Handling of Case Reopening and Long-Term Storage

Cases may require reopening or extended review years or decades after the initial examination for various reasons: new evidence emerging in previously unresolved investigations; identification of previously unidentified decedents; new appellate proceedings arising from earlier convictions; new information about the decedent's health context; or specific research use requiring access to the historical records. Long-term case file preservation with organized systematic documentation supports these subsequent uses. Cases from decades earlier may still require access; some notable cold cases have been resolved through examination of preserved specimens and documentation from earlier examinations. The retention discipline supports both the immediate case function and the very long-term function that cannot always be predicted at the initial examination.

### The Role of Case Documentation in Aggregate Professional Knowledge

Case documentation across the aggregate forensic pathology practice contributes substantially to the ongoing development of professional knowledge. Case reports and case series in the professional literature draw on documented cases from individual practices. Systematic reviews and meta-analyses synthesize documented case findings across multiple sources. Training programs use case examples from documented practice to illustrate specific patterns. Professional guidance development draws on case series documentation for the evidence base. Attention to documentation quality at individual case preparation supports the aggregate professional knowledge; abbreviated or inconsistent documentation limits the aggregate contribution. The individual pathologist's documentation practice thus contributes not only to the specific case but to the ongoing professional knowledge development. This aggregate contribution is a specific professional responsibility.

### SCENE-TO-CERTIFICATION DECISION SYSTEM — Documentation Determination Arcs

**The Report Function:** The autopsy report provides comprehensive documentation of the forensic examination supporting the death certificate summary. The report serves individual case documentation, legal proceedings, quality assurance, and aggregate professional function. Attention to report quality supports each of these functions.

**Systematic Documentation:** External and internal examination documentation follows systematic approach with attention to positive and negative findings, dimensional detail, and specific characterization of pathologic findings. Injury documentation follows specific standards supporting the forensic significance of each injury.

**Photographic Standards:** Photographic documentation supports the written examination with multiple levels of detail (overall, regional, close-up with scale) and specialized techniques as case circumstances warrant. Systematic photography protocols support consistency and adequate documentation across the practice.

**Case File Preservation:** The case file encompasses complete case documentation with systematic organization, appropriate retention, and access control preserving confidentiality while enabling legitimate access. The file supports individual case function and subsequent review through legal proceedings, family requests, and quality assurance.

**Quality and Peer Review:** Quality standards from professional organizations support consistent practice. Peer review systems support both individual case quality and aggregate practice improvement. Accreditation through external inspection provides validation of practice standards. Continuous quality improvement integrates individual and aggregate practice.

## Summary and Key Concepts

The autopsy report provides comprehensive documentation of the forensic examination supporting the death certificate summary. The report supports individual case documentation, legal proceedings, quality assurance, and aggregate professional function.

External and internal examination documentation follows systematic approach with attention to positive and negative findings. Injury documentation follows specific standards supporting the forensic significance of each injury.

Photographic documentation supports the written examination with multiple levels of detail and standardized technique. Scale reference and consistent standards support subsequent measurement and comparison.

Ancillary study integration and consulting specialist findings are incorporated into the aggregate case documentation. The report integrates the specific findings into the systematic case reasoning.

The case file encompasses complete case documentation with systematic organization, appropriate retention, and access control preserving confidentiality while enabling legitimate access.

Quality standards from professional organizations, peer review systems, and accreditation through external inspection support both individual case quality and aggregate practice improvement.

# CHAPTER 24: COURTROOM TESTIMONY AND EXPERT WITNESS

**Learning Objectives**

1. Articulate the role of the forensic pathologist as expert witness in criminal and civil legal proceedings.
2. Perform systematic pretrial preparation including case review, expert report preparation, and coordination with counsel.
3. Deliver effective direct examination testimony with attention to clarity, accuracy, and defensibility.
4. Respond effectively to cross-examination with attention to professional composure and honest engagement with legitimate challenges.
5. Apply the Daubert standard and related frameworks governing admissibility of expert testimony.
6. Recognize and maintain ethical standards and professional boundaries specific to expert witness practice.

## The Forensic Pathologist as Expert Witness

The forensic pathologist frequently serves as expert witness in legal proceedings arising from cases the office has investigated. Criminal cases including homicide prosecutions, drug-related death prosecutions, and terrorism cases commonly involve testimony by the certifying pathologist. Civil cases including wrongful death actions, insurance disputes, and product liability litigation similarly involve pathology testimony. Administrative proceedings including workers compensation, disability determinations, and licensing actions may involve testimony. The role of expert witness is a substantial component of forensic pathology practice, requiring specific skills and preparation distinct from the case examination itself.

The expert witness role differs fundamentally from the fact witness role. A fact witness testifies to specific observations — what the witness saw, heard, or experienced directly. An expert witness testifies to opinions and interpretations based on specialized knowledge, education, training, and experience that the witness brings to the case findings. The forensic pathologist testifies as an expert witness because the specialized medical knowledge required to interpret autopsy findings is beyond the general knowledge of the jury; the expert witness provides the interpretive framework the jury needs to understand the specific case findings.

The forensic pathologist testifying about a case they personally examined is both a fact witness (to their own observations during the examination) and an expert witness (in the interpretation of those observations). The dual role affects specific elements of the testimony: the pathologist testifies about specific findings observed during the examination as fact testimony, and about the interpretation of those findings as expert testimony. In cases where the pathologist is testifying about findings documented by another pathologist (as reviewing expert rather than examining expert), the role is expert testimony without the personal fact witness component. Understanding the specific role in each case supports effective preparation and delivery.

### Retention as Expert Witness

Retention as expert witness occurs through several patterns. For medicolegal cases the pathologist examined at the medical examiner's office, the pathologist typically testifies as a subpoenaed witness at the request of the prosecution or one of the parties, without specific retention arrangement or compensation beyond regular office responsibilities. For consulting expert work outside the pathologist's office jurisdiction, formal retention as expert witness with specific compensation arrangements applies; consulting cases may involve either prosecution or defense retention in criminal matters, or either party in civil matters. Both patterns of practice have specific characteristics and ethical requirements; the pathologist typically develops experience with both patterns over time.

**KEY POINT:** The forensic pathologist testifies both as fact witness to observations during their own case examination and as expert witness in interpretation of those findings. Understanding the specific role in each case supports effective preparation and delivery. Expert witness practice is a substantial component of forensic pathology practice requiring specific skills distinct from the case examination itself.

## Pretrial Preparation

Effective testimony depends on systematic pretrial preparation. The specific preparation activities support both the substantive content of the testimony and the presentation approach.

### Case Review

Case review before testimony includes: careful re-reading of the autopsy report and associated case documentation; review of photographs and other visual evidence; review of ancillary study reports and their interpretation; review of any subsequent findings or investigations affecting the case; and review of any related cases or comparative findings relevant to the testimony. The pathologist testifying about a case examined years earlier requires substantial review to refresh recall of the specific findings and reasoning; testimony without adequate review risks inaccuracy or apparent uncertainty that reduces credibility. The specific time required for review depends on the case complexity and the time since examination; complex cases from years earlier may require several hours of review.

### Coordination With Counsel

Coordination with counsel before testimony is standard and appropriate. The pathologist typically meets with the calling attorney to discuss: the specific topics expected to be covered in the testimony; the anticipated questions and the responses; specific case elements the attorney plans to highlight; any potential cross-examination challenges anticipated; and logistical arrangements for the testimony. This coordination is not coaching about what to say — the substantive content of the testimony reflects the pathologist's independent professional judgment — but rather coordination about how to communicate the professional findings effectively in the specific legal context. The specific coordination content is not privileged and may be inquired into during cross-examination; testimony should reflect the case findings, not a scripted narrative developed with counsel.

### Expert Report Preparation

In consulting expert cases, an expert report is typically prepared before deposition or trial testimony. The report documents the specific opinions the expert intends to offer, the basis for the opinions (methodology, materials reviewed, specific reasoning), and the credentials of the expert. Federal Rule of Civil Procedure 26 governs expert report requirements in federal civil cases; state rules govern state proceedings with similar general requirements. The expert report anchors the testimony — the testimony must be consistent with the report, and opinions not disclosed in the report may be excluded from testimony under specific rules. Preparation of the expert report requires substantial time and attention to accuracy; the report is subject to discovery and cross-examination review.

### Deposition Preparation

Deposition testimony in civil cases and specific criminal contexts requires specific preparation. The deposition is testimony under oath in a specific procedural context, typically at the office of one of the attorneys with a court reporter recording the testimony. Depositions can range from brief testimony on specific issues to extended examinations covering the full case content. Deposition testimony is preserved and can be used in subsequent trial testimony including cross-examination based on the deposition record. Careful preparation for deposition supports both the immediate deposition function and the subsequent trial use.

**Figure 24.1: Expert Testimony Process: From Case Preparation to Trial**

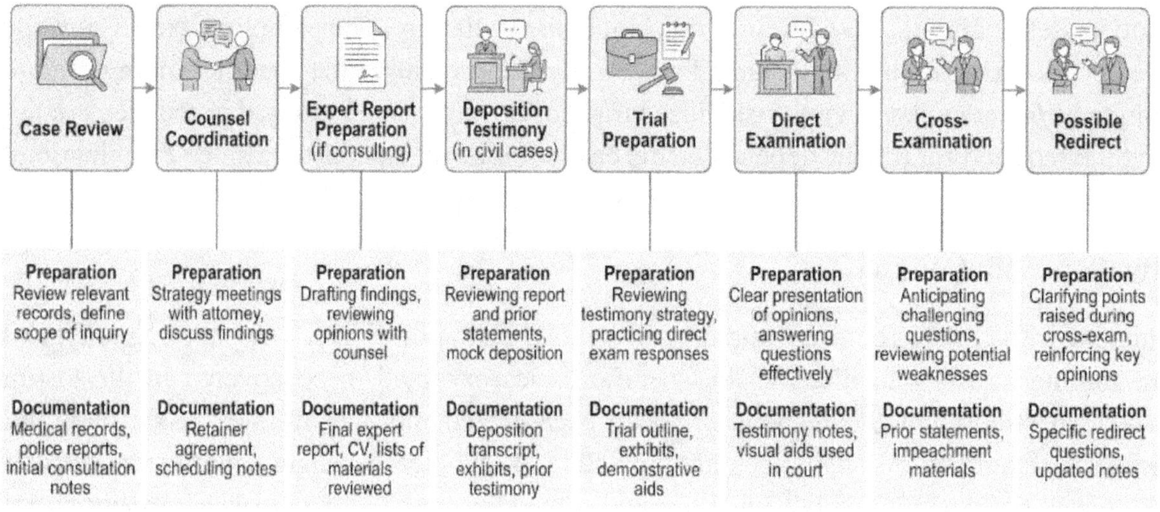

## Direct Examination and Testimony Delivery

Direct examination is the testimony delivered in response to questions from the party who called the witness. For the certifying pathologist testifying about a case examined at their office, direct examination typically comes from the prosecutor (in criminal cases) or the plaintiff's attorney (in civil cases). The pathologist responds to specific questions with substantive testimony about the case findings and their interpretation.

### Establishing Credentials

Direct examination typically begins with establishing the pathologist's credentials qualifying them as an expert witness. Questions address education, training, board certification, professional experience, publications, and prior expert testimony experience. The court formally qualifies the witness as an expert in the specific field before substantive testimony proceeds. The credential establishment supports the jury's assessment of the expert's qualifications; excessive elaboration is unnecessary but adequate documentation is important. Curriculum vitae is typically provided in advance and referred to during the credential examination.

### Explaining Findings to the Jury

The core of direct examination is explaining the case findings and their interpretation to the jury. The pathologist speaks in accessible language that jurors without medical background can understand, defines medical terms as they are used, and uses visual aids (photographs, diagrams, models) where they support the jury's understanding. Complex concepts are broken down into understandable elements. The testimony demonstrates the systematic case reasoning that supports the specific conclusions. Speaking directly to the jury (rather than to the calling attorney or to the court) supports the communication function. The specific style develops through experience and reflection on effective testimony.

### Use of Visual Evidence

Visual evidence including photographs, diagrams, and specific case materials supports the testimony. The pathologist references specific visual materials during testimony, explains what each shows, and integrates the visual with the verbal testimony. Photographs of injuries typically require careful presentation given the potentially disturbing content; the pathologist may work with counsel to identify appropriate photograph selection that supports the testimony without unnecessary emphasis on graphic content. Diagrams and models can support the jury's understanding of spatial relationships and specific mechanisms. The use of visual evidence is a professional communication skill developed through practice.

**SCENE-TO-CERTIFICATION DECISION SYSTEM — Testimony Preparation Arc**

**Presenting Death Scenario:** A homicide case is proceeding to trial approximately 18 months after the initial autopsy. The pathologist who performed the examination has received a subpoena from the prosecution to testify. The case involved multiple gunshot wounds with substantial reconstruction complexity. The pathologist has been in continuous practice since the examination but has managed hundreds of subsequent cases. Preparation for the specific case testimony requires substantial review and coordination.

**Autopsy Signature:** The pathologist retrieves the case file and conducts systematic review: the autopsy report documenting the specific gunshot wounds and their reconstruction; photographs documenting each wound at multiple levels of detail; ancillary study reports; and any subsequent case documentation. The pathologist meets with the prosecutor to discuss: the specific topics expected to be covered; anticipated defense cross-examination themes; specific case findings the prosecutor plans to emphasize; and logistical arrangements. The pathologist refreshes recall of the specific case reasoning including the wound track reconstructions and the aggregate case documentation. Preparation identifies specific elements requiring particular focus: the trajectory reconstruction and its supporting evidence, the systematic exclusion of alternative mechanisms, and the identification of specific injuries as fatal versus incapacitating.

**Cause Determination:** The multiple gunshot wound cause determination is confirmed through review.

**Manner Determination:** Homicide (as originally certified).

**Trap Logic:** The trap in testimony preparation is either inadequate review (arriving for testimony without adequate refresh of specific case details, risking inaccuracy or apparent uncertainty) or overrehearsal (creating scripted testimony that appears artificial or that fails to accommodate specific cross-examination challenges). Systematic preparation: reviews the systematic case documentation thoroughly; identifies specific case elements requiring particular attention; coordinates with counsel about the specific topics and approach without scripting the substantive content; and prepares for both direct and cross-examination. The specific preparation approach reflects the case complexity and the specific proceedings.

**Certification Anchor:** Testimony preparation involves systematic case review, coordination with counsel, and specific attention to the elements the specific proceeding will address. Preparation supports both the substantive content and the effective delivery of the testimony.

## Cross-Examination Strategies

Cross-examination by opposing counsel tests the specific case reasoning, the pathologist's methodology, and the aggregate credibility of the testimony. Effective cross-examination response requires specific approaches distinct from direct examination.

### Professional Composure

Professional composure during cross-examination is essential. Cross-examination questions may be aggressive, challenging, or apparently critical of the case work; the effective response is composed, professional, and substantive. Reactive responses (defensive body language, argumentative tone, emotional reactions) reduce credibility even when the substantive content of the testimony is correct. The pathologist maintains a professional demeanor throughout, treats opposing counsel with the same respect as the calling counsel, and responds to questions substantively rather than reactively. Composure develops through experience and reflection; new pathologists benefit from mentorship and observation of experienced witnesses.

### Honest Engagement With Legitimate Challenges

Honest engagement with legitimate challenges strengthens credibility. When opposing counsel identifies a valid limitation of the case reasoning — a specific finding that could support an alternative interpretation, a specific methodology limitation, an unresolved uncertainty — the effective response acknowledges the specific point honestly rather than deflecting or minimizing. Acknowledgment of legitimate limitations does not concede the case; systematic case reasoning includes recognition of limitations, and the pathologist who honestly acknowledges limitations demonstrates the systematic reasoning approach. Attempts to hide or minimize legitimate limitations damage credibility when the limitations are identified through further examination.

Figure 24.2: Testimony Delivery: Communication with the Jury

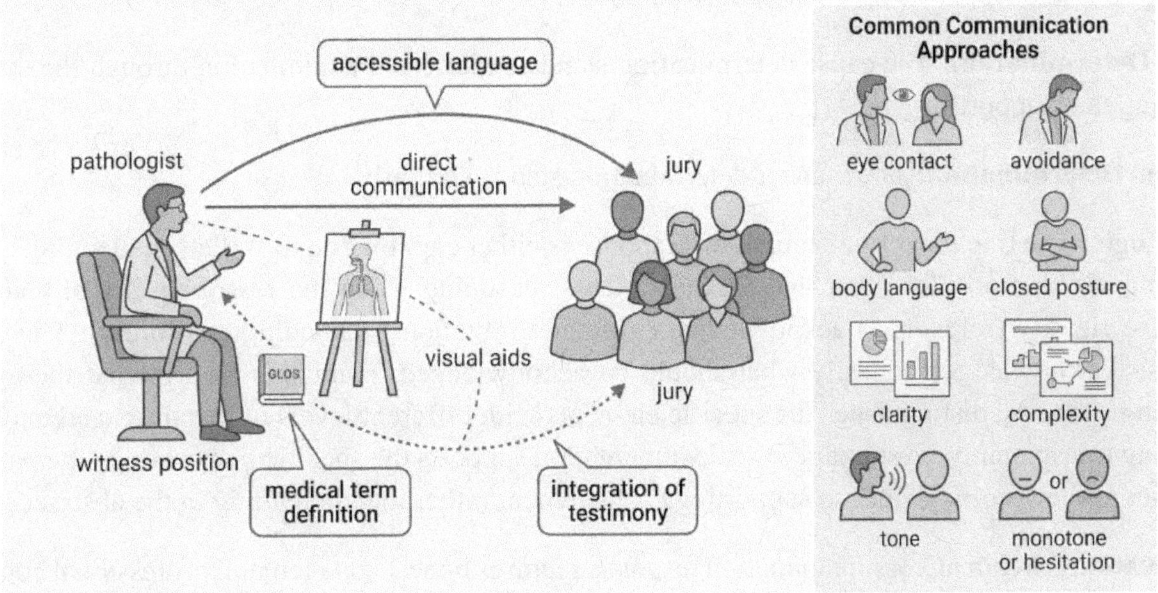


### Recognizing and Responding to Improper Questions

Some cross-examination questions are improperly framed, contain false premises, or attempt to elicit responses beyond the pathologist's expertise. Recognizing these questions and responding appropriately is a professional skill. Responses to false-premise questions may correct the premise before answering ("The question assumes X, but that's not accurate. What actually happened was Y."). Responses to questions beyond expertise acknowledge the limits ("I can't speak to that specific question; it's beyond my expertise as a forensic pathologist."). Responses to compound questions may separate the elements

("You've asked several things; let me address each."). The specific responses reflect the substantive content and the limits of appropriate testimony.

**SCENE-TO-CERTIFICATION DECISION SYSTEM — Cross-Examination Response Arc**

**Presenting Death Scenario:** During cross-examination in the homicide trial, defense counsel challenges the pathologist's wound trajectory reconstruction. The specific challenge suggests that the reconstruction is uncertain and that alternative interpretations could support the defense theory of the case. The cross-examination is skilled and identifies specific limitations of the reconstruction methodology. The pathologist must respond effectively while maintaining professional composure and honest engagement.

**Autopsy Signature:** The pathologist responds to the specific questions: acknowledges honestly the specific methodology used for the reconstruction and its recognized limitations; explains the specific evidence supporting the primary reconstruction; distinguishes between what the evidence establishes with high confidence and what elements have specific uncertainty; and integrates the aggregate case reasoning supporting the specific conclusions despite the acknowledged limitations. The pathologist maintains composure throughout the challenging questioning, does not become defensive or reactive, and treats the defense counsel with professional respect. When the defense counsel presents an alternative interpretation the pathologist believes is inconsistent with the evidence, the pathologist explains specifically why the alternative is not supported by the aggregate findings.

**Cause Determination:** The cause determination stands under cross-examination through the systematic reasoning that supports it.

**Manner Determination:** The manner determination stands similarly.

**Trap Logic:** The trap in cross-examination response is either capitulation to skilled challenging questions (agreeing with propositions that undermine the case reasoning when the reasoning actually stands) or defensive rigidity (refusing to acknowledge legitimate limitations, damaging credibility). The effective response: acknowledges honestly what should be acknowledged; maintains firmly what the aggregate reasoning supports; distinguishes the specific elements with different levels of certainty; and explains the reasoning transparently. Systematic case documentation supports the specific responses — the pathologist can point to the specific evidence supporting each element rather than defending in the abstract.

**Certification Anchor:** Cross-examination response requires honest engagement, professional composure, and substantive engagement with the specific challenges. The systematic case documentation supports specific responses; the systematic case reasoning supports the aggregate conclusions.

## The Daubert Standard and Admissibility of Testimony

The Daubert standard governs the admissibility of expert testimony in federal court and in most state courts that have adopted the framework. Understanding the standard supports both the preparation of admissible testimony and the response to admissibility challenges.

### The Daubert Framework

Under Daubert v. Merrell Dow Pharmaceuticals (1993), expert testimony must be based on scientific methodology that meets specific requirements. The trial judge acts as gatekeeper, evaluating whether proposed expert testimony meets the admissibility threshold. Key factors include: whether the methodology has been tested and is testable; whether it has been subjected to peer review and publication; the known error rate of the methodology; and general acceptance in the relevant scientific community. Additional factors developed through subsequent cases and Federal Rule of Evidence 702 amendments further refine the framework. The Daubert standard aims to exclude expert testimony that lacks scientific reliability while admitting testimony based on established scientific methodology.

### Forensic Pathology Methodology Under Daubert

Forensic pathology methodology generally meets Daubert requirements when properly practiced. Autopsy examination methodology is established through decades of practice and professional consensus. Toxicological interpretation methodology is documented in peer-reviewed literature. Injury interpretation follows established scientific principles. Cause and manner determination follows systematic reasoning documented through professional guidance. Testimony that clearly describes the specific methodology used, references the professional practice supporting the methodology, and provides transparent reasoning generally satisfies Daubert requirements. Testimony that appears speculative, that lacks methodological transparency, or that reaches beyond the pathologist's expertise may face admissibility challenges.

### Specific Areas of Daubert Challenge

Certain forensic pathology topics have faced specific Daubert challenges in recent litigation. Interpretation of specific pattern injuries (bite marks, tool marks in some contexts) has faced challenges based on questions about methodology reliability. Certain reconstruction methodologies (specific blood spatter analysis approaches) have faced challenges. Interpretation of specific findings in pediatric cases (particularly shaken baby syndrome and specific interpretations) has faced challenges in some jurisdictions. Understanding the specific areas of active challenge supports preparation for admissibility questions in relevant cases. The professional community engages with these challenges through evidence review, methodology refinement, and specific practice guidance.

### Preparing for Admissibility Challenges

Preparation for potential admissibility challenges includes: familiarity with the specific admissibility framework in the jurisdiction; ability to articulate the methodology used with reference to the professional literature; documentation of the specific reasoning supporting the opinions; and coordination with counsel regarding specific admissibility concerns. Response to Daubert challenges typically occurs in pretrial motions with the specific issue litigated before the substantive testimony proceeds; the pathologist may be called for the specific admissibility hearing to explain the methodology. Effective preparation supports admissibility outcomes when the methodology is properly established.

## Ethical Standards and Professional Boundaries

Expert witness practice involves specific ethical standards and professional boundaries. Attention to these standards supports both individual practice integrity and the aggregate credibility of the specialty.

### Objectivity and Independence

The forensic pathologist testifies as an independent expert based on the professional judgment about the case findings, not as an advocate for the retaining party. The testimony reflects what the case findings support, not what the retaining party wishes the testimony to support. This objectivity is fundamental to the professional role; testimony that appears to bend to the retaining party's preferences damages both individual credibility and the aggregate credibility of the specialty. In consulting cases where retention is by a specific party, the objectivity principle requires the pathologist to reach the honest conclusion regardless of the retaining party's preference. If the honest conclusion does not support the retaining party's case, the appropriate response is to communicate that finding rather than to modify the conclusion to fit the retention.

Figure 24.3: The Expert Witness Framework: Roles and Standards

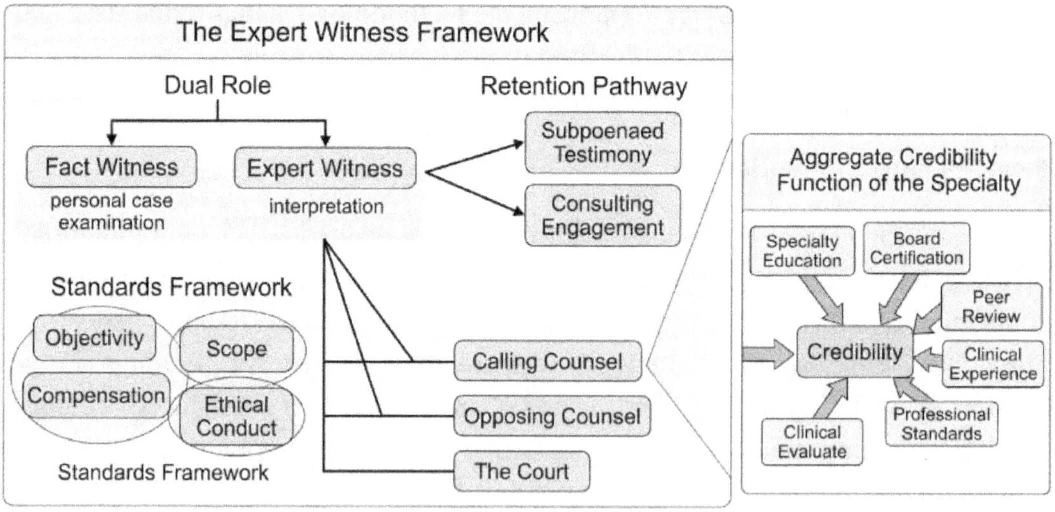


### Scope of Testimony

Testimony should remain within the scope of the pathologist's expertise and the specific case work. Questions outside the specific expertise (specific engineering questions, specific psychological questions, specific legal questions) warrant acknowledgment that the response is outside the pathologist's expert competence. Questions beyond the specific case work (interpretation of findings the pathologist did not personally review, hypothetical scenarios not grounded in the case) warrant careful response with clear identification of the specific basis. The professional boundary supports both the credibility of the specific testimony and the aggregate credibility of expert testimony.

### Compensation Standards

Compensation for expert witness work in consulting cases follows specific ethical standards. Compensation is for the pathologist's time and expertise regardless of the outcome of the case; contingent-fee arrangements (compensation dependent on outcome) are prohibited under professional standards because they compromise the objectivity of the testimony. Reasonable compensation reflects the specific time required for review, report preparation, and testimony. Disclosure of the specific compensation is appropriate during testimony when asked, and there is no ethical issue with reasonable compensation for professional expertise. Excessive compensation or specific compensation patterns suggesting bias may compromise credibility.

### Communication With Colleagues

Communication with colleagues about ongoing cases follows specific standards. Discussion of case specifics with pathologists retained by opposing parties is generally not appropriate during active proceedings; communication occurs through the formal legal process. Discussion of general methodology and reasoning with colleagues supporting professional development is appropriate. Peer review of specific opinions when authorized by the retaining party supports opinion quality. The specific communication standards vary with the specific case context; the general principle is transparency with the retaining party and appropriate confidentiality regarding the specific case content.

### The Pathologist's Aggregate Practice

The pathologist's aggregate expert witness practice is subject to review through both individual case testimony and broader patterns. Testimony history including prior expert engagements is subject to discovery and cross-examination. Patterns suggesting bias (testifying almost exclusively for one side, testifying beyond expertise, specific inconsistencies with prior testimony) can be identified through this review. Maintaining a professional practice with attention to objectivity, appropriate scope, and consistent reasoning supports the aggregate credibility over the extended career. Some pathologists develop specific consulting subspecialty (specific case types where they have particular expertise); others maintain general consulting practice; still others limit consulting work to focus on office practice. Each approach has its specific implications.

### Testimony in the Broader Professional Context

Individual expert testimony contributes to the aggregate professional standing of forensic pathology. Testimony that reflects systematic reasoning, honest engagement with challenges, and appropriate professional boundaries supports the aggregate credibility of the specialty. Testimony that reflects poorly on the professional standards — through inadequate preparation, apparent bias, methodology weakness, or ethical lapses — damages both the individual practitioner and the aggregate specialty standing. The professional community engages with concerns about problematic testimony patterns through peer review, professional discipline where applicable, and educational activities supporting improved practice. Maintaining professional standards in individual testimony contributes to the aggregate professional standing.

### Testimony in Specific Case Types

Different case types have specific testimony considerations. Homicide testimony typically involves substantial jury attention to specific injury details, wound reconstruction, and cause of death reasoning; visual evidence including photographs plays a central role. Drug-related death testimony involves the specific toxicological interpretation, the reasoning about specific mechanism, and the manner determination reasoning; jurors may be less familiar with the toxicological framework than with injury patterns. Pediatric testimony (particularly non-accidental injury cases and SUID cases) carries emotional weight requiring particular care in delivery; the specific findings supporting or excluding inflicted mechanism require careful explanation. Sexual assault case testimony involves specific findings and their interpretation with attention to preserving the dignity of both the decedent and the surviving parties. Each case type benefits from specific preparation aligned with the specific reasoning most relevant to the case.

### Grand Jury Testimony

Grand jury testimony precedes formal criminal charges in many homicide investigations. The forensic pathologist typically appears before the grand jury without opposing counsel present (grand jury proceedings are typically ex parte with only the prosecutor and the grand jurors present). Testimony explains the specific case findings supporting the criminal charges under consideration. The testimony is preserved through court reporter documentation and may be used in subsequent proceedings. Grand jury testimony has specific procedural characteristics distinct from trial testimony but similar preparation considerations. The grand jury testimony often provides an early opportunity to organize the case narrative that will subsequently be developed at trial.

### Media Attention and Public Communication

High-profile cases involve substantial media attention that affects the testimony context. Media coverage may develop before trial with substantial public interest in the specific case elements. The pathologist typically does not communicate directly with media about specific cases; office public information officers or the calling attorney manage media communication. The pathologist maintains professional composure with respect to media presence in the courtroom or nearby during testimony. Post-testimony media inquiries are typically declined or referred to the office public information officer. The specific media approach reflects office policy and the specific case circumstances. Managing the media context supports both the specific case testimony and the aggregate professional standing.

### Personal Safety and Security

Personal safety and security in expert witness practice is a specific consideration in some cases. High-profile testimony (particularly in cases involving organized criminal activity, terrorism, or specific threat contexts) may involve safety concerns for the testifying pathologist. Office security measures, court security, and specific personal security arrangements support safety when concerns exist. Threats received in response to testimony are documented and referred to appropriate law enforcement for evaluation. Continuing testimony practice despite specific safety concerns requires the aggregate support of the office, court system, and law enforcement. Most testimony proceeds without safety concerns, but recognition of the specific pattern in high-risk cases supports appropriate response when concerns arise.

### International Expert Witness Practice

International expert witness practice occurs when American forensic pathologists testify in foreign proceedings or when foreign forensic pathologists testify in American proceedings. The practice occurs in specific case contexts including international litigation, war crimes proceedings, and specific cross-border cases. The specific procedural framework differs across jurisdictions; American testimony conventions may not directly translate to foreign proceedings and vice versa. Preparation for international testimony includes familiarity with the specific procedural framework, coordination with the retaining party about the specific expectations, and attention to translation and cultural considerations. The professional community engages with international practice through international professional organizations and specific training opportunities.

### Emerging Challenges: AI Evidence and Novel Methods

Emerging challenges in expert witness practice include the increasing integration of artificial intelligence into evidence analysis, the development of novel scientific methods with specific admissibility questions, and the ongoing evolution of the specific admissibility framework. Testimony involving AI-generated findings (image analysis results, pattern recognition outputs, specific analytical AI systems) faces specific admissibility questions about methodology, error rates, and reliability. Novel scientific methods (novel DNA techniques, novel imaging modalities, novel toxicological analytical platforms) face similar questions when introduced. The pathologist engaging with emerging methodology maintains familiarity with the specific admissibility framework and prepares testimony that supports admissibility when the methodology is properly established. The professional community engages with emerging challenges through professional guidance, methodology validation studies, and specific practice recommendations.

### Career Longevity and Managing Testimony Practice

Career longevity in forensic pathology practice with substantial expert witness engagement requires attention to both professional and personal management. Sustained expert witness practice can be demanding; specific cases may involve substantial emotional weight, and the aggregate practice may accumulate over the career. Maintaining balance across office practice, expert testimony, and personal life supports sustained engagement. Some pathologists limit consulting testimony to focus on office practice;

others develop substantial consulting practice as a significant component of professional activity. Recognition of personal limits and appropriate professional boundaries supports sustained practice. Mentorship relationships and peer support contribute to sustainable practice patterns.

### Public Health and Aggregate Testimony

Some testimony extends beyond individual case content to aggregate public health issues. Forensic pathologists testifying about specific case patterns (drug overdose trends, homicide patterns, specific injury patterns) may extend testimony to the aggregate patterns their office has documented. Legislative testimony (before state and federal legislative committees on public health matters) similarly extends beyond individual cases to aggregate patterns. Testimony in class action civil litigation may involve specific patterns across multiple cases. These broader testimony contexts require preparation drawing on aggregate office data, published research, and the specific public health framework. The forensic pathology contribution to public health function includes not only case work but also aggregate testimony supporting evidence-based policy development.

### Legacy and Historical Perspective

The forensic pathology community has developed substantial legacy of expert witness practice contributing to legal proceedings and public policy over generations. Historical figures in the specialty including pioneering forensic pathologists have contributed to specific case investigations and to the aggregate development of practice standards. Contemporary practice builds on this historical development and contributes to future practice through the ongoing development of methodology, standards, and professional community. Individual pathologists engaging with the specialty legacy through professional community engagement, contribution to guidance development, and mentorship of subsequent practitioners contribute to the aggregate legacy their careers represent. The specific historical context provides framework for understanding contemporary practice and the ongoing evolution of the specialty.

### Training Programs and Testimony Skill Development

Training in expert witness testimony is a specific component of forensic pathology fellowship. Fellows observe experienced pathologists testifying in specific cases when possible, participate in mock testimony exercises, and receive instruction on the specific skills of testimony delivery. The National Association of Medical Examiners and other professional organizations offer specific courses on testimony skills for both new and experienced practitioners. Mock trial exercises with practicing attorneys serving as examining counsel provide practical experience in a controlled setting. Continued professional development through observation of specific proceedings, participation in mock exercises, and reflection on individual testimony experiences supports ongoing skill development. Testimony skills, like case examination skills, benefit from continued practice and reflection throughout the career.

## Curriculum Vitae Maintenance for Expert Witness Practice

The curriculum vitae serves specific functions in expert witness practice. It documents the credentials qualifying the expert for testimony, provides the basis for the credential-establishing portion of direct examination, and supports the retained party's pretrial evaluation of expert qualifications. Maintenance of a current, accurate curriculum vitae is essential; outdated or inaccurate CVs can cause admissibility problems and credibility damage during cross-examination. Standard elements include: education and training with specific dates and institutions; board certifications with specific dates; positions held with specific dates and responsibilities; professional society memberships; publications with complete citations; prior expert testimony experience (some jurisdictions require detailed disclosure of prior testimony); teaching activities; and specific areas of expertise. Regular updates and specific attention to accuracy in each element support the CV's function in expert practice.

## Courtroom Demeanor and Physical Presentation

Courtroom demeanor and physical presentation affect testimony reception. Professional attire (business dress, typically suit or professional equivalent) supports the credibility of the expert role. Posture during testimony (upright, engaged with the jury) supports the communication function. Voice modulation and pacing (clear speech, appropriate speaking pace, adequate volume) support jury reception. Handling of case materials during testimony (appropriate reference to reports, careful handling of photographs) reflects the professional standards. Non-verbal communication elements (eye contact with the jury, facial expression, gestural communication) contribute to the aggregate reception. The specific demeanor develops through practice; new pathologists benefit from observation of experienced testifying pathologists and from feedback about specific demeanor elements. Formal training in courtroom demeanor is available through some professional development programs.

## Redirect Examination and Rebuttal Testimony

Redirect examination following cross-examination allows the calling counsel to address specific issues raised during cross. The pathologist's redirect testimony typically clarifies specific points that may have been left ambiguous during cross-examination, addresses specific challenges raised by opposing counsel, and reinforces the aggregate case reasoning. Redirect testimony has specific procedural limits (typically limited to matters raised during cross-examination) but can substantially strengthen the aggregate testimony. Rebuttal testimony (testimony introduced after the opposing party has presented its case) may involve response to specific expert testimony from opposing witnesses. Preparation for redirect and rebuttal requires attention to the anticipated cross-examination themes and the potential need for specific clarification. Effective redirect and rebuttal testimony can significantly influence the aggregate reception of the specific case reasoning.

### The Case After Testimony

The case after testimony continues to develop through jury deliberation, verdict, and potential appellate proceedings. The pathologist's testimony contributes to the case outcome but does not determine it; jury deliberation integrates the pathologist's testimony with all other evidence and reaches the specific verdict. Appellate proceedings may raise specific issues related to the expert testimony including admissibility challenges, sufficiency of evidence questions, and specific procedural issues. The pathologist may be called for additional testimony in appellate proceedings or in new trials following successful appeals. The pathologist's specific case work continues to be part of the case record throughout the proceedings and may be reviewed for years or decades after the initial testimony. Attention to systematic preparation and delivery of the initial testimony supports the aggregate case record throughout its subsequent history.

### SCENE-TO-CERTIFICATION DECISION SYSTEM — Expert Testimony Determination Arcs

**The Expert Witness Role:** The forensic pathologist serves as both fact witness to personal case observations and expert witness in interpretation of case findings. Expert witness practice is a substantial component of forensic pathology practice requiring specific skills distinct from case examination. The role differs fundamentally from fact witness testimony and involves specific ethical standards.

**Pretrial Preparation:** Systematic pretrial preparation includes case review, coordination with counsel, expert report preparation in consulting cases, and specific preparation for deposition and trial testimony. Preparation supports both substantive content and effective delivery of the testimony.

**Direct and Cross-Examination:** Direct examination establishes credentials and delivers case findings in accessible language with visual support. Cross-examination requires professional composure, honest engagement with legitimate challenges, and appropriate response to improper questions. Both phases benefit from systematic preparation and experience.

**The Daubert Standard:** The Daubert standard governs admissibility of expert testimony with focus on methodology reliability. Forensic pathology methodology generally meets Daubert requirements when properly practiced. Preparation for admissibility challenges supports specific practice areas facing active challenge.

**Ethical Standards:** Objectivity and independence, appropriate scope of testimony, ethical compensation standards, and appropriate communication with colleagues form the ethical framework of expert witness practice. Attention to these standards supports both individual credibility and aggregate professional standing of the specialty.

## Summary and Key Concepts

The forensic pathologist frequently serves as expert witness in legal proceedings, testifying both as fact witness to personal case observations and as expert witness in interpretation of findings. The role requires specific skills distinct from case examination.

Effective testimony depends on systematic pretrial preparation including case review, coordination with counsel, expert report preparation in consulting cases, and specific preparation for deposition and trial phases.

Direct examination delivers case findings in accessible language with credentials established and visual evidence supporting the testimony. Cross-examination requires professional composure, honest engagement with legitimate challenges, and appropriate response to improper questions.

The Daubert standard governs admissibility of expert testimony. Forensic pathology methodology generally meets Daubert requirements when properly practiced with methodology transparency and reference to professional practice.

Ethical standards for expert witness practice include objectivity and independence, appropriate scope, ethical compensation, and appropriate professional boundaries. These standards support both individual credibility and aggregate professional standing.

The aggregate expert witness practice of the forensic pathology community contributes to the professional standing of the specialty. Maintaining professional standards in individual testimony supports both individual practice and aggregate specialty credibility.

# THE SCENE-TO-CERTIFICATION MASTER ATLAS

This Atlas consolidates the Scene-to-Certification Decision System across the full text into a single indexed reference. Every determination arc developed in the chapters is represented here as a compact scene-to-certification anchor entry organized by death category. Each entry captures the presenting scene signature, the autopsy signature that identifies the pattern, the decision anchor that locks the cause determination, the trap logic that distinguishes the pattern from its look-alikes, and the chapter cross-reference where the full arc is developed. The Atlas is a scanning reference — designed for the pathologist reviewing a case at the scene, during autopsy, or during report preparation. It reads as a structured reference navigator, indexed by death category and cross-referenced back to the originating chapter.

## Part I: Foundational Investigation and Scene Reconstruction

### The Medicolegal Death Investigation Framework

Scene Signature: unexpected death, unwitnessed death, injury of any mechanism, custody death, or specific jurisdictional category. Autopsy Signature: systematic examination integrating scene, history, and physical findings. Decision Anchor: the specific determination reflects the aggregate case reasoning; systematic evaluation supports each determination. Trap Logic: incomplete investigation on any element (scene, history, autopsy, ancillary studies) compromises the aggregate reasoning. Chapter Cross-reference: Chapter 1.

### Scene Investigation

Scene Signature: the location where the decedent is found, with position, environment, associated materials, and specific circumstances. Autopsy Signature: findings consistent or inconsistent with the scene reconstruction. Decision Anchor: scene evidence provides context supporting the case reasoning; inconsistency between scene and autopsy findings requires investigation. Trap Logic: assumption that scene appearance necessarily reflects the actual mechanism, without systematic evaluation of alternatives. Chapter Cross-reference: Chapter 2.

### Postmortem Changes and Time of Death

Scene Signature: livor mortis pattern (with attention to position dependence), rigor mortis stage, decomposition status, ambient temperature effects. Autopsy Signature: aggregate postmortem changes integrated for time-of-death estimation. Decision Anchor: time-of-death estimates are reported in broad ranges consistent with the interpretive limits of the postmortem change framework. Trap Logic: overconfident narrow time-of-death estimates from single findings without integration of the aggregate pattern. Chapter Cross-reference: Chapter 3.

### The Forensic Autopsy

Scene Signature: acceptance of jurisdiction with case circumstances warranting autopsy examination. Autopsy Signature: systematic external and internal examination with documentation, specimen collection, and ancillary studies. Decision Anchor: the systematic approach ensures completeness and supports the aggregate case reasoning. Trap Logic: abbreviated examination missing findings that later prove important, or excessive workup obscuring the specific significant findings. Chapter Cross-reference: Chapter 4.

## Part II: Trauma Death Categories

### Blunt Force Injury Deaths

Scene Signature: fall from height, motor vehicle collision, assault with blunt object, industrial injury. Autopsy Signature: contusions, abrasions, lacerations, fractures, and specific internal injuries (visceral lacerations, cardiac contusion, aortic injury) reflecting the specific mechanism. Decision Anchor: aggregate injury pattern integrated with scene reconstruction supports the specific mechanism reasoning. Trap Logic: overreliance on single-injury interpretation without the aggregate pattern reasoning; failure to distinguish antemortem from postmortem injuries. Chapter Cross-reference: Chapter 5.

### Sharp Force Injury Deaths

Scene Signature: knife or other sharp implement at scene, specific wound patterns visible externally, blood pattern at scene consistent with sharp force mechanism. Autopsy Signature: incised wounds and stab wounds with specific characteristics (edge morphology, depth, tract direction, presence of hesitation marks). Decision Anchor: wound characteristics support the specific mechanism reasoning including self-inflicted versus assault distinction. Trap Logic: assuming that hesitation marks alone confirm self-infliction without the aggregate reasoning; missing subtle wound patterns supporting specific weapon characteristics. Chapter Cross-reference: Chapter 6.

### Gunshot Wound Deaths

Scene Signature: firearm or spent projectile at scene, gunshot wounds evident on external examination. Autopsy Signature: entrance wound with specific range indicators (contact, close, intermediate, distant), exit wound if present, wound track through body with associated injuries, retained projectile if no exit. Decision Anchor: range determination integrated with wound track reconstruction supports the specific event reconstruction; systematic imaging (postmortem CT) preserves wound track spatial documentation. Trap Logic: contact wound features (searing, muzzle imprint) confused with close-range features; failure to systematically document each wound track. Chapter Cross-reference: Chapter 7.

### Asphyxial Deaths

Scene Signature: ligature, plastic bag, evidence of restraint, drowning circumstance, choking mechanism. Autopsy Signature: petechial hemorrhages (conjunctival, facial), specific neck injuries (hyoid or thyroid cartilage fracture, deep neck hemorrhage), pulmonary edema, other specific findings by mechanism.

Decision Anchor: aggregate findings support the specific asphyxial mechanism; layered anterior neck dissection is standard for suspected strangulation. Trap Logic: absence of petechial hemorrhages does not exclude asphyxial mechanism; presence in specific circumstances (severe congestion, resuscitation) does not confirm it. Chapter Cross-reference: Chapter 8.

### Thermal, Electrical, and Chemical Deaths

Scene Signature: fire scene with body position and environmental context, electrical apparatus or exposure history, chemical exposure with specific agent identifiable at scene. Autopsy Signature: burn injury pattern with specific characteristics distinguishing antemortem from postmortem, elevated carboxyhemoglobin and cyanide in antemortem fire exposure, electrical injury with entrance and exit marks, chemical exposure findings with specific agent effects. Decision Anchor: antemortem fire exposure supported by elevated carboxyhemoglobin and soot in airways; electrical death identified by specific injury pattern and circumstance. Trap Logic: pugilistic posture (postmortem thermal contraction) confused with defensive posturing; postmortem burns confused with antemortem injury. Chapter Cross-reference: Chapter 9.

## Part III: Sudden Natural Death Categories

### Sudden Cardiac Death

Scene Signature: sudden collapse of previously well individual, exercise-associated collapse, syncope preceding collapse, or unwitnessed sudden death. Autopsy Signature: coronary atherosclerosis with acute lesion, hypertrophic cardiomyopathy, dilated cardiomyopathy, specific structural cardiac disease, or, in some young decedents, normal autopsy with molecular findings supporting inherited arrhythmia syndrome. Decision Anchor: structural findings support the specific mechanism; negative autopsy with age and circumstance appropriate for inherited arrhythmia warrants postmortem genetic evaluation and family screening. Trap Logic: coronary atherosclerosis as automatic cause without evidence of acute lesion; failure to consider inherited arrhythmia syndromes in young sudden death. Chapter Cross-reference: Chapter 10.

### Sudden Death From Neurological, Pulmonary, and Other Natural Causes

Scene Signature: sudden collapse, brief prodromal symptoms, or unwitnessed sudden death without cardiac substrate. Autopsy Signature: intracranial hemorrhage (specific vascular anomaly, hypertensive vascular disease), pulmonary embolism (thrombus in pulmonary arteries with source in deep venous system), specific pulmonary disease, or other identified structural cause. Decision Anchor: the specific natural cause supported by the systematic examination. Trap Logic: attributing sudden death to a specific finding without systematic exclusion of alternative causes. Chapter Cross-reference: Chapter 11.

## Part IV: Pediatric and Special Populations

### Pediatric Death and SUID

Scene Signature: infant found unresponsive during sleep, in specific sleep environment, with specific circumstances. Autopsy Signature: systematic examination with attention to sleep-related asphyxial findings, developmental pathology, infection screening, and specific findings supporting or excluding alternative causes. Decision Anchor: the SUDI framework integrates scene, history, and autopsy for the specific determination; SIDS is the specific diagnosis when the systematic evaluation supports it. Trap Logic: automatic SIDS diagnosis without systematic exclusion; missing subtle findings supporting specific alternative causes. Chapter Cross-reference: Chapter 12.

### Abusive Head Trauma and Child Abuse

Scene Signature: infant or child with unexplained collapse, history inconsistent with mechanism, delayed presentation for care, or specific concerning circumstances. Autopsy Signature: subdural hematoma (particularly bilateral and thin-film), retinal hemorrhages (with attention to layers and distribution), cerebral edema, associated injuries including specific fracture patterns (metaphyseal corner, posterior rib), and specific pattern of injuries at different ages. Decision Anchor: the aggregate injury pattern supports the specific mechanism reasoning; the pattern of injuries at different ages supports repeated inflicted mechanism. Trap Logic: attributing findings to unrelated pathology (birth trauma, medical intervention, unrecognized coagulopathy) without systematic evaluation; missing the pattern that supports the inflicted mechanism. Chapter Cross-reference: Chapter 13.

### Elder Abuse and Neglect

Scene Signature: elderly decedent with unexplained injuries, evidence of neglect (untreated pressure ulcers, malnutrition, poor hygiene), suspicious circumstances of death, or specific concerning circumstances of the care environment. Autopsy Signature: injuries inconsistent with reported mechanism, pressure ulcers of specific severity, evidence of dehydration or malnutrition, medication mismanagement findings. Decision Anchor: the aggregate findings supported by systematic evaluation of the care context; specific patterns support inflicted injury or systematic neglect. Trap Logic: automatic attribution of findings to natural decline of aging without systematic evaluation; missing specific patterns that support abuse or neglect. Chapter Cross-reference: Chapter 14.

### Sexual Assault Deaths

Scene Signature: specific evidence of sexual contact at scene, victim positioning, evidence of restraint or force, associated injuries. Autopsy Signature: evidence of sexual contact with specific findings, anogenital injuries (with attention to specific injury patterns), associated injuries from restraint or force, specific findings supporting mechanism. Decision Anchor: systematic sexual assault evidence collection with proper chain of custody supports the case reasoning. Trap Logic: absence of anogenital injuries does not exclude sexual assault; presence in specific circumstances may reflect consensual contact requiring specific reasoning. Chapter Cross-reference: Chapter 15.

### Deaths in Custody and Restraint

Scene Signature: death during law enforcement encounter, during restraint, during transport, or during custody. Autopsy Signature: restraint injuries (specific patterns), asphyxial findings (specific to positional or mechanical asphyxia in restraint context), specific injuries from law enforcement mechanisms (specific injuries from weapon deployment), or specific mechanism of death in custody circumstances. Decision Anchor: aggregate findings support the specific mechanism; the intersection of restraint circumstances with substrate conditions (cardiovascular disease, substance intoxication) supports the specific reasoning. Trap Logic: attribution of custody death to substance intoxication alone without recognition of restraint contribution; missing the pattern supporting positional or mechanical asphyxia. Chapter Cross-reference: Chapter 16.

## Part V: Toxicology and Drug Deaths

### Postmortem Toxicology Interpretation

Scene Signature: scene evidence of substance use, prescription medication containers, drug paraphernalia, or specific circumstances suggesting substance involvement. Autopsy Signature: findings supporting specific substance mechanism (pulmonary edema in opioid overdose, cardiovascular findings in stimulant overdose, specific findings by substance), toxicological results from systematic specimen collection. Decision Anchor: peripheral blood concentrations interpreted with reference to the specific drug's redistribution behavior; central blood concentrations of redistribution-affected drugs do not by themselves establish antemortem toxic exposure. Trap Logic: overinterpretation of elevated central blood levels without recognition of redistribution behavior; underinterpretation of positive findings without integration with case context. Chapter Cross-reference: Chapter 17.

### Drug and Alcohol Deaths

Scene Signature: opioid overdose scene evidence (syringes, foil residue), stimulant scene evidence, alcohol containers, or specific substance-related circumstances. Autopsy Signature: pulmonary edema and foam cone in opioid overdose, cardiovascular findings in stimulant overdose, hepatic pathology in chronic alcohol use, specific findings by substance category. Decision Anchor: opioid deaths certified with specific reference to substances involved (combined fentanyl and heroin toxicity, etc.); manner determination reflects the specific case circumstances (accident dominant in current epidemic, suicide requiring evidence of intent). Trap Logic: single-substance attribution when combinations are present; failing to identify fentanyl contamination pattern; missing the tolerance context that affects interpretation. Chapter Cross-reference: Chapter 18.

## Part VI: Postmortem Imaging and Identification

### Postmortem Imaging

Scene Signature: gunshot wound cases, pediatric cases, sudden death cases with structural cause consideration, decomposed body cases, or specific case requiring imaging. Autopsy Signature: postmortem CT identifying skeletal injuries, retained projectiles, wound tracks, structural pathology, and specific findings supporting the case reasoning. Decision Anchor: postmortem CT supplements autopsy examination with three-dimensional documentation preserved for later review; specific findings guide the autopsy dissection and support the aggregate case documentation. Trap Logic: overreliance on imaging without tissue-level examination; misinterpretation of normal postmortem findings (decomposition gas, blood pooling) as pathologic. Chapter Cross-reference: Chapter 19.

### Human Identification and Skeletal Remains

Scene Signature: unidentified decedent, severely damaged remains, skeletal remains without identifying context, or specific identification challenge. Autopsy Signature: biological profile from skeletal analysis (sex, age, ancestry, stature with appropriate confidence intervals), specific identification-supporting findings (surgical implants, distinctive dental features, specific findings), specimens for DNA analysis. Decision Anchor: scientific identification through fingerprint, DNA, or forensic odontology provides higher certainty when circumstances warrant beyond presumptive identification. Trap Logic: acceptance of presumptive identification when circumstances warrant scientific comparison; overinterpretation of biological profile without appropriate confidence intervals. Chapter Cross-reference: Chapter 20.

### Mass Fatality Response

Scene Signature: multi-decedent event exceeding local capacity (aircraft crash, terrorism, natural disaster, pandemic surge, industrial disaster). Autopsy Signature: systematic mass fatality protocols with scaled processing while preserving identification rigor; specific mechanism findings appropriate to the event type. Decision Anchor: coordinated multi-agency response through DMORT and state emergency management supports the aggregate response; parallel analytical streams for identification maximize efficiency; prioritization framework balances family concerns, investigative priorities, and preservation. Trap Logic: individual case processing pace producing case backlogs, or excessive acceleration producing quality problems; failure to preserve identification rigor at scale. Chapter Cross-reference: Chapter 21.

## Part VII: Certification, Documentation, and Testimony

### Death Certification

Scene Signature: completed case investigation supporting cause and manner determination. Autopsy Signature: systematic case documentation supporting the certification. Decision Anchor: cause-of-death cascade documents immediate cause, intermediate causes, and underlying cause with contributing conditions in Part II; manner of death (natural, accident, suicide, homicide, undetermined) reflects systematic case reasoning. Trap Logic: overcomplicating the cascade with non-distinct intermediate causes; undersimplifying with generic terminal events (cardiopulmonary arrest, multiorgan failure); vague certification limiting the aggregate value. Chapter Cross-reference: Chapter 22.

### The Autopsy Report and Case Documentation

Scene Signature: completed case examination requiring documentation supporting the certification and subsequent uses. Autopsy Signature: systematic external and internal examination documentation with photographs, ancillary study integration, and aggregate case reasoning documentation. Decision Anchor: the report supports the certificate summary with underlying documentation; the case file with systematic organization supports the range of subsequent uses (legal proceedings, family requests, quality review, aggregate research). Trap Logic: abbreviated documentation missing findings that later prove important; excessive documentation obscuring the specific findings and reasoning; inadequate photographic support. Chapter Cross-reference: Chapter 23.

### Expert Witness Testimony

Scene Signature: legal proceedings arising from the case (criminal prosecution, civil litigation, administrative proceedings) requiring expert testimony. Autopsy Signature: the underlying case documentation supporting the testimony. Decision Anchor: systematic pretrial preparation, effective direct examination with accessible language and visual support, honest engagement with cross-examination while maintaining composure, methodology consistent with Daubert standard requirements. Trap Logic: inadequate preparation risking inaccuracy; overrehearsal producing scripted testimony; capitulation to skilled cross-examination when reasoning stands; defensive rigidity refusing to acknowledge legitimate limitations. Chapter Cross-reference: Chapter 24.

## Part VIII: Second-Arc Anchors and Cross-Reference Index

The chapters develop two rhythm arcs each. Part I above catalogued the first arc from each chapter organized by category. Part VIII below catalogues the second arc from each chapter, developing the additional decision anchor patterns the framework identifies. Together, Parts I and VIII index the full set of Scene-to-Certification anchors developed in the text.

### Injury Documentation Systematic Approach (Chapter 4 Second Arc)

Scene Signature: multiple injury case requiring systematic documentation. Autopsy Signature: sequential injury documentation with dimensional detail, photographic support, and specific characterization. Decision Anchor: systematic sequence supports the aggregate reasoning; each injury characterized before proceeding. Trap Logic: documenting injuries in aggregate without individual characterization; missing subtle findings by inadequate sequential approach. Chapter Cross-reference: Chapter 4.

### Fall From Height Reconstruction (Chapter 5 Second Arc)

Scene Signature: decedent found at location consistent with fall from height with specific circumstances. Autopsy Signature: injury pattern consistent with the specific fall mechanism (impact site, deceleration injuries, specific fracture patterns). Decision Anchor: the aggregate injury pattern supports reconstruction of the fall mechanism; specific findings distinguish fall from height from other blunt trauma mechanisms. Trap Logic: attributing to fall when injuries suggest alternative mechanism; missing evidence of assault preceding or during fall. Chapter Cross-reference: Chapter 5.

**Sharp Force Self-Infliction Determination (Chapter 6 Second Arc)**

Scene Signature: sharp force injury case with question of self-infliction versus assault. Autopsy Signature: hesitation marks (superficial parallel injuries in accessible areas), lack of defensive wounds, wound pattern accessible to the decedent, specific location consistent with self-infliction. Decision Anchor: aggregate pattern of hesitation, accessibility, and location supports self-infliction reasoning; absence of these features raises assault as differential. Trap Logic: hesitation marks alone without aggregate reasoning; failing to consider self-inflicted assault-mimicking patterns. Chapter Cross-reference: Chapter 6.

**Gunshot Range Determination (Chapter 7 Second Arc)**

Scene Signature: gunshot wound case with specific reconstruction requirement including range. Autopsy Signature: contact wound (searing, muzzle imprint, soot deposit), close-range wound (soot deposit, gunpowder stippling), intermediate range wound (gunpowder stippling without soot), distant wound (no soot or stippling, entrance wound features alone). Decision Anchor: range determination based on specific findings systematically identified; documentation supports subsequent reconstruction. Trap Logic: contact and close-range features confused; failure to identify contact wound features on skin cleaned during initial care. Chapter Cross-reference: Chapter 7.

**Layered Neck Dissection (Chapter 8 Second Arc)**

Scene Signature: suspected strangulation, hanging, or specific asphyxial case. Autopsy Signature: systematic layered dissection identifying deep neck hemorrhage, hyoid or thyroid cartilage fracture, and specific tissue findings. Decision Anchor: layered approach identifies findings that surface examination cannot; documentation supports subsequent reasoning. Trap Logic: superficial examination missing deep findings; identifying hemorrhage without systematic layer-by-layer approach missing specific patterns. Chapter Cross-reference: Chapter 8.

**Carboxyhemoglobin Interpretation in Fire Deaths (Chapter 9 Second Arc)**

Scene Signature: fire scene with decedent recovered. Autopsy Signature: elevated carboxyhemoglobin supporting antemortem exposure; cyanide levels supporting inhalation exposure; soot in airways and lungs supporting active breathing during fire. Decision Anchor: carboxyhemoglobin above threshold levels supports antemortem exposure; low or absent levels with fire exposure suggest death preceded fire or rapid death without exposure. Trap Logic: postmortem exposure at fire scenes producing low-level carboxyhemoglobin misinterpreted; specific case scenarios producing atypical patterns. Chapter Cross-reference: Chapter 9.

**Coronary Reconstruction (Chapter 10 Second Arc)**

Scene Signature: sudden collapse with cardiac substrate consideration. Autopsy Signature: systematic coronary examination with cross-sectioning, identification of acute lesions (thrombosis, plaque rupture), and characterization of underlying atherosclerosis severity and distribution. Decision Anchor: acute coronary event identified through specific findings; atherosclerosis without acute event characterizes substrate but does not identify acute mechanism. Trap Logic: attributing sudden death to atherosclerosis alone without specific acute findings; missing subtle acute lesions through inadequate systematic approach. Chapter Cross-reference: Chapter 10.

**Pulmonary Embolism Recognition (Chapter 11 Second Arc)**

Scene Signature: sudden collapse with pulmonary consideration. Autopsy Signature: thrombus in pulmonary arterial system with source in deep venous system, right heart strain findings, associated risk factors identified. Decision Anchor: specific thrombus location and character supports the mechanism; source identification supports the aggregate reasoning. Trap Logic: postmortem clot confused with antemortem thrombus; failure to identify subtle findings supporting the mechanism. Chapter Cross-reference: Chapter 11.

**SUID Scene Reenactment (Chapter 12 Second Arc)**

Scene Signature: infant death during sleep with sleep environment reconstruction. Autopsy Signature: findings supporting or excluding sleep-related asphyxial mechanism, developmental pathology considerations, infection screening. Decision Anchor: aggregate scene reenactment with autopsy findings supports the specific determination within the SUDI framework. Trap Logic: dismissing scene environment factors without reenactment; automatic SIDS diagnosis when specific findings support alternative causes. Chapter Cross-reference: Chapter 12.

**The Timing Reconstruction in Abusive Head Trauma (Chapter 13 Second Arc)**

Scene Signature: pediatric collapse with abusive head trauma consideration and timing question. Autopsy Signature: characterization of subdural hematoma age (fresh, subacute, chronic), retinal hemorrhage findings and their expected persistence, associated injuries at different ages. Decision Anchor: timing reconstruction integrates specific findings with expected evolution; multiple ages of injury support repeated inflicted mechanism. Trap Logic: overconfident narrow timing without recognition of variability; missing evidence of multiple episodes through inadequate timing assessment. Chapter Cross-reference: Chapter 13.

**Pressure Ulcer Evaluation in Elder Abuse (Chapter 14 Second Arc)**

Scene Signature: elderly decedent with pressure ulcers requiring evaluation of severity and care context. Autopsy Signature: pressure ulcer staging (I through IV), location documentation, evidence of infection or complications, correlation with care history. Decision Anchor: stage III and IV pressure ulcers in expected care contexts warrant systematic evaluation of neglect; distribution and severity pattern supports specific reasoning. Trap Logic: dismissing all pressure ulcers as expected in decline; attributing all pressure ulcers to neglect without care context evaluation. Chapter Cross-reference: Chapter 14.

**Sexual Assault Evidence Collection (Chapter 15 Second Arc)**

Scene Signature: suspected sexual assault death requiring evidence collection. Autopsy Signature: systematic sexual assault evidence collection with specimens for DNA analysis, documentation of anogenital and other injuries, specific findings supporting mechanism. Decision Anchor: proper collection with chain of custody supports subsequent investigation; systematic approach ensures completeness. Trap Logic: incomplete evidence collection compromising subsequent investigation; specimens without proper chain of custody unusable in prosecution. Chapter Cross-reference: Chapter 15.

**Positional Asphyxia in Restraint (Chapter 16 Second Arc)**

Scene Signature: death during physical restraint with position that compromised respiration. Autopsy Signature: asphyxial findings (petechial hemorrhages, congestion) in restraint context, evidence of positional mechanism, aggregate case reconstruction supporting the specific mechanism. Decision Anchor: positional asphyxia identified through the specific pattern; substrate conditions (obesity, cardiac disease, substance intoxication) may contribute to the aggregate mechanism. Trap Logic: attributing custody death only to substrate condition without positional recognition; overinterpreting positional finding without adequate substrate consideration. Chapter Cross-reference: Chapter 16.

**Toxicology-Autopsy Integration (Chapter 17 Second Arc)**

Scene Signature: substance-related death requiring integration of toxicological findings with autopsy findings. Autopsy Signature: findings consistent with specific substance mechanism, toxicological results in appropriate specimens, aggregate case reasoning. Decision Anchor: the specific determination reflects the integration; positive toxicology alone does not establish substance-related death, negative toxicology alone does not exclude it. Trap Logic: automatic attribution to substance based on positive toxicology without integration; automatic exclusion based on negative toxicology in specific mechanism types. Chapter Cross-reference: Chapter 17.

**Alcohol-Related Determination (Chapter 18 Second Arc)**

Scene Signature: alcohol-related death across categories (acute intoxication, chronic disease, withdrawal). Autopsy Signature: findings specific to the alcohol-related mechanism, integration with toxicological findings, evidence of chronic use. Decision Anchor: category-specific reasoning for each pattern; the specific mechanism determines the certification approach. Trap Logic: single generic "alcohol-related" classification without specificity; missing withdrawal pattern in individuals with prior chronic use. Chapter Cross-reference: Chapter 18.

**Virtopsy Approach Decision (Chapter 19 Second Arc)**

Scene Signature: case with family or religious objection to invasive autopsy, or specific case where imaging alone may support reasoning. Autopsy Signature: postmortem CT and where indicated MRI documenting findings, targeted specimen collection under image guidance. Decision Anchor: virtopsy adequate for specific case types where imaging supports the case reasoning; full autopsy required when specific findings would benefit from tissue-level examination. Trap Logic: applying virtopsy in cases requiring full autopsy; failing to offer virtopsy when appropriate. Chapter Cross-reference: Chapter 19.

**Skeletal Injury Interpretation (Chapter 20 Second Arc)**

Scene Signature: skeletal remains with injuries identified. Autopsy Signature: systematic injury identification on skeletal elements, distinguishing perimortem from taphonomic changes, characterization of specific mechanisms. Decision Anchor: skeletal injury interpretation within specific framework with appropriate confidence intervals; integration with case context supports mechanism reasoning. Trap Logic: overinterpreting scavenger damage as inflicted; missing subtle perimortem injuries. Chapter Cross-reference: Chapter 20.

**Mass Fatality Case Prioritization (Chapter 21 Second Arc)**

Scene Signature: mass fatality event with prioritization requirement. Autopsy Signature: systematic mass fatality protocols with specific attention to identification streams, evidence preservation, and family communication. Decision Anchor: prioritization balances family concerns, investigative priorities, and preservation considerations transparently. Trap Logic: routine processing pace producing backlogs; excessive acceleration producing quality problems; unclear prioritization causing family concern. Chapter Cross-reference: Chapter 21.

**Manner-of-Death Determination Reasoning (Chapter 22 Second Arc)**

Scene Signature: case requiring specific manner determination. Autopsy Signature: findings supporting the specific manner reasoning integrated with scene evidence and antecedent history. Decision Anchor: each manner category (natural, accident, suicide, homicide, undetermined) has specific reasoning framework; the determination reflects systematic case reasoning. Trap Logic: single-element manner determination without integration; overuse of undetermined; misclassification through inadequate systematic reasoning. Chapter Cross-reference: Chapter 22.

**Documentation Chain Integrity (Chapter 23 Second Arc)**

Scene Signature: case with subsequent legal proceedings requiring systematic documentation. Autopsy Signature: comprehensive case documentation with photographs, ancillary studies, and reasoning documentation supporting subsequent uses. Decision Anchor: attention to documentation quality at case preparation supports subsequent legal proceedings, family requests, quality review, and aggregate research. Trap Logic: abbreviated documentation compromising subsequent uses; inadequate photographic support for specific findings. Chapter Cross-reference: Chapter 23.

### Cross-Examination Response Framework (Chapter 24 Second Arc)

Scene Signature: cross-examination testimony with substantive challenges to the case reasoning. Autopsy Signature: the underlying case documentation supporting responses to specific challenges. Decision Anchor: honest engagement with legitimate challenges, professional composure throughout, substantive response to specific questions. Trap Logic: capitulation to skilled challenges when reasoning stands; defensive rigidity refusing to acknowledge legitimate limitations. Chapter Cross-reference: Chapter 24.

## Part IX: Category-Level Cross-Reference Index

The following cross-reference index groups the arc entries by clinical category for scanning by presentation type.

### Sudden Unexpected Death Category

Cardiac substrate (Chapter 10 arcs), non-cardiac natural (Chapter 11 arcs), pediatric SUID (Chapter 12 arcs). Systematic evaluation of substrate versus acute mechanism supports the specific determination.

### Traumatic Death Category

Blunt force (Chapter 5 arcs), sharp force (Chapter 6 arcs), gunshot wound (Chapter 7 arcs), asphyxial (Chapter 8 arcs), thermal/electrical/chemical (Chapter 9 arcs). Mechanism reconstruction through injury pattern integrated with scene and history.

### Non-Accidental Injury Category

Abusive head trauma (Chapter 13 arcs), child abuse patterns (Chapter 13 arcs), elder abuse (Chapter 14 arcs), sexual assault (Chapter 15 arcs), deaths in custody with restraint (Chapter 16 arcs). Specific pattern recognition integrated with systematic evaluation of alternative causes.

### Substance-Related Death Category

Toxicological framework (Chapter 17 arcs), specific drug and alcohol patterns (Chapter 18 arcs). Integration of toxicology with autopsy findings and case context; specific attention to redistribution behavior.

### Identification and Documentation Category

Postmortem imaging integration (Chapter 19 arcs), human identification and biological profile (Chapter 20 arcs), mass fatality response (Chapter 21 arcs), certification (Chapter 22 arcs), documentation (Chapter 23 arcs), testimony (Chapter 24 arcs).

## Part X: The Integrated Framework

The Scene-to-Certification Decision System developed across the chapters of this text integrates the scene, autopsy, and certification phases of forensic pathology practice into an aggregate reasoning framework. The scene provides the initial context; the autopsy identifies the specific findings; the certification documents the aggregate reasoning supporting the specific determination. Each phase supports the others; abbreviated engagement with any phase compromises the aggregate reasoning.

The framework applies across the full spectrum of forensic pathology practice: routine natural death cases, complex trauma cases, pediatric death investigation, drug-related deaths, deaths in custody, mass fatality events, unidentified decedents, and the specific challenges each case category presents. The systematic approach supports both the individual case function and the aggregate professional standing of the specialty.

This Atlas serves as reference scaffolding for the forensic pathologist applying the framework in individual cases. The scanning entries above support recognition of specific patterns and the associated reasoning framework; the full development in the referenced chapters supports the aggregate understanding. Together, the Atlas and the chapters provide the aggregate reference for systematic forensic pathology practice.

### Using the Atlas in Practice

The Atlas is designed for scanning reference during active case work. The pathologist encountering a case at scene, at autopsy, or during report preparation can identify the relevant death category, review the compact anchor entry for the specific pattern, and, where the aggregate case reasoning warrants, review the full framework development in the referenced chapter. The Atlas supports both immediate case recognition and the aggregate professional practice through systematic reference organization.

### The Aggregate Contribution

The individual case work supported by this framework contributes to the aggregate forensic pathology practice: the individual certifications support the aggregate vital statistics; the individual investigations support the aggregate criminal justice and civil justice functions; the individual identifications support the family and legal purposes; the individual case documentation supports the aggregate professional knowledge development. Attention to systematic practice in individual cases supports each of these aggregate functions.

### Continuing Practice Development

Forensic pathology practice continues to evolve. New techniques, new substance patterns, new understanding of specific mechanisms, and new challenges emerge continuously. The systematic framework provides the aggregate approach that adapts to the evolving practice; the specific findings and reasoning are updated as understanding develops. The pathologist maintaining engagement with the professional community, the professional literature, and the developing practice continues to support both individual case work and aggregate professional development throughout the career. This text provides the foundation for that continuing engagement.

# CONCLUSION

A textbook cannot teach a practice. It can lay out the framework, catalog the patterns, describe the reasoning, and index the categories. The practice itself — the way a pathologist stands at the table on a Tuesday morning with a decedent nobody yet knows the name of, and works through what happened — that has to be built over years, one case at a time. This closing chapter is not another chapter of content. It is a reflection on what the framework in this text is actually for, on the work the reader will do with it, and on the specialty the reader is entering or continuing.

## What the Framework Is For

The Scene-to-Certification Decision System developed across these twenty-four chapters is a scaffold, not a substitute. It is not a checklist that produces certifications when the boxes are filled. It is not an algorithm that removes judgment from the work. It is a habit of mind — a way of moving through a case that keeps the reasoning honest across the phases of investigation, so that the pathologist ends up in the right place for the right reasons and can explain, years later, exactly why.

The framework asks the same questions of every case, in the same order. What does the scene tell you? What does the body tell you? What do the ancillary studies tell you? What is the aggregate reasoning that ties them together? What is the decision anchor that locks the determination? What is the trap logic that keeps the determination from being the wrong one? These are not novel questions. Every experienced forensic pathologist has developed some version of them through years of practice. The value of the framework is that it makes the questions explicit, gives them names, and organizes them so that the reader entering practice does not have to reinvent the discipline from scratch.

The framework will fail the reader in some cases. There are cases that do not fit the patterns, cases in which the scene and the autopsy and the toxicology and the history all point in different directions, cases in which the honest answer is undetermined and no amount of systematic reasoning will move it. The framework is not designed to force determinations on such cases. It is designed to make the reasoning transparent — so that when the pathologist arrives at undetermined, the record shows the systematic evaluation that led there, and the family and the court and the profession can see the work.

## The Habit of Discipline

Forensic pathology is a discipline in the older sense of that word — a set of practices repeated until they become automatic, and then repeated some more so that the automatic practices are still questioned when the automatic answer is wrong. The layered anterior neck dissection in every suspected strangulation. The peripheral blood specimen in every toxicology case. The photograph with scale next to every injury. The documentation of negative findings, not just positive ones. The systematic sequence through every organ system, on every case, even the ones that seem obvious. These are not exciting practices. They are the practices that separate defensible forensic pathology from indefensible forensic pathology when a case turns unexpectedly complicated three years after the certification was signed.

The reader entering practice should understand that the discipline is what protects them. A case done systematically, documented systematically, and reasoned systematically will withstand review by opposing experts, appellate courts, professional peers, and the pathologist's own future self reviewing the case in preparation for testimony a decade later. A case done in a hurry, documented in shorthand, and reasoned informally will not. There is no shortcut past the discipline, and the discipline is what makes the professional practice possible over the long career.

## The People Behind the Cases

A textbook of forensic pathology necessarily focuses on the mechanisms — the wound tracks, the toxicology levels, the biological profiles, the certification cascades. But every case in this text represents, in the actual practice, a specific person: someone who had a name, a history, a family, a life that came to an end in the circumstances now under investigation. The forensic pathologist works among the dead, but the work is for the living: for the families who need to know what happened, for the communities that need public health surveillance, for the legal system that needs the documented findings, for the specific individuals whose deaths would otherwise pass without accounting.

This is worth naming explicitly because it is easy, over the years, to lose sight of it. The volume of cases in a busy office produces a rhythm in which the individual case can become just another case, another number, another entry in the daily list. Attention to the specific person — reading the case history carefully, communicating carefully with the family, treating the decedent with the same care whether the death was noteworthy or unremarkable — is part of the professional practice. It is also part of what makes the work sustainable over a career. Pathologists who lose the connection to the human dimension of the work tend not to stay in the specialty. The connection to the people behind the cases is not a distraction from the technical work; it is what gives the technical work its meaning.

This is particularly true in the cases that carry substantial emotional weight — the pediatric deaths, the deaths involving abuse or neglect, the deaths of individuals with substance use disorder whose families have been living with the illness for years, the deaths in circumstances that involve public controversy. In these cases the pathologist is not only performing a technical function; the pathologist is contributing to the specific human resolution that the family and the community are working toward. The certification, the report, the testimony — all of these carry meaning beyond the immediate case documentation.

## The Profession and Its Community

Forensic pathology is a small specialty. The community of practicing forensic pathologists in the United States numbers in the low thousands; the community of board-certified forensic pathologists is smaller still. This creates both challenges and opportunities. The challenge is that the specialty faces persistent workforce shortages, that many offices operate below their optimal capacity, and that the aggregate American death investigation system remains substantially heterogeneous with substantial variation in practice standards. The opportunity is that the small community is unusually collegial. Pathologists know each other across offices and states. The professional organizations — the National Association of Medical Examiners, the American Academy of Forensic Sciences, the College of American Pathologists —

actually function as communities of practice. Individual practitioners can meaningfully contribute to the aggregate professional development.

The reader entering practice will find that engagement with the professional community pays back substantially over the career. Mentorship relationships — with senior pathologists during and after fellowship, with peers in other offices, with colleagues in adjacent specialties (radiology, toxicology, anthropology, odontology) — support both the individual professional development and the aggregate quality of practice. Participation in professional organizations supports both the individual's continuing education and the aggregate development of standards. Contribution to the professional literature through case reports, case series, and specific research supports the aggregate knowledge base that the specialty draws on.

The specialty is also facing substantial evolution. Postmortem imaging continues to develop. Analytical toxicology continues to expand into novel psychoactive substances and evolving drug patterns. Molecular pathology and genetic testing continue to add capability. Artificial intelligence and computational approaches are beginning to enter the workflow. The framework in this text will remain useful across these developments, but the specific applications will evolve. The pathologist entering practice today can reasonably expect the specialty at retirement to look substantially different from the specialty at fellowship completion. Continued engagement with the evolving practice is part of what sustains the career.

## On Sustaining the Work

Forensic pathology is demanding work. The case volume in a busy office is substantial. The subject matter includes death in every category, including categories that carry substantial emotional weight. The professional demands include not only case examination but also administrative responsibilities, family communication, legal proceedings, professional development, and, in many cases, teaching or mentorship. The specialty attracts pathologists who are drawn to the intellectual challenge, the public health function, the legal and criminal justice engagement, and the specific character of investigative pathology practice. It also asks a great deal of those who enter it.

Sustaining the work over the long career requires attention to balance. Some pathologists develop specific case-type expertise (pediatric, cardiovascular, toxicology, mass fatality); others maintain broad practice. Some develop substantial teaching and academic engagement; others focus on office practice. Some maintain active consulting expert practice; others limit consulting engagement to focus on the day-to-day office work. There is no single right way to structure the practice; different pathologists find their sustainable pattern through experience. What is common across sustainable practice is attention to the whole person of the pathologist — physical health, mental and emotional wellbeing, relationships outside work, engagement with life beyond the specialty. Pathologists who sustain long careers in forensic pathology invariably attend to these dimensions, even when the demands of the work make it hard.

## The Standing Charge

This text closes with a reflection rather than a summary because a summary would repeat what the chapters and the Atlas have already delivered. The framework is on the page. The patterns are catalogued. The reasoning is explicit. What remains is the reader's practice — the actual work of applying the framework, case by case, for the years and decades ahead.

That work is worth doing. The forensic pathology community serves a specific and irreplaceable function in the aggregate response to death, injury, and violence in the population. The individual case work supports the specific families, the specific investigations, the specific communities. The aggregate case work supports the vital statistics, the public health surveillance, the criminal justice system, the civil justice system, the research and policy development that draws on the aggregate documentation. The specialty is not glamorous. The rewards are not immediate. The work happens largely out of public view. But the specialty is substantial in what it produces and in what it makes possible.

The reader entering practice or continuing in practice with this text as reference is joining, or continuing in, a community of practice that goes back generations and that continues forward into the future. The framework in these pages is one contribution to the aggregate development of that community. What each pathologist brings to the practice — the specific case work, the specific documentation, the specific reasoning, the specific engagement with families and communities and the professional community — is what sustains and develops the specialty for the pathologists who will come next.

The work is systematic. The work is documented. The work is defensible. The work is honest. The work matters. Go do it well.

www.ingramcontent.com/pod-product-compliance
Lightning Source LLC
LaVergne TN
LVHW060441061126
851857LV00016B/1685